# Frames of Reference for
## Pediatric
## Occupational
## Therapy

# Frames of Reference
## for
# Pediatric
# Occupational
# Therapy

**PAULA KRAMER, MA, OTR, FAOTA**
Associate Professor
Occupational Therapy Department
Kean College of New Jersey
Union, New Jersey

**JIM HINOJOSA, PhD, OTR, FAOTA**
Associate Professor
Department of Occupational Therapy
School of Education, Health, Nursing and
Arts Professions
New York University
New York, New York

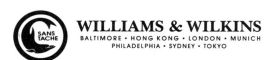

**WILLIAMS & WILKINS**
BALTIMORE · HONG KONG · LONDON · MUNICH
PHILADELPHIA · SYDNEY · TOKYO

*Editor:* John P. Butler
*Managing Editor:* Linda Napora
*Copy Editor:* Patricia J. Grayson
*Designer:* Norman W. Och
*Illustration Planner:* Ray Lowman
*Production Coordinator:* Anne Stewart Seitz
*Cover Designer:* Norman W. Och

Copyright © 1993
Williams & Wilkins
428 East Preston Street
Baltimore, Maryland 21202, USA

Accurate indications, adverse reactions, and dosage schedules for drugs are provided in this book, but it is possible that they may change. The reader is urged to review the package information data of the manufacturers of the medications mentioned.

*Printed in the United States of America*

**Library of Congress Cataloging-in-Publication Data**

Frames of reference for pediatric occupational therapy / [edited by] Paula Kramer, Jim Hinojosa.
    p.    cm.
    Includes index.
    ISBN 0-683-04779-5
    1. Occupational therapy for children.    I. Kramer, Paula.
II. Hinojosa, Jim.
    [DNLM: 1. Occupational Therapy—in infancy & childhood.
2. Occupational Therapy—methods.    WS 368 F813]
RJ53.025F73  1993
615.8'515—dc20
DNLM/DLC
for Library of Congress                         92-4912
                                           CIP

92 93 94 95 96
1 2 3 4 5 6 7 8 9 10

*To the children and families with whom we have worked, who have changed our lives and perspectives; and to those children whose lives may be changed by this book, we dedicate our collaborative efforts.*

# Foreword

There are two vital tenets set forth in this text: first, it is only through knowledgeable use of frames of reference that therapists are able to assist clients in an organized and systematic manner; second, it is only through employing frames of reference that therapists have a clear understanding of what they are doing, why they are doing it, and what theoretical rationale they have for their actions. In other words, frames of reference are essential to good practice.

The student reader may well ask, "Why do these tenets need to be emphasized?" "Why are they not automatically accepted as given?" Perhaps these questions are answered most succinctly by taking a step back in time, through a short history lesson, if you will. Until recently, practice in occupational therapy consisted primarily of the use of a collection of techniques, the majority of which had no articulated theoretical foundation. Yes, theoretical information was taught in school, but it remained separate from technique. If there were any relationships between theory and technique, students were rarely assisted in identifying them.

In addition, the profession had few specific statements concerning how a therapist should go about selecting the techniques likely to be effective in assisting a client. Assessment with a client often was not related directly to the intervention process that followed. Practice was guided primarily by intuition or, conversely, by the idea that only one invariant solution existed for each given problem.

It was out of the situation just outlined that the entity, now referred to as frame of reference, came into being. Its development was prompted by two interrelated needs of the profession—the need to link theory with practice and practice with theory; and the need for theoretically based guidelines to use as the foundation for problem identification and problem remediation with clients.

Although the structure and requisite content of a frame of reference were first presented in 1968, it has only been in the past few years that the profession has given studied attention to the clear articulation of frames of reference and to their conscious and regular use in practice. This delay is somewhat understandable. The process of developing a frame of reference requires sophisticated, rigorous thinking. The skilled use of frames of reference in practice demands knowledgeable, disciplined action. In addition, occupational therapy, like most professions, is relatively conservative, and old ways of thinking and doing are slow to change. Also, the profession, as a whole, needed to learn a great deal more before adequate frames of reference could be developed and used consistently in practice.

All these things say to the student reader, "You have come to occupational therapy at a good time, a time when the profession is in a far better position than previously to assist you in becoming a knowledgeable and skilled therapist." Nowhere is that more evident than in this text. Following the path of my work, Jim and Paula and their contributing authors have prepared an excellent source for understanding the frames of reference that are integral parts of occupational therapy with pediatric clients. This text should serve you well in the process of becoming a therapist. That is not where the usefulness of this text ends, however; it also points to future work to be done. Some of the frames of reference presented here, as well as they are stated, need further refinement. In addition, all of these frames of reference require study with regard to their safety, effectiveness, efficiency, and the client population for which they are more or less useful. Also, there are areas of pediatric practice for which additional frames of reference still need to be developed.

The student reader should note that the competent therapist uses the frames of reference described in this text and elsewhere, but that is only the beginning. The next step is to develop, refine, and assess the adequacy of these and future frames of reference.

Anne Cronin Mosey, PhD, OTR, FAOTA
Professor of Occupational Therapy
New York University

# Preface

Occupational therapy's major area of growth in the past decade has been in pediatrics. Job opportunities have been excellent as practice settings have expanded to include school systems, private practice, neonatal units, and well baby clinics. Because of the increased need for skilled therapists in this area, curricula throughout the country have begun to place greater emphasis on teaching theory and on developing practice materials relevant to pediatrics. The advent of laws that mandate occupational therapy services in early intervention programs and educationally related services in the school system has added to the need for increased academic preparation. With the changing practice arena, it is essential that entry-level curricula provide a foundation for shifting occupational therapy service delivery demands, emerging theories, and alternative practice settings.

This text provides comprehensive information regarding pediatric practice for the entry-level occupational therapy student. To accomplish this, essential information for the student is organized according to various frames of reference currently in use. As set forth by Anne Cronin Mosey, PhD, OTR, FAOTA (1970), the frame of reference provides a methodical organization of theoretical and practical material in the sequence necessary for identification of and solutions for problems in practice. It provides an outline of essential theoretical material in particular areas of function, a guideline for assessing functional capacities in an individual, a method of conceptualizing and initiating intervention—in essence, a blueprint for practice.

State-of-the-art skills necessary for the entry-level occupational therapist are concerned with improving the functional performance of clients. The mechanism of a frame of reference has become an acceptable vehicle for organizing theoretical material in occupational therapy and for moving it into practice through a functional perspective. Frames of reference, therefore, enable the practitioner to use theory in actual practice.

This text is unique because it provides comprehensive pediatric materials organized through the structure of frames of reference. To use frames of reference as the structural scheme differs from the prevalent use of diagnostic categories seen in most occupational therapy textbooks (e.g., Banus, 1979; Pratt & Allen, 1989; Hopkins & Smith, 1985; Pedretti & Zoltan, 1985; Trombly, 1989). Although a child's diagnosis may provide some insight into that child's disabilities, occupational therapists are primarily concerned with functional capacities. A text organized around diagnostic categories, therefore, does not address the essential focus of the occupational therapy process. In addition, a child may exhibit various functional disorders not addressed through specific diagnostic categories but essential to intervention. In so far as a frame of reference is designed first to highlight the functionally related information in traditionally used theories and, second, to relate that information for intervention strategies, it provides a blueprint for approaching such a child.

The frame of reference is an accepted tool used extensively in many occupational therapy curricula. Numerous textbooks on occupational therapy theory and mental health have been organized successfully around the frame of reference structural scheme (e.g., Bruce and Borg, 1987; Mosey, 1970, 1986).

*Frames of Reference for Pediatric Occupational Therapy* is intended primarily for use in entry-level occupational therapy education programs. It is appropriate for adoption in courses that focus on pediatric practice, developmental dysfunction, and neurobehavioral treatment approaches. It also is useful in courses on occupational therapy theory and functional disorders of childhood. Graduate students who wish to specialize in pediatric practice will find this book to be a basic text that provides an overview of commonly used frames of reference.

Practicing therapists will find the book helpful in understanding the theoretical concepts that underlie intervention and the development of treatment planning according to a frame of reference approach. As such, therapists will be able to use this text to analyze their current practices. Those who want to enter pediatric specialty areas from other areas of practice will find this text useful for updating their basic knowledge. Although the text is intended for occupational therapy education, anyone who works with children will find it to be an informative resource.

In the conceptualization of this book, we decided to include those frames of reference most commonly used in pediatric practice. We chose not to include those frames of reference based on commonly understood theories of the profession. Frames of reference that deal with the acquisition of general developmental skills, such as hand function and activities of daily living, therefore, are not presented.

*Frames of Reference for Pediatric Occupational Therapy* is designed to be a teaching tool devoted to instructional/lecture material and, to that end, presents seven of the more complicated and frequently used frames of reference for pediatric practice. In addition, three case studies illustrate the use of the frames of reference. Each chapter is a discrete unit, designed to be integrated easily into existing pediatric practice or neurobehavioral courses, and each unit is set at a reasonable length for students to read and digest over the span of one week. Each chapter serves as the reading material for one week, delineating and supplementing the central topic covered in class. The case study chapters, with accompanying study questions, can be used as examples and inserted into the course as best suits the instructor. At the end of each frame of reference chapter, a comprehensive outline of the frame of reference is provided for study purposes. Also, several didactic chapters cover important aspects of pediatric practice.

Finally, a word about the language used in the book. After considerable deliberation, we chose to refer to the therapist consistently as "she" and the child consistently as "he." We apologize to anyone who might be offended by this seemingly sexist language. It is not our intent to be sexist; however, on early drafts of the manuscript, reviewers found the use of "he/she" to be confusing, especially when reading theoretical material. We therefore settled on "she" for the therapist and "he" for the child and sacrificed "nonsexist" language for clarity and ease of understanding.

Paula Kramer, MA, OTR/L, FAOTA
Jim Hinojosa, PhD, OTR/L, FAOTA

### References

Banus, B. S. (1979). *The developmental therapist* (2nd ed.). Thorofare, NJ: Slack.

Bruce, M. A. & Borg, B. (1987). *Frames of reference in psychosocial occupational therapy.* Thorofare, NJ: Slack.

Hopkins, H. L. & Smith, H. D. (Eds.). (1988). *Willard and Spackman's occupational therapy* (7th ed). Philadelphia, PA: J. B. Lippincott.

Mosey, A. C. (1986). *Psychosocial components of occupational therapy.* New York: Raven Press.

Mosey, A. C. (1970). *Three frames of reference for mental health.* Thorofare, NJ: Slack.

Pedretti, L. W. & Zoltan, B. (Eds.). (1985). *Occupational therapy: practice skills for physical dysfunction* (2nd ed.). St. Louis, MO: C. V. Mosby.

Pratt, P. N. & Allen, A. S. (1989). *Occupational therapy for children* (2nd ed.). St. Louis, MO: C. V. Mosby.

Trombly, C. A. (Ed.). (1989). *Occupational therapy for physical dysfunction* (3rd ed.). Baltimore, MD: Williams and Wilkins.

# Acknowledgments

First and foremost we thank our parents, Ray and Rose Hinojosa and Samuel and Rosalia Kramer. We also thank Elaine Kramer, who always wanted to be a writer and would have been proud of this effort.

We acknowledge with gratitude our mentor, Dr. Anne Cronin Mosey, who taught us to structure our thinking so that it made sense and who has strongly influenced our professional development in innumerable ways.

A special thanks goes to all the authors who contributed to this book, and to their spouses, lovers, families, and friends who were understanding and assisted them to turn in quality work. It is a tribute that they still consider us to be their friends.

Paula wishes to recognize her husband David L. Hunt, for his love and support throughout this project.

Thanks to Steven A. Smith, who not only kept us fed and comfortable when we worked long hours in New York City but also supported our efforts continually.

To our friends and professional colleagues who encouraged us to grow personally and who contributed to our understanding of children we give special thanks: Jill Anderson, Cheryl Colangelo, Ann Grady, Judy Grossman, Stephanie Hoover, Adele Kapp, Jane Korczynski, John D. O'Brien, Gary Ranum, and Jenifer Thuell. Paula also wishes to acknowledge Jerome Margolis and colleagues at the Toddler-Infant Program for Special Education who enhanced her understanding of families and culture and their impact on the therapeutic process.

To all our colleagues at Kean College and New York University, we thank you for your encouragement during this seemingly endless project and for your gracious tolerance of our unavailability and our exhaustion.

We also appreciate the efforts of John Butler, Linda Napora, Anne Stewart Seitz, and the entire team at Williams & Wilkins, who made this book a reality.

Finally, we wish to thank the children and their parents who allowed their pictures to be used to illustrate this text and especially all the special children who have taught us so much.

# Contributors

JILL ANDERSON, MS, OTR/L
Private Practice
Occupational Therapy Supervisor Step-by-Step Infant Development Center

Clinical Assistant Professor
State University of New York
Health Science Center at Brooklyn
Brooklyn, New York

GARY BEDELL, MA, OTR/L
Private Consultant in Early Intervention and Pediatrics

Doctoral Candidate and Part-time Instructor
Department of Occupational Therapy
New York University
New York City

CHERYL ANN COLANGELO, MS, OTR/L
United Cerebral Palsy of Westchester
Purchase, New York

Clinical Assistant Professor
State University of New York
Health Science Center at Brooklyn
Brooklyn, New York

JIM HINOJOSA, PhD, OTR/L, FAOTA
Associate Professor and Director of Advanced Graduate Programs
Department of Occupational Therapy
New York University
New York, New York

MARGARET T. KAPLAN, MA, OTR/L
Assistant Professor
State University of New York
Health Science Center at Brooklyn
Occupational Therapy Department
Brooklyn, New York

JUDITH GIENKE KIMBALL, PhD, OTR/L, FAOTA
Professor and Chair
University of New England
Biddeford, Maine


PAULA KRAMER, MA, OTR/L, FAOTA
Associate Professor and Chair
Occupational Therapy Department
Kean College of New Jersey
Union, New Jersey

Doctoral Candidate
New York University
Department of Occupational Therapy
New York, New York


MARY MUHLENHAUPT, OTR/L
Coordinator of Occupational and Physical Therapy Services
The Board of Cooperative Educational Services #2
Patchogue, New York


SUSAN NESBIT, MS, OTR
Pediatric Occupational Therapy Consultant
New Jersey

Doctoral Candidate
New York University
New York, New York


SHIRLEY PEGANOFF O'BRIEN, MS, OTR/L FAOTA
Associate Professor
Occupational Therapy Department
Eastern Kentucky University
Lexington, Kentucky


LAURETTE OLSON, MA, OTR/L
Occupational Therapy Consultant
Mamaroneck Public Schools
Mamaroneck, New York

formerly:
Therapeutic Activities Program Coordinator
Child and Adolescent Psychiatry
New York Hospital—Cornell Medical Center
Westchester Division
White Plains, New York

SARAH A. SCHOEN, MA, OTR/L
Supervisor, Occupational Therapy
Rose F. Kennedy Center
Children's Evaluation and Rehabilitation Clinic
Albert Einstein College of Medicine
Bronx, New York

Clinical Assistant Professor
State University of New York
Health Science Center at Brooklyn
Brooklyn, New York

Pediatric Occupational Therapy Consultant
New York Metropolitan Area


MARGERY A. SZCZEPANSKI, MA, OTR/L
Coordinator of Clinical Services
Williamsburg Infant and Early Childhood Center
Brooklyn, New York

Part-time Instructor
New York University
Department of Occupational Therapy
New York, New York


VALORIE RICCIARDONE TODD, MA, OTR/L
Pediatric Occupational Therapy Consultant
Ulster County, New York


G. GORDON WILLIAMSON, PhD, OTR/L, FAOTA
Director, Social Competence Project
Pediatric Rehabilitation Department
John F. Kennedy Medical Center
Edison, New Jersey


SHIRLEY ZEITLIN, EdD
Psychologist
Private Practice
Loch Arbour, New Jersey

# Contents

Foreword.............................. vii
Preface ................................ ix
Acknowledgments ............. xiii
Contributors........................ xv

## Section I / THEORY

**1** Developmental Perspective: Fundamentals of Developmental
Theory ................................................................................. 3
*Jim Hinojosa and Paula Kramer*

**2** Domain of Concern of Occupational Therapy Relevant to Pediatric
Practice................................................................................. 9
*Paula Kramer and Jim Hinojosa*

**3** Legitimate Tools of Pediatric Occupational Therapy ............................ 25
*Jim Hinojosa and Paula Kramer*

## Section II / FRAMES OF REFERENCE

**4** Structure of the Frame of Reference ......................................... 37
*Paula Kramer and Jim Hinojosa*

**5** Neurodevelopmental Treatment Frame of Reference........................... 49
*Sarah Shoen and Jill Anderson*

**6** Sensory Integrative Frame of Reference................................... 87
*Judith Gienke Kimball*

**7** Visual Perceptual Frame of Reference: An Information Processing
Approach ............................................................................. 177
*Valorie Ricciardone Todd*

8  Biomechanical Frame of Reference............................................ 233
    *Cheryl Ann Colangelo*

9  Human Occupation Frame of Reference............................... 307
    *Shirley Peganoff O'Brien*

10 Psychosocial Frame of Reference........................................ 351
    *Laurette Olson*

11 Coping Frame of Reference ................................................. 395
    *G. Gordon Williamson, Margery Szczepanski, and Shirley Zeitlin*

# Section III / PRACTICE APPLICATION

12 From Frames of Reference to Actual Intervention............................. 439
    *Jim Hinojosa and Paula Kramer*

13 Alternative Applications of Frames of Reference ............................. 447
    *Paula Kramer and Jim Hinojosa*

14 Influence of Settings on the Application of Frames of Reference ....... 455
    *Mary Mulhenhaupt*

15 Influence of the Human Context on the Application of Frames
    of Reference ............................................................... 475
    *Jim Hinojosa and Paula Kramer*

# Section IV / CASE STUDIES

16 Case Study: Neurodevelopmental Treatment Frame of Reference ...... 485
    *Margaret Kaplan and Gary Bedell*

17 Case Study: Biomechanical Frame of Reference................................. 511
    *Cheryl Ann Colangelo*

18 Case Study: Combined Sensory Integrative and Neurodevelopmental
    Treatment Frame of References........................................... 525
    *Susan Nesbit*

Index................................................................................. 547

# THEORY

# Developmental Perspective: Fundamentals of Developmental Theory

JIM HINOJOSA / PAULA KRAMER

As set forth by Anne Cronin Mosey, PhD, OTR, FAOTA (1970), frames of reference provide methical organization of theoretical and practical material in sequences needed for problem identification and solution in practice. In the pediatric arena, the frame of reference offers an outline of fundamental theoretical concepts relative to particular areas of function. It likewise serves as a guideline for assessing functional capacities in the client and offers a method for conceptualizing and initiating intervention.

The frame of reference has become an acceptable vehicle for organizing theoretical material in occupational therapy and for translating it into practice through a functional perspective. Frames of reference, therefore, enable the practitioner to shift theory into practice.

The presentation of theoretical material frequently is organized around diagnostic categories. As a structural scheme, the frame of reference differs from this. Although a diagnosis may provide insight into a child's disabilities, occupational therapists are concerned primarily with functional capacities. Material organized around diagnostic categories does not always address the essential focus of the occupational therapy process. In addition, a child may exhibit several other functional disorders not described in the diagnostic category but still essential to intervention. The frame of reference is designed first to highlight traditionally used theories, then to relate that information to function, and, finally, to organize that information into intervention. The frame of reference essentially is a blueprint for approaching the child.

# Developmental Perspective

Occupational therapy intervention with a child is based upon an understanding and appreciation of normal development. Differences exist in the perceptions of development, yet everyone tends to describe patterns or sequences of development that are accepted as being characteristic for all children everywhere. In other words, there is a sequential nature to all theories of child development. Some theorists support the idea of linear progression—that is, several components of a process must occur before the skill as a whole is acquired or learned (Freud, 1966; Gesell & Armatruda, 1947; Kohlberg, 1969). This is similar to the links in a chain, where each link provides an important piece toward the strengths of the whole chain. Other theorists view progression as being more pyramidal in nature (Ayres, 1972, 1979; Erikson, 1963; Llorens, 1976; Piaget, 1963; Reilly, 1974)—that is, there must be a basic foundation from which skill development evolves. In this perspective, all blocks at the base of the pyramid must be strong and placed securely to provide support.

Those therapists who view development as linear are called reductionists. Their main concern is with the components of a process and the resultant conditional responses. As the child develops, behavior represents a continual set of sequences. Other theories that support this perspective have been proposed by Pavlov (1927), Skinner (1974), and Kaluger and Kaluger (1984). Behaviorism and learning theory are included in this philosophy.

Those therapists who view development as pyramidal are called nonreductionists. Their concern is with the development of each level of function to provide the foundation for higher level skills. Processes that take place at lower levels only provide the foundation on which more sophisticated processes may develop. Inherent in this view is the idea that skills are stage specific—that is, a skill that evolves in one stage forms a component part for the behaviors that take place at a later stage. These ideas have been proposed by Piaget (1963), Gagne (1970), and Maslow (1970). This perspective is summarized by Travers (1977):

> The development of complex behavior is analogous to the construction of a building. First the foundation has to be laid. The form of the foundation has much to do with the kind of building that can be constructed on it; a round building cannot be readily erected on a square foundation. The size and strength of the foundation

has much to do with the structure that can be built. The walls determine the kind of roof that can be used to crown the structure (p. 25).

The reductionist viewpoint generally is not thought of as developmental in nature. Instead, the component parts of a process are considered first, followed by the conditional response. Some occupational therapists tend to think of this as creating a "splinter skill"—which has a negative connotation—whereas others see it as creating learned or acquired behavior—a more positive connotation. Despite the negative or positive outlook, both groups believe that a certain set of conditions and skills exist before a new skill can be obtained. From our vantage point, this can be considered as developmental because there is a specified sequence that must take place, or that must be developed, before the actual skill can occur. When a child requires a specific piece of adaptive equipment, the therapeutic intervention usually not only involves choosing the appropriate device but also teaching the child how to use it. The child's subsequent use of this device generally is thought of as learned behavior. In a pediatric setting, a therapist could not facilitate the successful use of a therapeutic device unless the child previously had obtained specific abilities that set the stage for using the particular piece of equipment. The sequential nature of the reductionist process, therefore, may be seen as one type of developmental process.

The viewpoint that sees function as a pyramidal process, where each stage depends on the skills that have been preestablished, is traditionally considered to be developmental.

Within the pediatric context, the linear and pyramidal processes both qualify as developmental, even though each differs in its perspective of what development actually means. Development may occur through learning and skill acquisition, or it may occur through maturation, where subsequent skills are created based on preestablished foundations. Both viewpoints involve an attempt to understand the patterns of progression. Each of these theoretical perspectives describes a particular pattern of progression in a child's development differently, yet each shares the generally accepted principles of human development (Daub, 1988).

Rates of development vary from child to child, with no two children being exactly alike. There is a range of normalcy within progression and rates of development. For example, it generally is accepted that a child creeps before walking. Usually, children spend several months mastering creeping, but some children progress very quickly through this stage and begin to attempt to walk soon after they have started to creep. When viewing normal development, however, it usually is orderly, predictable, and sequential. To be sure, there always is some degree of individuality with a child, with one aspect at times being more important than another. For instance, at an earlier stage in life, motor performance may be more imperative than cognitive performance. Finally, development does not always occur at a consistent rate, but rather, in spurts that alternate with rest periods, at which time consolidation of skills takes place. As a child begins to ambulate, he usually starts to ignore previous favored toys that required him to be sedentary. Instead, he now wants to explore his environment with his new found freedom.

A child does not develop in a vacuum. He is part of an everchanging, dynamic process because changes occur continuously in the internal and external environments. A child's body and mind represent the internal environment and they are greatly influenced by growth and maturation. Human and nonhuman objects are part of the external environment. These two worlds influence the child's development separately and together. The importance of each environment varies with each child's capabilities, the specific demands of a situation, the objects involved, and the performance required. Although a child is considered to have many separate areas that develop independently, motor, psychological, and social development all are interrelated and interdependent. In reality, although a child's motor development may be discussed in isolation, it cannot be considered to be independent of the child's whole life. Some variables that affect the motor development also involve the neurophysiological status, the orthopaedic status, early sensory and cognitive experiences, and the family situation. The child who is unable to walk may have limited access to interaction with his peers and, therefore may have difficulty with age-appropriate social development.

Although occupational therapists learn about all aspects of development, their major concern is with the child's ability to translate development into action. Pediatric occupational therapists share a unique viewpoint in their concern for development of performance skills. That is, occupational therapists are concerned with children being able to function within their own environments to the best of their abilities. This viewpoint requires consideration of the many different factors that can influence a child's overall development. Therapists, therefore, are inherently concerned with the child's abilities and how the human and nonhuman influences affect the development of these abilities. The child's abilities may be seen as a composite of various specific performance skills. To address the development of these performance skills, therapists concentrate first on ascertaining the child's developmental level, which refers to a determination of each child's patterns and sequences of development and then on an evaluation of the level that has been attained.

Once a child's pattern, sequence and level of development are determined, an occupational therapist can address needs in two ways. First, the therapist can establish the performance skills a child has or can develop at his current level of function. The child who cannot walk or talk still may be able to participate actively in his self-feeding. Second, based on a pattern or sequence of development, a therapist can determine a child's deficits and the possible influencing factors. Based on some hypothesis, a therapist uses knowledge about normal growth and development, anatomy, neurophysiology, and life tasks to develop an intervention plan that is sensitive to any sequela of disease or to any known data about the development of the particular systems in which a child has deficits. In addition, occupational therapists are concerned with other areas, such as family life, educational program, and other factors, that may influence development. Knowledge about the characteristic pattern of the development of a particular performance component must be balanced by the particular child's direction, rate, and sequence of development.

Perhaps the easiest area to understand is motor progression which, usually is presented in a format that identifies the sequence in which the child acquires the ability to move. This progression, like those of other systems, inherently includes the acceptance of two basic assumptions: (1) development has natural order and (2) development is sequential. Although affected by environment, stimulation, and the child's personal characteristics, motor development has a natural order that is consistent from child to child. Furthermore, the sequential order of each child seems to follow the same basic sequence to achieve similar basic skills. Some children develop faster in one area, some slower, but each child basically follows the same sequence.

Mechanisms of the performance component cannot be observed directly, but evidence that change has occurred is obvious from developing skills.

### References

Ayres, A. J. (1972). *Sensory integration and learning disorders*. Los Angeles, CA: Western Psychological Services.

Ayres, A. J. (1979). *Sensory integration and the child*. Los Angeles, CA: Western Psychological Services.

Daub, M. M. (1988). Occupational therapy—base in the human development process. In H. L. Hopkins & H. D. Smith (Eds.) *Willard and Spackman's occupational therapy* (7th ed.). Philadelphia, PA: J. B. Lippincott.

Erikson, E. H. (1963). *Childhood and society* (2nd ed.). New York: Norton & Co.

Freud, S. (1966). *Standard edition of the complete psychological works of Sigmund Freud*. London: Hogarth Press.

Gagne, R. M. (1970). *The conditions of learning* (2nd ed.). New York: Holt, Rinehart, & Winston.

Gesell, A., & Armatruda, C. S. (1954). *Developmental diagnosis* (2nd ed.). New York: Harper & Brothers.

Kaluger, G., & Kaluger, M. F. (1984). *Human development: the span of life* (3rd ed.). St Louis, MO: C. V. Mosby.

Kohlberg, L. (1969). Stage and sequence: The cognitive developmental approach to socialization. In D. Groslin (Ed.) *Handbook of socialization theory and research.* Chicago, IL: Rand McNally.

Llorens, L. A. (1976). *Application of developmental theory for health and rehabilitation.* Rockville, MD: American Occupational Therapy Association.

Maslow, A. H. (1970). *Motivation and personality* (2nd ed.). New York: Harper & Row.

Mosey, A. C. (1970). *Three frames of reference for mental health.* Thorofare, NJ: Charles B. Slack.

Pavlov, I. P. (1927). *Conditioned reflexes* (trans. by G. V. Andrep). London: Oxford.

Piaget, J. (1963). *Psychology of intelligence.* Paterson, NJ: Littlefield, Adams & Co.

Reilly, M. (1974). *Play as exploratory learning.* Beverly Hills, CA: Sage.

Skinner, B. F. (1974). *About behaviorism.* New York: Vintage Books.

Travers, R. M. W. (1977). *Essentials of learning.* New York: Macmillan.

## 2

# Domain of Concern of Occupational Therapy Relevant to Pediatric Practice

PAULA KRAMER / JIM HINOJOSA

In most professions, a continuous evolution of the concerns within the profession defines its focus and explains why it is important to society. Society rarely stays the same, so, as society changes, the professions need to respond accordingly. All helping professions evolve and change to meet a unique need of the society that they serve.

It is virtually impossible to define a profession in discrete terms because of this constant change. To remain viable, a profession must be dynamic, continuously developing and modifying to meet the changing needs of society. Those persons who study or enter a profession may struggle, however, with this concept, because they usually strive for one constant definition of their profession.

One group of caretakers, the health professions, must adapt to changes in social priorities and in the ways that they deliver health care. Society tends to have different trends during different eras, when one age group or particular category of disability receives more attention than others. This leads to an increased professional focus on those particular groups and may lead to specialized practice. This has been the case in occupational therapy in the United States. For example, pediatric occupational therapists have been affected dramatically by societal changes. In the early 1970s, federal laws emphasized and supported the educational needs of special children and required

9

that occupational therapy be a related service (Gilfoyle & Hayes, 1979; Hanft, 1990; Ottenbacher, 1982). This idea was expanded during the 1980s when the needs of infants and toddlers became an area of concern, and occupational therapy was identified as a primary service (Hanft, 1990). In response, occupational therapy practice has evolved to address and focus on these priorities. This has led not only to an increase in the number of occupational therapists who work in education-based practice but also to a change in the site of practice, with more services provided in schools and community settings.

# Domain of Concern

The domain of concern in occupational therapy defines its expertise. The profession has categorized and defined itself as one that encompasses human performance components that serve as the basis for occupational performance areas. It is beyond the scope of this book to identify the entire domain of concern for the profession of occupational therapy. This chapter focuses, therefore, on the domain of pediatric practice.

The profession has identified the performance components that comprise occupational performance. Again, these may change over time, depending on the needs of society and the focus of practice as it adapts to societal change. In 1979, to develop a uniformity of definition for practice within the profession, a document called Uniform Terminology was approved by the American Occupational Therapy Association (AOTA) Representative Assembly. To respond to the evolution of practice, AOTA then recognized the need to update the document continually to reflect current practice and to reemphasize the need for uniformity of definitions. It currently is recognized that Uniform Terminology defines the domain of concern for the profession of occupational therapy. To continue to reflect the needs of society, in 1992, the Commission on Practice of AOTA again revised this document to develop a third edition of Uniform Terminology. This edition encompasses performance context to define more accurately the domain of concern of the profession.

Performance components and occupational performance areas are influenced strongly by a person's age, stage of development, sociocultural background, and environment. Particularly relative to children, the age and stage of development are critical factors. The domain of concern for pediatric occupational therapists therefore incorporates a description of all areas of life that concern therapists when working with a child and his family.

# Performance Components

Performance components are arbitrary divisions of human functioning with sensory motor component, cognitive integration and cognitive component, and psychosocial skills and psychological components being the areas of major concern for occupational therapy (American Occupational Therapy Association, 1989). Separating human function into basic parts allows the occupational therapist to understand the individual sections that make up the whole. By looking at the small sections, a therapist gains a better understanding of how the client processes information in these discrete areas. Through this specific examination of each discrete area or performance component, a more comprehensive understanding of the child's skills and deficits can be gained. By examining and understanding the component parts, a therapist's knowledge and understanding of the complex human organism increases.

Performance components are closely interrelated. Each performance component embodies an area of a child's development that occupational therapists are expert in. Understanding performance components and their interrelation provides basic information about the child. From this point, the occupational therapist can develop appropriate interventions after considering the child's biological potential and developmental status.

Pediatric occupational therapy tends to emphasize particular aspects of each performance component—that is, a subset of each performance component. As a growing human being, a child matures and develops skills in each of the performance areas, making him more sensitive to any condition that may interfere with his development. It is important then that a therapist also understand the various subparts of each performance component. For example, the sensory motor performance component is divided into three units: sensory integration, neuromuscular, and motor. Based on the condition of the child who is being treated, the therapist may need to focus on only one or two of these subcomponents. For example, with a child who has cerebral palsy, the therapist might be more concerned with the neuromotor and motor subcomponents than with the sensory integrative subcomponent.

## Sensory Motor Performance Component

A child's sensory motor performance component includes those parts of human function that depend on the processing of sensory input. It encompasses sensory integration, neuromuscular, and motor performances. Motor skills are included because refined motor function is considered to be based in the adequate processing of sensory information.

**Sensory integration** involves skills and performance in the development and coordination of sensory input, motor output, and sensory feedback. Sensory integrative functioning is based on the status of the central nervous system (CNS) and the child's neurophysiological responses. Sensorimotor responses are thought to develop from a generalized response to a more sophisticated, discrete response to specific stimuli. The tactile system, for example, develops the ability to recognize internal as opposed to external sensation, discrimination between objects, and, finally, identification. The visual system likewise develops more sophisticated responses through recognition of pattern, form, and constancy, up to and including the ability to deal with spatial relations. Accordingly, sensory integration subsumes sensory awareness, sensory processing, and perceptual skills (American Occupational Therapy Association, 1989).

**Neuromuscular** involves areas of development that underlie the motor aspects of behavior. This depends on the maturity of the CNS and the neurophysiological system. Neuromuscular subsumes reflex, range of motor, muscle tone, strength, endurance, postural control, and soft-tissue integrity (American Occupational Therapy Association, 1989).

**Motor** involves performance of the motor aspects of behavior. Generally, motor performance is viewed as sequential development with generalized rules: cephalo to caudal, proximal to distal, and gross control to fine control (Fig. 2.1). Motor functioning subsumes activity tolerance, gross motor coordination, crossing the midline, laterality, bilateral integration, praxis, fine motor coordination/dexterity, visual-motor integration, and oral-motor control (American Occupational Therapy Association, 1989).

## Cognitive Integration and Cognitive Components

For children, cognitive integration and cognitive components involve the mental processes needed to comprehend or understand. At the basic level, this involves the child's conscious awareness and knowledge of objects through perception, memory, and reasoning. Included within this extensive performance component are level of arousal, orientation, recognition, attention span, memory, sequencing, categorization, concept formation, intellectual operations in space, problem solving, generalization of learning, integration of learning, and synthesis of learning (American Occupational Therapy Association, 1989).

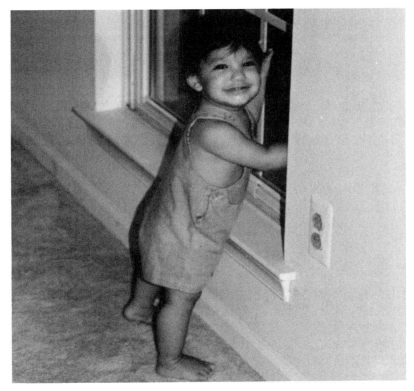

**Figure 2.1**  Child just beginning to stand with support

## Psychological Skills and Psychological Components

Psychological skills and psychological components combine the child's psychological, social aspects, and self-management functions. **Psychological functions** involve skill and performance in developing a self-concept and the ability to handle life situations. Roles, values, interests, initiation of activity, termination of activity, and self-concept are especially important in the psychological performance component (American Occupational Therapy Association, 1989). The development of adequate psychological abilities allows a child to express and control himself.

**Social** involves the child's developing abilities and skills in relation to other people (Fig. 2.2). Included in this area are social conduct, conversation, and self-expression (American Occupational Therapy Association, 1989).

**Self-management** skills allow the child to deal with his daily life routines in a way that supports his psychological and social development. Involved

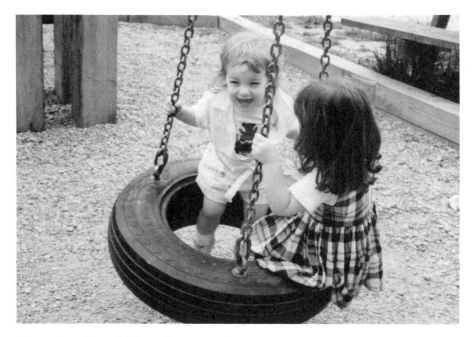

**Figure 2.2**   Two children playing together on a tire swing

in this are the child's coping skills, time management, and self-control (American Occupational Therapy Association, 1989).

## Performance Components and Intervention

The pediatric occupational therapist keeps several things in mind when viewing children. These involve looking at children relative to normal development and understanding their mastery of developmental milestones. Another important consideration is the relationship between the child's skills and his chronological and developmental age. Sometimes a child appears to have mastered part of the task but not the whole task. The therapist first needs to look at the task and then must analyze the component parts needed to master the whole task. For example, a child may be able to move himself from sitting into a quadruped position but then cannot move himself forward to begin creeping. The therapist needs to analyze the task and understand what parts of the task have been mastered. The child can move from one position to another but has difficulty weightshifting to begin reciprocal movement of the limbs. This analysis also involves identifying what parts of the task a child still needs to develop to master the whole task. In essence, this is a process of understanding the status of the child's performance component.

Occupational therapists must know about the characteristics and developmental aspects of the performance components that often are important in determining intervention. Pediatric therapists are responsive to the developmental status of a child with regard to each performance component. This responsiveness is possible because of the therapist's understanding and appreciation for the development of each performance component based on the appreciation for normal development. Therapists know that performance components do not develop in isolation. In fact, each performance component depends on another for the child to grow and learn.

As defined by Uniform Terminology (2nd ed.), the performance components are rather broad categories, and, sometimes, they are too broad for dealing with a specific child. Because of the specific types of intervention, therapist need to divide these performance components into even smaller entities. When a therapist deals with a child who has grasp problems for example, the categories of gross and fine coordination are not sufficient to understand and analyze these deficits. In this situation, the therapist needs to divide the child's motor performance into even more discrete and specific aspects of performance.

This extended division may be a result of specific areas of practice or of a particular frame of reference. When an occupational therapist uses a specific frame of reference, a certain performance component may become more important, and the therapist then focuses on that particular performance component. When this happens, therapists may reorganize the performance components in a more sophisticated way, often dividing them into smaller segments. For example, therapists who work with infants who have cerebral palsy are concerned primarily with neuromuscular and motor development. They therefore may develop sophisticated subsections related to the sensory motor performance component. Furthermore, if the neurodevelopmental frame of reference is used, the therapist may develop even more explicit subsections related to the importance of postural tone, righting reactions, and equilibrium responses—things that the frame of reference considers to be important for the development of motor skills.

Although individual therapists may divide human function in different ways, what remains important is that the whole of what is considered to be human function still remains the same. More discrete and specific performance components serve a specific need for the therapists' understanding of the children with whom they work. Performance components are only arbitrary divisions of human function that allow therapists to understand the parts of the whole to which children respond and then interact with their own environments. By understanding the component parts, a therapist has a better perspective for analyzing the child's overall function. On a more global level, this information gives the therapist a clear picture of how the child responds to situations and interacts with his environment.

# Occupational Performance Areas

Occupational performance areas are arbitrary divisions or classifications of the purposeful activities in which people engage. Occupational performance is defined as the accomplishment of tasks related to occupational performance areas (Llorens, 1991). For children, occupational performance areas include activities of daily living, work activities, and play or leisure activities. The extent to which each of the occupational performance areas is important and to which occupational performance can be achieved depends on the child's environmental and cultural demands based on his age and stage of development (Llorens, 1991). The occupational therapist is concerned with the child's ability to perform life tasks. Life tasks refer to all those activities that must be accomplished to meet these goals or needs and to be a contributing member of a community (Mosey, 1981).

## Activities of Daily Living

Activities of daily living include the child's ability to perform the tasks needed for self-care. These include grooming, oral hygiene, bathing, toilet hygiene, dressing, feeding and eating, medication routines, socialization, functional communication, functional mobility, and sexual expression (American Occupational Therapy Association, 1989) (Fig. 2.3). The extent to which each of these areas is important to the child depends on his cultural background, environmental demands, particular age, and stage of development.

## Work Activities/Education

Llorens uses the term *work activities* in combination with the term *education*, to form the term *work activities/education* (Llorens, 1991). This is particularly pertinent for relating this occupational performance area to children. Work activities/education refers to involvement and accomplishment of activities in the home, in school, and in the community.

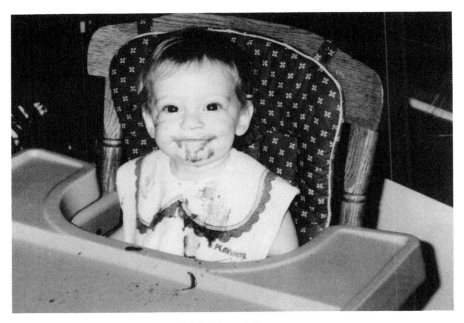

**Figure 2.3**   Child developing self-feeding skills

Work activities include home management, care of others, educational activities, and vocational activities (American Occupational Therapy Association, 1989). Again, it is important to emphasize that the relevancy of each subcategory depends on cultural background and environment, as well as on age and stage of development. For children, home management may relate to household chores, maintaining one's room, and keeping clothes neat. Care of others may include looking after a younger sibling or care of a pet. Educational activities may include day care, nursery and preschool routines or afterschool learning activities, such as religious education as well as traditional school involvements around classroom performance. The term *vocational activities* generally does not apply to young children. It may relate to older children who begin to be involved in work activities, such as paper routes, mowing lawns, or shoveling snow.

## *Play or Leisure Activities*

Although Uniform Terminology refers to this area as play or leisure activities, the term *leisure* does not generally apply to younger children. Play or leisure activities are those things in which a child *chooses* to engage. They are

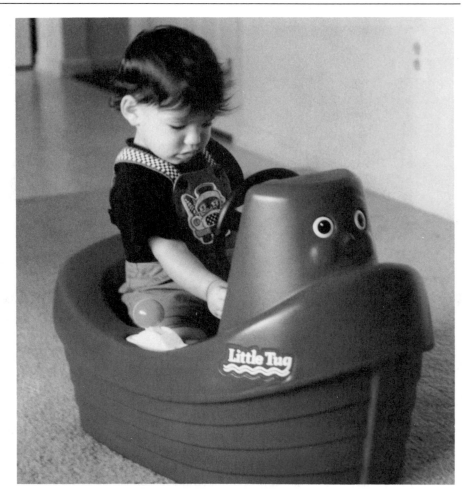

**Figure 2.4**   Child amusing himself in play

selected for a child's amusement, enjoyment, or self-expression (Fig. 2.4). Intrinsically, play should be pleasurable, promoting the child's enjoyment or relaxation. Play should encourage skill development through involvement with objects and interaction with others. Professionally speaking, play is divided into two parts: play exploration and play performance. Play exploration relates to the identification of play interests that promote skills and opportunities. Play performance includes physical and social activities that are inherently gratifying.

# Occupational Performance Areas and Intervention

Occupational therapists are always concerned with the occupational performance of their clients. With children, the focus is to enable the child to function effectively within various environments: family, school, and community. To address the child's ability to function effectively within the occupational performance areas, the therapist should become sensitive to the child's life situation. As discussed under performance components, occupational therapists usually are aware of the child's developmental levels. It is also necessary, however, for the therapist to develop a sensitivity to the child's cultural and social background. The cultural and social background affect the child's everyday routines through parental and societal expectations, and it is to the therapist's advantage to understand each case at these levels, to ensure a good therapist-client association (with optimal outcome).

## Culture

Whenever occupational performance areas are addressed, it is important for the therapist to become familiar with the child's culture. This may have an impact on the child's expectations of himself and the parents' expectations of the child. Subsequently, this may reflect on the child's performance. For example, in some cultures, it is acceptable for a child to use a bottle until he is ready to enter preschool, whereas in other cultures a child is weaned from the bottle once he becomes a toddler. This would impact on the child's exposure to a cup and his ability to drink from it. This is an example of a cultural expectation that affects performance. Throughout life, culture influences what a person considers to be normal and what constitutes expected patterns of behavior. Within the process of intervention, the therapist needs to be aware of and sensitive to the cultural background of each child encountered.

## Temporal Adaptation

When occupational performance is at issue, a major concern is temporal adaptation (Mosey, 1986). Temporal adaptation encompasses three major areas: first, the child's learned ability to structure himself to accomplish tasks and to interact with others; second, the ability to structure daily activities to fulfill social roles; and third, the ability to assume responsibility for the organization of time, allowing the child to enjoy being a family member and taking on the culturally expected roles of work and play. Each of these three areas is determined by the child's cultural background and environment.

Temporal adaptation that involves the child's ability to structure himself to accomplish tasks and to interact with others relates to the understanding of time as an external factor that regulates daily activities. As determined by his culture, the child learns that each day has its own cycle. This includes proscribed times to eat, to engage in activities, and to sleep. This structure gives the child a routine that allows him to predict what will happen each day and how to construct his interaction with others.

The ability to structure daily activities to fulfill social roles builds on the child's learned ability to structure himself (i.e., his behavior). Through his understanding of time, the child is now able to behave according to his needs and personal priorities. Very often, however, the structure is controlled by external factors such as family or school.

Again, building on the previously discussed areas, the child develops the ability to assume responsibility for the organization of his time, allowing him to enjoy family, work, and play. As the child matures, he develops his own time plan based on the influences of his family, community, and school. As these routines develop, the child takes more responsibility for organizing his time and for developing and refining his roles as a family member, peer, student, and worker. The child now can take into account his internal needs, as well as the demands of his culture, environment, and society. He also has to establish a balance between those needs and the demands of those around him (Pratt, 1989).

Within the intervention process, it is important for the therapist to take temporal adaptation into account so that the child will develop appropriate age and cultural routines, as well as patterns of behaviors, and will be able to satisfy his needs while becoming a responsible member of his community.

## Activities of Daily Living

Activities of daily living represent a primary area of concern for occupational therapy intervention. The therapist is dedicated to developing the child's ability to engage in self-care activities. Another aspect of activities of daily living is working with the child's care providers so that they are able to care for the child as well as foster independence in the child. Activities of daily living involve aspects of personal care, such as toileting and personal hygiene activities that provide the child with a sense of personal dignity (Fig.

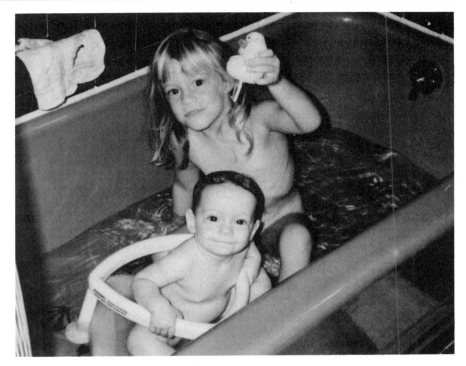

**Figure 2.5**   Two children engaging in a personal care activity

2.5). Although it may be difficult for therapists to work with these areas, it is critical that they do so because this may enable the child to become as independent as possible and to develop a positive sense of self. Although some frames of reference in this text do not address this area directly, it is understood that they are laying the foundation that allows the child to become independent in activities of daily living.

## Work/Education Activities

As previously discussed, when dealing with children, work encompasses education and selected activities (such as household chores and afterschool jobs). Occupational therapists usually address these areas through their concern with the interrelated foundational components of work/education.

## Play or Leisure Activities

Play or leisure activities are those things chosen by the child, because they are amusing, enjoyable, relaxing, or self-expressive. Play often promotes skill development and interaction with others. The occupational therapist uses play in two separate ways. First, the therapist tries to facilitate play exploration, so that the child can try out various types of play and decide which ones he finds enjoyable. Second, the therapist uses play as a therapeutic modality, to facilitate not only the performance but also the development of the child. This aspect of play is addressed later (as part of the legitimate tools of occupational therapy).

## Summary

All helping professions evolve and change to meet the needs of society. Within these professions, their areas of expertise are considered their domain of concern. Occupational therapy's domain of concern encompasses human performance components that serve as the bases for occupational performance areas. Performance components and occupational performance areas are influenced strongly by a person's age, stage of development, sociocultural background, and environment.

Performance components include sensory motor, cognitive integration and cognitive, and psychosocial skills and psychological. Performance components are significant in the way in which the occupational therapist views intervention. Although these component parts are essential to intervention, it is important for the therapist to maintain the perspective of the total child.

Activities of daily living, work activities/education, and play or leisure activities constitute the occupational performance areas. Occupational therapists are always concerned with the occupational performance of their clients. The focus in pediatric occupational therapy is the child's ability to function within a variety of environments. The child's culture provides that setting for intervention and must be taken into account by the therapist. A major concern in intervention is temporal adaptation, so that the child is able to develop age and culturally appropriate routines.

### References

American Occupational Therapy Association. (1979). *Occupational therapy output reporting system and uniform terminology for reporting occupational therapy services.* Rockville, MD: Author.

American Occupational Therapy Association. (1989). *Uniform terminology for occupational therapy - Second edition.* Rockville, MD: Author.

Gilfoyle, E. & Hayes, C. (1979). Occupational therapy roles and functions in the education of the school-based handicapped student. *American Journal of Occupational Therapy, 33,* 565–576.

Hanft, B. E. (1991). Impact of Federal policy on pediatric health and education programs. In W. Dunn (ed.) *Pediatric occupational therapy: Facilitating effective service provision.* (pp. 273–284). Thorofare, NJ: Slack.

Llorens, L. A. (1991). Performance tasks and roles throughout the life span. In C. Christiansen & C. Baum (eds.) *Occupational therapy: Overcoming human performance deficits.* (pp. 45–66). Thorofare, NJ: Slack.

Mosey, A. C. (1986). *Psychosocial component of occupational therapy.* New York: Raven.

Mosey, A. C. (1981). *Occupational therapy: Configuration of a profession.* New York: Raven.

Ottenbacher, K. (1982). Occupational therapy and special education: Some issues and concerns related to PL 94–142. *American Journal of Occupational Therapy, 36,* 81–84.

Pratt, P. N. (1989). Occupational therapy in pediatrics. In P. N. Pratt, & A. S. Allen, (Eds.) *Occupational therapy for children* (2nd ed.) (pp. 121–131). St. Louis, MO: C. V. Mosby.

# 3

# Legitimate Tools of Pediatric Occupational Therapy

JIM HINOJOSA / PAULA KRAMER

As previously stated, the frame of reference provides organized theoretical and practical material in a methodical and sequential way so that therapists can use it for intervention. It is an outline of essential theoretical concepts relative to particular areas of function, a guideline for assessing those areas of function and a method for conceptualizing intervention. In its exploration of a particular area of function, the frame of reference tends to be more global and general so that it is applicable to larger groups or populations. It is not specific; it generally proposes *how* the therapist can create an environment to promote change. Although the frame of reference discusses the tools available to the therapist in a general sense, it is **assumed** that the therapist has a firm understanding of the various tools and is competent in their use. Tools are defined as those items, means, methods, or instruments used in the practice of a profession.

## Legitimate Tools

Every health profession has a specific set of tools or instruments to use in bringing about change. These are referred to as the profession's legitimate tools. Society accepts the professional as that person who is expert in the use of these specific legitimate tools. Legitimate tools change over time, based on the knowledge of the profession, technological advances in society, and the needs and values of the profession and society. To bring about change, occupational therapists use various legitimate tools.

Most professions hold their legitimate tools in high regard. For some practitioners, they are symbolic of the profession. Because legitimate tools are used daily as a means of interacting with clients, they may be considered more tangible than the body of knowledge or domain of concern (Mosey, 1986). Many practitioners feel that the tools of their professions are unique, and, in some cases, this may be true. In most situations, however, this is not the case; rather, the way in which the tools are used in the application of the frame of reference makes them unique.

Each frame of reference addresses the process of change or the way in which the therapist promotes change in the client. Occupational therapy has many frames of reference that relate to many types and areas of practice. Legitimate tools are chosen by the therapist to fit the particular frame of reference that she has determined to be appropriate for the particular client. Furthermore, specific legitimate tools are chosen based on their compatibility with the client's developmental level and the environment in which intervention is provided. Some legitimate tools are used by the profession as a whole but may be applied uniquely in pediatric occupational therapy. There have been extensive discussions about the tools of the profession as they relate to the profession as well as about specific areas of practice (Ayres, 1979; Christiansen & Baum, 1991; Hopkins & Smith, 1988; Mosey, 1986; Pedretti & Zoltan, 1990; Trombly, 1989). This chapter presents an overview of selected legitimate tools for pediatric practice, including the nonhuman environment, conscious use of self, activity analysis and adaption, purposeful activities, activity groups, and the teaching/learning process. In addition to the tools presented here, others exist that are very specialized and often are specific to only one frame of reference. These may be discussed in the theoretical base of the frame of reference. Often, however, such specialized tools require advanced education and training and, therefore, are beyond the scope of this chapter.

## The Nonhuman Environment

The nonhuman environment includes everything that the child comes in contact with that is not human (Mosey, 1986; Searles, 1960). This includes the community, the school, and the home. It also includes pets, objects, play things, and transitional objects (a blanket, preferred stuffed animal, favored doll, or a diary), which can be anything that is not human that has meaning for the person. A child's nonhuman environment is influenced, to some extent, by cultural background and developmental level. For example, it may be considered unacceptable for a male child of Italian or Hispanic culture to play with kitchen utensils or pots and pans, because that is not considered appropriate to the role for a male child in these cultures in which gender roles are clearly delineated for children.

When working with children, particular aspects of the nonhuman environment are significant to the pediatric therapist. The first is that the physical, nonhuman environment changes as the child grows. The child starts out primarily in the crib, and, in some cultures, in an infant seat. As the child grows older, he may have a more varied nonhuman environment, moving onto the floor, into a playpen or in a walker. The facets of the child's physical, nonhuman environment vary, depending on culture. Some parents are eager to expose their children to a wide variety of environments, whereas others feel more secure in limiting their children's environment. The child's interaction and awareness of the nonhuman environment changes as his physical environments change and as he adapts to the different things around him.

As the child develops, he relates differently to toys and other objects that are part of his nonhuman environment. At first, he may be unaware of a stuffed animal placed in his crib. As he matures, however, he becomes aware that the same stuffed animal, a teddy bear perhaps, is always in his crib and that the animal has become important to him, separate from the environment of the crib. Regardless of his surroundings, that animal is important, and the child may be reluctant to engage in any new tasks without the presence of "Teddy" at his side. In this case, the stuffed animal may be a transitional object, helping the child move from one stage to another. Transitional objects often help to make a child feel secure, especially in a new environment. For example, a young child will often take a favorite toy with him when moving from a crib to a bed.

Toys are particularly important learning tools in the nonhuman environment. They provide the child with basic stimulation, enjoyment, and an initial sense of mastery over his environment. The child learns a sense of competency from toys; he learns that he is able to do things. The child develops his initial understanding of task performance through interaction with toys. The occupational therapist is skilled at the use of toys in intervention and at matching toys with the child's developmental level (Proctor, 1989).

Pets also are significant parts of the nonhuman environment, especially for children at the preschool level and older. They may serve a function similar to transitional objects. Pets also may help the child to develop nurturing qualities and assist in the move away from the natural egocentrism of early childhood. Pets likewise can be a source of pleasure and companionship.

In today's world, technology—assistive devices and computers—is becoming increasingly important in occupational therapy in terms of nonhuman objects. This includes low technology—devices that are not electronically powered—and high technology alike. Examples of low technology include new writing devices (such as markers), Velcro® fasteners and bathtub books. High technology includes computer systems, recording equipment, and talking toys.

The nonhuman environment often is used by pediatric occupational therapists in the intervention process. The therapist selects objects appropriate to the child's age, developmental level, and culture as part of the intervention. The therapist works to facilitate the child's mastery of the nonhuman environment. This mastery involves the child's ability to learn from his toys and to experiment with objects in his physical environment. The therapist also uses the nonhuman environment to facilitate the child's development of performance component skills. For example, a specific toy used in therapy may contribute to improvement in fine motor coordination.

Although the nonhuman environment is often thought of in an emotional context, it can be considered in a physical sense as well. The therapist may adapt or manipulate the physical nonhuman environment to use it in the process of intervention. Examples of this include changing the child's equipment, using adaptive devices, or positioning. Low technology (such as assistive devices for feeding and writing, and adaptive and positioning equipment) would be used for such purposes. High technology devices for intervention include adapted computers, page-turning devices, environmental controls, and augmentative communication devices.

Whether the nonhuman environment is used from an emotional or physical perspective, it always should be taken into account when planning intervention so that the intervention is meaningful to the child within the context of his environment.

## Conscious Use of Self

Conscious use of self involves the therapist's use of herself as an agent to effect change within the therapeutic process. The establishment of a positive therapeutic relationship between therapists and client is a major part of the conscious use of self. An important characteristic of this relationship is the therapist's ability to develop a comfortable rapport, that is, to make the child aware that the therapist cares about him and to accept the child at his current level of performance. In addition, it requires that the therapist controls her own responses, so that she acts in a way that promotes the child's ability to function or operate in his world.

Like the nonhuman environment, the conscious use of self can also be thought of in a physical context. Therapists can consciously use themselves physically in the intervention process. Examples of this would be handling and some of the neuromuscular facilitation techniques.

The pediatric occupational therapist continually uses herself as an agent for positive change in the child, which involves entering the child's world. The therapist needs to relate to the child at his own level, emotionally, physically, and developmentally. If the child is at the developmental level at which he spends most of his time on the floor, then the therapist needs to work with the child on the floor. For the same child, objects and directions may have to presented in a specific and concrete manner, so that the child can understand them and respond. The conscious use of self in this example is the therapist's awareness of the child's level and her ability to adapt her posture and behavior to that level. Toys and therapeutic tools also need to be at the child's developmental level, or slightly higher, to stimulate the child's growth. In essence, the therapist has to have a clear understanding of the child's developmental level and skills so that she can intervene at that same level or above. Otherwise, the intervention may be less than successful.

The therapist's conscious use of self can be extended to interactions with the family and with other care providers. The therapist needs to gauge the family's understanding of the child to be able to collaborate successfully. She cannot dictate to them or talk down to them; she needs to interact with them positively. This entails language, posture, gestures, and tone of voice that engages family members—things that they can understand—so that all family members can play an effective part in the therapeutic process. The conscious use of self in this sense therefore may mean that the therapist provides an appropriate role model for the family. The therapist's role with the family is flexible and needs to be able to change over time depending on need.

The skillful application of the conscious use of self develops with practice. To the master clinician, this becomes a natural part of her repertoire.

## Activity Analysis and Adaptation

Activity analysis is the identification of the component parts of an activity. Occupational therapists are continually fascinated by the parts that make up an activity. Even activities that seem simple because of their familiarity may actually be complex. The occupational therapist analyzes activities so that they can be used to treat a client. Through the use of this tool, the therapist can identify whether the child has the necessary skills to perform or complete the activity. Activity analysis also enables the therapist to teach the activity more successfully, through a clear understanding of its component parts.

When working with children, activity analysis is a constant focus of the intervention process. The pediatric occupational therapist continually divides activities into component parts to determine which skills are necessary to complete the task or activity. This is just the first step in the intervention process. The next step involves observation of how the child reacts and interacts with the activity or its component tasks. The therapist then analyzes the activity as well as the child's actions with or participation in it. This process provides the therapist with the information she needs to adapt, grade, or combine activities to make them effective in intervention (Hinojosa, Sabari, & Rosenfeld, 1983).

The complexity of the activity analysis process is illustrated in the simple activity of stacking blocks. The preliminary analysis entails gaining an understanding of the skills required for the child to stack blocks. The child needs to have beginning fine motor skills, the ability to grasp the blocks, and controlled release for stacking the blocks. Then, as the child begins to stack the blocks, the therapist observes the child's behavior and response to the blocks. The next step involves analyzing the child and activity in combination. The questions that follow are examples of what the therapist might ask to start this analysis:

1. What is the level of the child's fine motor skills in this task?
2. Can he pick up the blocks?
3. Can he place the blocks neatly on the stack?
4. Does he have difficulty letting go of the blocks?
5. Does he exhibit other compensatory body movements when engaged in the task?
6. Is he more interested in building the tower or knocking it down?

The therapist answers these questions based on her preliminary analysis combined with the knowledge gained from observing the child perform the activity. The therapist needs to look at the answers to all these questions before she proceeds, to know how to modify this activity to make it therapeutic for the child. Furthermore, the same activity might be different with another child, because the reactions of the child and the answers to the previously stated questions would be different. Any activity becomes modified by the way a particular child interacts with the environment and how he performs the activity.

The next step in the use of this tool involves adaptation. Activity adaptation means that elements of the activity are modified to meet the needs of the client and to facilitate positive change. Activities are adapted by modifying the child's position, the presentation of the materials, or the characteristics of the materials (shape, size, weight, or texture). Adaptation may also involve modifying the procedure or sequence of events for the activity and the nature and degree of interpersonal contact (Hinojosa, Sabari, & Rosenfeld, 1983).

In pediatric practice, the therapist continually adapts activities for the child. As discussed previously, an example of adaptation is the modification of stacking blocks. The therapist might use larger blocks, seat the child at a small table rather than on the floor, present one block at a time, or add Velcro® to the blocks so that they may be attached more easily to each other. The possibilities of adaptation for this activity are endless, limited only by the therapist's creativity.

## Purposeful Activities

Purposeful activities are those that have meaning to the child and that involve interaction with the human and nonhuman environments (King, 1978). Many purposeful activities for children revolve around play and schoolwork. Erikson (1963) proposed the idea that play is the work of the child. Play is one category available among the tools of purposeful activity. Children learn through play. The various types of play include sensorimotor play, constructional play, imaginary play, and group play. Sensorimotor play is characterized by the use of a sensory stimulation along with a motor component. Constructional play promotes pleasure through building and creating things. Imaginary play entails cognition combined with fantasy and creativity. Group play is an interactional process where children work together with a relatively common theme. Based on the developmental level, culture, and needs of the child, the pediatric occupational therapist uses and adapts the types of therapeutic experiences to the benefit of that child. Through the skilled therapeutic use of play as a tool, the therapist can enhance the child's enjoyment and success in therapy.

Purposeful activities need to be viewed within the context of the child and his environment. Some contextual aspects of a purposeful activity are culture, temporal adaptation, and socioeconomic climate. Each activity becomes modified because of how the child interacts with and performs that activity. Purposeful activities are an inherent part of occupational therapy. The pediatric occupational therapist must take care in selecting activities so that they

are meaningful to the child. The activities should be developmentally appropriate and motivating to the child, meshing comfortably with the child's
lifestyle and environment.

## Activity Groups

Activity groups are those that have a common goal that involves purposeful activities. As a tool, activity groups are used more often in some frames
of reference than in others. Mosey (1986) has clearly described activity groups
and their various levels.

In pediatric occupational therapy, activity groups are used as a tool to
promote age-appropriate peer interaction in a therapeutic environment. Occupational therapists draw from their knowledge of child development, group
dynamics, and a firm understanding of activities. Activity groups are used to
develop play, task, social, and physical skills. The involvement of peers can
be useful for facilitating motivation. The occupational therapist fosters group
interaction in a safe and supportive environment.

## Teaching/Learning Process

The teaching/learning process as a legitimate tool consists of two parts.
Teaching gives instruction to a child or shows him how to do something,
whereas learning promotes acquisition of knowledge or information from
instruction, observation, or experience. Learning results in a relatively permanent change in behavior. As a tool, the teaching/learning process is more
commonly used in some frames of reference than in others. A therapist
facilitates learning through the creation of an environment that encourages
a positive change in the child.

A pediatric occupational therapist teaches through the careful selection
of activities reflective of the child's developmental level, age, abilities, and
interests. The learning process is enhanced through the use of positive reinforcement and feedback to the child based on his performance. The child is
more likely to learn from therapeutic interventions that are enjoyable and
interesting. Important aspects of learning include trial and error, shaping,
modelling, repetition, and practice. The learning environment should be supportive and appropriate for the chosen activity.

# Summary

This chapter has outlined the current major legitimate tools for pediatric
occupational therapy. Other legitimate tools exist that have not been pre-

sented here but that are specific to one frame of reference and may be highly specialized. These specialized tools often require advanced education and training. The tools of the profession can change over time, just as practice changes over time. Because these tools are used within a frame of reference to create an environment for change, each frame of reference has tools that are more relevant and acceptable to it than to others. Within each frame of reference, the change process is outlined, delimiting the tools that are viable.

### References

Ayres, A. J. (1979). *Sensory integration and the child*. Los Angeles, CA: Western Psychological Services.

Christiansen, C., & Baum, C. (Eds.) (1991). *Occupational therapy: overcoming human performance deficits*. Thorofare, NJ: Slack.

Erikson, E. H. (1963). *Childhood and society* (2nd ed.). New York: Norton.

Hinojosa, H., Sabari, J., & Rosenfeld, M. S. (1983). Purposeful activities. *American Journal of Occupational Therapy*, *37*, 805–806.

Hopkins, H. L., & Smith, H. D. (Eds.) (1988). *Willard & Spackman's Occupational therapy* (7th Ed.). Philadelphia, PA: J. B. Lippincott.

King, L. J. (1978). Towards a science of adaptive responses. *American Journal of Occupational Therapy*, *7*, 429–437.

Mosey, A. C. (1986). *Psychosocial components of occupational therapy*. New York: Raven Press.

Pedretti, L. W., & Zoltan B. (Eds.) (1990). *Occupational therapy practice skills for physical dysfunction* (3rd ed.) St. Louis, MO: C. V. Mosby.

Proctor, S. A. (1989). Adaptations for independent living. In P. N. Pratt & A. S. Allen (Eds.). *Occupational therapy for children* (pp. 335–357). Baltimore, MD: C. V. Mosby.

Searles, H. F. (1960). *The nonhuman environment*. New York: International Universities Press.

Trombly, C. A. (Ed) (1989). *Occupational therapy for physical dysfunction* (3rd ed.). Baltimore, MD: Williams and Wilkins.

# FRAMES OF REFERENCE

# 4

# Structure of the Frame of Reference

PAULA KRAMER / JIM HINOJOSA

There are various ways to intervene with any particular child. Each therapist uses clinical judgment to select an approach that will be beneficial and meaningful to the child. In occupational therapy one way to organize intervention approaches is the frame of reference.

Anne Cronin Mosey, PhD, OTR, FAOTA (1970) proposed the frame of reference as a method of organizing knowledge so that it could be used for planning intervention. She presents the frame of reference as a linking structure between theory and application. Dr. Mosey's original components of a frame of reference are the theoretical base, function/dysfunction continua, evaluation, and postulates regarding change. Expanding on Mosey's work, we have added another component, application for intervention. The purpose of this component is to articulate for the therapist how the frame of reference is used for treatment. This component is meant to clarify how a therapist moves clinically from a theoretical perspective through the process of evaluation and the identification of specific problem areas to clinical intervention.

The challenge to any therapist is the application of theoretical knowledge to practice. Moving from theory to practice is a complex process; it entails taking ideas that are abstract and bringing them to a level at which they can be used. When choosing a frame of reference, the occupational therapist looks at the child's needs, strengths, limitations, and environment. With a comprehensive understanding of all these issues, the therapist chooses the most appropriate approach to the child. The frame of reference **delineates** the perspective of the occupational therapist when approaching the child.

These concepts are abstract and can be understood best through the use of examples. Examples are presented that are intended to clarify some of the ideas introduced while adding a note of levity to this complex topic. Our example of a frame of reference deals with adolescents making contact with persons of the opposite sex. It is not intended to be a completely developed frame of reference but, rather, a brief sample that exemplifies the various parts needed to understand the structure. This "frame of reference" can be found in marked sections throughout the chapter.

# Theoretical Base

Basic professional education provides occupational therapists with a broad knowledge base. One aspect of this educational process is the study of various theories. "A theory is concerned with how and under what circumstances those events happen and how they are related. The purpose of theory is to make predictions about the relationships between events or phenomena" (Mosey, 1981, p. 30). Theories provide therapists with ways of understanding the effects of their actions on the subsequent reactions of the child.

If intervention is based on theory, a therapist is able to understand the relationship between the treatment and the subsequent reactions of the child. For example, if the theory states a relationship between tickling and laughter, when a child is tickled the therapist should then expect the child to laugh. If the child does not laugh, then the theory also should provide a means for the therapist to understand the lack of response. Intervention should be based on theory, because the therapist should be able to describe the link between the intervention and the expected changes in the child.

Sometimes therapists have difficulty in moving from theory to practice. It is as if the theoretical knowledge is in one sphere and the practical knowledge constitutes a separate set of specific skills or techniques. Theoretical and practical levels of knowledge must be integrated. An organized, consistent treatment plan for the child flows from the clear understanding of the underlying theories. The underlying reasons for any intervention have to be clearly understood. The therapist's actions do not come from intuition but from a well thought out theoretical understanding. The frame of reference, therefore, provides the cohesion between theory and intervention in a practical manner; and the theoretical base provides the framework for the actual intervention.

The theoretical base provides the foundation of the entire frame of reference. The theoretical base may draw from one or more theories. If more than one theory is used, the theories must be consistent internally or be operating from the same basic premises (Mosey, 1981). Included in the base are assumptions, concepts, definitions, postulates, and hypotheses. Furthermore, the theoretical base states the relationships between all these elements.

### Making Contact with Persons of the Opposite Sex as an Adolescent: Theoretical Base

Interest in developing relationships with the opposite sex generally begins around the preadolescent or early adolescent stage of development. It is normal and natural in early adolescence to begin to get interested in the opposite sex. It is somewhat difficult and uncomfortable, however, to make initial contact with an unknown person of the opposite sex. As one grows older, one usually finds it easier to initiate and maintain contacts with members of the opposite sex. Furthermore, as one gains more experience relating to the opposite sex, one becomes more interested in and comfortable with the idea of choosing a life mate. Persons become more focused about who they are and what they want, expect, and need from others.

The theoretical base of this frame of reference is drawn from several developmental theorists, including Blos (1962), Erikson (1968, 1982), Freud (1966), Rogers (1961), and Elkind (1967). Erikson (1968) describes development in terms of stages. The stages during preadolescence and early adolescence are industry versus inferiority and self identity versus role diffusion. Blos (1962) states that at the preadolescent stage, it is normal to begin to get interested in the opposite sex, although this interest may be expressed first in an inappropriate and somewhat hostile manner; however, this is still a means of making contact. Erikson (1968, 1982) further states that the beginning of interest in the opposite sex is a preparatory step toward young adulthood (intimacy and solidarity versus isolation), when one becomes involved in choosing a life partner. Elkind (1967) reinforces the concept that it is initially difficult to make contact with the opposite sex for the adolescent because he/she feels self-conscious. He states that adolescents presume that everyone around them is an "imaginary audience" and that they are the center of attention. Adolescents believe that everyone is looking at them. This presents some conflict to the preadolescent or early adolescent. They want to make contact with the opposite sex and yet it is difficult for them. Freud's (1966) contribution to this theoretical base is his theories about sexual development and the natural state of relationships between opposite sexes. Rogers' (1961) contribution is his theories of interpersonal communication and the ability to establish relationships. All these theories take the position that making contact with the opposite sex is normal and natural. Furthermore, they assume that a heterosexual orientation is normal and natural at this stage of life and that other behaviors at this stage may represent deviance.

There are various ways that people begin to make contact with the opposite sex during this stage of life. One way is generally referred to as flirting. Flirting is an attempt to get the attention of someone, usually a person that you do not know well, and generally has an underlying sexual connotation. It involves making eye contact, smiling, acting in a coquettish manner, and making actual contact in a socially appropriate way. Flirting is frequently used to determine if the other party has any interest in the person doing the flirting. Making eye contact and smiling at the same time is an acceptable way of flirting. In many situations, flirting is a socially appropriate way of making contact with someone of the opposite sex. In some situations, however, it may be seen as forward, or socially inappropriate behavior. Socially appropriate behavior refers to actions that are acceptable in a public situation based on age, sociocultural values, and norms.

## Assumptions

Assumptions are ideas that are held to be true and are not questioned or tested in any way. In other words, they are basic beliefs. All theories used by occupational therapists have assumptions. If the theoretical base draws from several theories, then all the assumptions made must be accepted by all of those theories.

- Assumption: It is normal and natural during early adolescence and preadolescence to want to make contact with the opposite sex.
- Assumption: It is difficult initially to make contact with someone of the opposite sex.
- Assumption: Preadolescents and early adolescents feel conflict because they want to make contact with the opposite sex and yet find it difficult.
- Assumption: These theories assume that a heterosexual orientation is normal and natural at this stage of life and that other behaviors may represent deviance.

## Concepts

Concepts are ideas that the theorist has labeled as important. They generally describe a phenomenon that has been observed. The following are concepts identified in this frame of reference: **flirting** and **behaving in a socially appropriate way.**

## Definitions

Definitions explain the meaning of important concepts. Keep in mind that every concept in a theoretical base should be defined in terms of what it means to the particular frame of reference.

- Definition: *Flirting* refers to getting the attention of someone, usually a person that you do not know well, in a coquettish manner that generally has an underlying sexual connotation. Flirting is frequently used to determine if the other party has any reciprocal interest. In some situations, it may be seen as forward or socially inappropriate behavior.
- Definition: *Socially appropriate behavior* refers to actions that are acceptable in a public situation based on age, sociocultural values, and norms.

## Postulates

Postulates state the relationship between concepts. Within the theoretical base, all concepts are related in some way. The postulate serves as the linking mechanism between concepts.

- Flirting is usually a socially appropriate way of making contact with someone of the opposite sex.
- Making eye contact and smiling at the same time is an acceptable way of flirting.

## Hypotheses

Hypotheses state the suspected relationships between the postulates. These relationships may be tested. There usually is a design in the theoretical base that describes how each of the parts fit together to form a whole. All parts may be interrelated (as Mosey suggests): parts may be chained in a linear progression, or parts may build on each other in the form of a pyramid or hierarchy. When learning a frame of reference, it is important to understand its design or the way in which it is organized. The way that the theoretical base is organized should be reflected in all subsequent parts of the frame of reference. This format enables the therapist to see the design of the frame of reference and to apply the theoretical base to intervention. This again highlights the importance of the theoretical base.

When therapists begin to use a new frame of reference, they should be certain to understand the theoretical base and its component parts. The theoretical base sets the stage for the entire frame of reference.

The theoretical base usually is the most complex and abstract section in the frame of reference, but it is critical to understand it to move from theory to implementation of the frame of reference into practice.

When studying the theoretical base of a frame of reference, it may be helpful to keep the following questions in mind:

1. What are the assumptions?
2. What are the concepts?
3. What are the definitions of the concepts? Do you understand them?
4. What are the postulates? Do you understand these relationships?
5. How is the theoretical base organized? What is the design of the theoretical base? Do you understand the design?

The theoretical base broadly delineates the areas of concern of the frame of reference within the broader context of occupational therapy. The theoretical base also identifies the various theories on which the frame of reference is based. It identifies all assumptions being made, and it identifies the major concepts and defines them. Concepts are organized in a hierarchical manner, according to their importance to the frame of reference. In the sample frame of reference, a conceptual hierarchy related to flirting is making eye contact, smiling, acting in a coquettish manner, and, finally, making actual contact in a socially appropriate way.

Postulates are stated to identify clearly the relationship between the concepts. When a relationship exists between postulates, it is stated as an hypothesis. Hypotheses are unique in that they predict expected behaviors. When hypotheses are important to the frame of reference, they should be identified and stated clearly within the theoretical base.

# Function/Dysfunction Continua

The next section in a frame of reference is referred as the function/dysfunction continua. This section clearly identifies those areas of function with which the frame of reference is concerned. As you read through the theoretical base, you should be able to identify the specific areas of performance important to the child's development of skills and abilities. These are the areas that the therapist evaluates to determine whether the child is functional or dysfunctional. Concept labels and definitions of those concepts from the theoretical base identify what therapists who use this frame of reference consider to be function. Likewise, concept labels and definitions identify what represents dysfunction. Each function/dysfunction continuum covers one area of performance important to the particular frame of reference. A frame of reference generally has several function/dysfunction continua, which are labelled as such because human performance rarely can be classified as good or bad, abled or disabled. The situation usually is not so clear cut. Function is at one end of the spectrum and dysfunction is at the other, and human performance may fall at any point along this scale:

**Function**--------------------------**Dysfunction**

The functional end of the continuum represents what the therapist expects the child to be able to do, whereas the dysfunctional end of the continuum represents disability:

| Function--------------------------Dysfunction |
|---|
| **Expected ability**            **Disability** |

Function/dysfunction continua come directly from the theoretical bases of the frames of reference, and, thus, are specific to those frames of reference. They cannot be taken out of context.

**Nonverbal contact** and **verbal contact** are two function/dysfunction continua for the sample frame of reference.

## Nonverbal Contact

| Communicating Nonverbally | Difficulty Communicating Nonverbally |
|---|---|
| FUNCTION: Ability to communicate nonverbally with an unfamiliar person of the opposite sex. | DYSFUNCTION: Inability to communicate nonverbally with an unfamiliar person of the opposite sex. |

## Verbal contact

| Speaking Comfortably | Difficulty Speaking |
|---|---|
| FUNCTION: Ability to speak with an unknown person of the opposite sex. | DYSFUNCTION: Inability to speak with an unknown person of the opposite sex. |

## Behaviors Indicative of Function/Dysfunction

Underneath each function-dysfunction concept label are either lists of behaviors or some type of functional scale. These are called behaviors indicative of function or dysfunction. When the frame of reference uses lists of behaviors, there is one list of expected abilities. This is the functional end of the continuum. Another list identifies behaviors that are considered disabilities, which represent the dysfunctional end of the continuum. Evidence of these behaviors, or sometimes physical manifestation, are used by the therapist during evaluation.

Sometimes, a functional scale is used for evaluation. Some areas of human performance exhibit wide variations in acceptable performance. For example, grasping an object involves many motoric steps. A child may have developed only part of this and still be functional in relation to his age but may not have developed the whole sequence of grasping. This child, because he has not fully mastered grasping, still would not fall at the functional end of the continuum. In some frames of reference, a functional scale is used to identify acceptable ranges of behaviors or performance rather than specified abilities.

After the therapist performs an evaluation, she can then look at her results and check them against these descriptive lists or functional scales. The more behaviors that the child exhibits indicative of dysfunction, the closer the child will be to the dysfunctional end of the continuum, showing that he needs intervention. Likewise, the fewer characteristics indicative of dysfunction that the child exhibits, the closer the child will be to the functional end of the scale.

What follows are two function/dysfunction continuum concept labels (including the behaviors indicative of function/dysfunction) from the sample frame of reference:

## Nonverbal Contact

| Communicating Nonverbally | Difficulty Communicating Nonverbally |
| --- | --- |
| FUNCTION: Ability to communicate nonverbally with an unfamiliar person of the opposite sex | DYSFUNCTION: Inability to communicate nonverbally with an unfamiliar person of the opposite sex |
| BEHAVIORS INDICATIVE OF FUNCTION: | BEHAVIORS INDICATIVE OF DYSFUNCTION: |
| Making eye contact with the opposite sex | Uncontrolled blushing in the presence of people of the opposite sex |
| Smiling at the opposite sex | Difficulty in smiling at people of the opposite sex |
| Appearing physically comfortable with people of the opposite sex | Assuming childlike postures when in the presence of people of the opposite sex |

## *Verbal Contact*

| Speaking Comfortably | Difficulty Speaking |
|---|---|
| FUNCTION: Ability to speak with an unknown person of the opposite sex | DYSFUNCTION: Inability to speak with an unknown person of the opposite sex |
| BEHAVIORS INDICATIVE OF FUNCTION: | BEHAVIORS INDICATIVE OF DYSFUNCTION: |
| Talking openly and smoothly with a person of the opposite sex | Stuttering when trying to talk with a person of the opposite sex |
| Making sense when talking with a person of the opposite sex | Giggling when trying to talk with a person of the opposite sex |
| | Calling a person of the opposite sex and hanging up before he/she answers |

## *Guide for Evaluation*

The function/dysfunction continuum serves as an evaluation **guide**. This section may serve as an evaluation protocol in defining the areas of performance that the therapist should assess. It is not, however, an evaluation tool; it does not tell the therapist how to evaluate a child, but rather, it tells her the things she should be looking at to determine if the child needs intervention. The evaluation section serves as a guide to the therapist by defining the areas of concern of the frame of reference, following the function/dysfunction continuum.

Through the evaluation, the therapist determines where the child falls on the function/dysfunction continuum. Is the child closer to function, or does he have so much difficulty with this area of performance that he has to be considered in need of intervention?

Available evaluation instruments appropriate to this frame of reference are listed and discussed in this section. If there is one tool considered more appropriate than another, it may be recommended as the instrument of choice. All tools used for evaluation must address specifically the function/dysfunction continua that previously have been identified.

Many frames of reference do not have specific tools or recommended evaluation procedures. In these situations, the therapist usually devises a set of tasks or observations that allow her to determine the child's performance in the various function/dysfunction continua. This is perfectly acceptable, as long as the tasks or observations chosen are directly related to the specified continua. Although it is often difficult to choose or devise evaluative tasks, the therapist should avoid falling back on "old favorites." She needs to choose tasks that demonstrate the specific behaviors outlined. Tools should not be chosen based on the therapist's comfort level but on whether the tools follow the continua previously stated in the frame of reference.

Using the function/dysfunction continuum as the guideline for the evaluation, the therapist can determine whether the child can be considered functional or dysfunctional in terms of this specific frame of reference:

---

- In this sample frame of reference, observation of the early adolescent in a peer group situation could be used as an evaluation. This observation would provide the therapist with information about the adolescent's behavior and physical manifestations in a peer socialization experience.

---

## Postulates Regarding Change

Postulates state the relationship between two concepts from the theoretical base of a frame of reference. Postulates regarding change also relate two concepts; however, these postulates are the guidelines for how the therapist should intervene with the child. *Postulates regarding change, just like function/ dysfunction continua, must relate back to the important concepts in the theoretical base.* The thread of continuity must be present from one section to another.

Postulates regarding change are critical because they move the frame of reference farther from the abstract level of theory to the more concrete level of practice. It may make it easier to think of the postulates as **"if-then"** statements. They state that **if** the therapist does something, **then** a resultant effect should occur. The statements are descriptive and guide the therapist's behavior and actions. As action-oriented statements, they convey to the therapist the type of environment that should be created to produce change, or the type of technique needed to bring about change. The result can be a change in the child's behavior or an enhancement of normal growth and development that has been impeded by dysfunction.

The term environment within the context of a postulate regarding change encompasses more than the physical space of the intervention setting. It involves the emotional climate, the social interaction with the therapist, and the various activities to which the child is exposed. It is important to note that therapists do not actually create the change in the child, but they do create an environment that allows the change to take place (Mosey, 1981, 1986). The therapist may create an environment that should enhance normal growth and development by providing the child with specific activities that he has not engaged in previously.

When a postulate relates to the use of a specific therapeutic technique, it states the type of action the therapist should take to bring about an explicit response in the child. For example, if the therapist applies direct pressure to the insertion of a muscle, then the muscle should relax. Because an environment that allows for change is important, it is rare that a frame of reference will have only postulates that describe the use of specific techniques. Most frames of reference include postulates regarding change that discuss the environment as well as the therapist's direct actions.

Postulates regarding change are the turning points in the frame of reference. They apply the abstract material stated in the theoretical base to the practical actions that need to be taken by the therapists to facilitate change in the child. The postulates give the therapist a mechanism for using the frame of reference to plan the intervention.

Within the frame of reference for establishing a relationship with the opposite sex, postulates regarding change might be the following:

- The therapist creates an environment in which the adolescent will be in a social situation with members of the opposite sex.

- If the therapist creates a situation where the adolescent has more opportunity to talk with a member of the opposite sex, then he will begin to feel more comfortable.

- If the therapist puts male and female adolescents in a comfortable and natural social situation, then social interaction will be facilitated.

- If the therapist presents a group activity in which male and female adolescents have to work together, then they will learn to interact in a socially appropriate manner.

## *Application to Practice*

The postulates regarding change have stated the important concepts that should be used by the therapist to facilitate that change in the child. Some frames of reference require a more in-depth explanation of the key concepts used to promote functional performance. Other frames of reference require additional descriptions of the actions to be taken by the therapist. Other frames of reference may require specific examples. Often it is difficult for even the most experienced therapist to make the move from the theoretical stage to practical application without additional explanation. This section eases that movement from theory to practice. In other words, this section is meant to provide added information for the therapist to put this frame of reference into practice effectively. In addition, this section might suggest guidelines for the selection of appropriate activities and describe how these activities may be graded so that the client can begin to interact and move from a state of dysfunction to one of function.

- For example, within the sample frame of reference presented in this chapter, Making Contact with Persons of the Opposite Sex as an Adolescent, intervention would have to be done in an environment that uses small groups, because interaction could not be facilitated in individual treatment. An occupational therapist would select activities that foster interaction among the adolescents in the group.

This section is not meant to be a cookbook for application. Instead, it is meant to provide clarification, where necessary, by addressing the following questions:

1. Is there any additional information that the therapist needs to know to apply this frame of reference effectively?
2. Is there anything about the frame of reference that might not be immediately apparent?
3. Is there anything that has not been stated clearly, that the therapist should keep in mind when applying this frame of reference for intervention?

### References

Blos, P. (1962). *On adolescence.* Glencoe, IL: Free Press.
Elkind, D. (1967). Egocentrism in adolescence. *Child Development, 38*, 1025–1034.
Erikson, E. H. (1968). *Identity: youth and crisis.* New York: Norton.
Erikson, E. H. (1982). *The life cycle completed: a review.* New York: W. W. Norton.
Freud, S. (1966). *Standard edition of the complete psychological works of Sigmund Freud.* London: Hogarth Press.
Mosey, A. C. (1970). *Three frames of reference for mental health.* Thorofare, NJ: Slack.
Mosey, A. C. (1981). *Occupational therapy: configurations of a profession.* New York: Raven Press.
Mosey, A. C. (1986). *Psychosocial components of occupational therapy.* New York: Raven Press.
Rogers, C. R. (1961) *On becoming a person.* Boston: Houghton Mifflin Co.

# 5

# Neurodevelopmental Treatment Frame of Reference

SARAH SCHOEN / JILL ANDERSON

Neurodevelopmental treatment is a sensorimotor approach widely used by occupational therapists in the treatment of neuromuscular disorders. Sensory motor techniques are applied to remediate the neurological and developmental sequelae of dysfunction. These intervention techniques are designed to enhance the quality of the client's functional motor performance. The use of this frame of reference specific to occupational therapy requires a focus on functional goal-directed activities.

## History

Neurodevelopmental treatment (NDT) has evolved and developed over 30 years, largely from the clinical experiences and personal views of Berta Bobath, a physiotherapist, and her husband, Karel Bobath, a physician, at the Western Cerebral Palsy Center in London. The center is now known as the Bobath Center. This approach originally was developed and used in the treatment of neurologically impaired children, primarily those diagnosed with cerebral palsy. It later was used with adults who had hemiplegia that resulted from cerebral vascular accidents. Clinical application of NDT has expanded and currently is used for various dysfunctions, including children who have neuromuscular disorders, immature central nervous system (CNS) disorders, such as found in some premature infants, and other developmental disabilities.

Neurodevelopmental treatment has progressed through various phases, from the early 1940s to today. Mrs. Bobath described the NDT approach as a "living concept," constantly changing as a result of her observations of client reactions during treatment. An early focus was to decrease muscle tone through the use of reflex inhibiting postures (RIP). These postures were opposite to the primitive reflex patterns typically assumed by the child (Campbell, 1986). Later, the study of normal motor development led to the incorporation of hierarchical motor sequences into therapy, with one activity following another during facilitation (such as head control, rolling, sitting, quadruped, and kneeling). When this approach was used, the child was placed passively into these developmental positions. A major difficulty with this approach was that the child was unable to move actively from one position to another.

The primary focus in the next phase of NDT emphasized the facilitation of automatic movement sequences as opposed to isolated developmental skills. The development of righting and equilibrium reactions were considered essential for the ability to move against gravity. The therapeutic approach had two important components. The first was the reduction of the therapist's control over the child's movement while facilitating the child's active control. This was alternated with the second component, the use of inhibitory techniques to reduce the effects of increased tone. The primary criticism of this intervention was that the motor outcomes were not generalized by the child. The movements, therefore, did not lead to increased functional abilities or to greater independence in activities of daily living (ADL).

The most current phase of NDT recognizes the need for treatment to be directed toward specific functional situations. That is, through the use of facilitation techniques, the child should be able to engage in functional and meaningful activities. The present approach focuses on the facilitation of normal movement patterns for functional activities.

In the evolution of NDT, other professionals in the field of pediatric rehabilitation have contributed extensively to the body of knowledge. Neurodevelopmental treatment continues to develop and be refined as therapists learn through their clients' reactions to intervention and through research.

# Theoretical Base of Neurodevelopmental Treatment

Neurodevelopmental treatment is a developmental frame of reference and makes the same assumptions as other developmental frames of reference— that is, its fundamental concepts constitute the building blocks of the theoretical base. It is expected that therapists who use this frame of reference have a comprehensive knowledge of normal development, a comprehensive understanding of abnormal development, a thorough understanding of the development of normal postural control, and an understanding of the components of movement. From this knowledge base, the occupational therapist can conceptualize how primitive or total movement patterns can be modified into more varied and select activities. The therapist relies on this information to understand and analyze how the abnormal deviates from the normal. This information also is critical to the development of an appropriate treatment plan.

According to this frame of reference, normal development is divided into four basic categories: (1) principles of normal development; (2) the sensory-motor-sensory feedback system; (3) components of movement; and (4) sequences in motor development.

## Principles of Normal Motor Development

General principles of normal motor development dictate that control precedes from cephalo to caudal, proximal to distal, and gross to fine. These principles provide a guide for the determination and sequencing of intervention. For example, if development proceeds from cephalo to caudal, then achievement of head control occurs before control of either the upper or lower extremities. In addition, control of large movements in transition from one position to another, such as rolling and creeping, proceeds control of the extremities, such as the use of the fingers for refined prehension. The hemiplegic child who attains control of the shoulder girdle before the elbow, wrist, and hand in the affected upper extremity illustrates the principle of proximal-distal control. In contrast to this principle, it recently has been hypothesized that there are two mechanisms of control: proximal and distal. This would be evidenced by a proximal system of control for the arms and a separate distal control system for the hand (Kuypers, 1963; Lawrence & Hopkins, 1972).

## Sensory-Motor-Sensory Feedback

It is assumed that children learn movement through a system of sensory-motor-sensory feedback. Developmentally, most movement is preceded by a sensory experience. A resulting motor response provides sensory feedback from the proprioceptors in the muscles and joints used to accomplish the specific movement. The initial sensory stimulus can be an internal event, an external event, or a combination of both. For example, the presentation of a colorful toy represents an external visual sensory stimulus that may activate a motor response. A primitive reflexive reaction, such as a change in head position that produces the asymmetrical tonic neck reflex (ATNR extension and abduction of the arm on the face side with elbow flexion and adduction of the arm on the skull side) can occur from an internal stimulus of the proprioceptors of the neck. Sensory feedback is provided by the resulting movement. The child senses something either internally or externally (or from both stimuli) and then responds, and this responsive movement provides the feedback to the central nervous system (CNS).

In addition, it is assumed that infants learn about themselves and their environments through sensory motor exploration with their mouths and hands. In this way, children learn about the texture, shape, and temperature of the objects that they explore. Then, through movement, they learn about space and their relation to the environment. Movement thus provides additional sensory-motor-sensory stimulation and feedback.

## Components of Normal Development

Four important components of normal movement are (1) the interplay between stability and mobility; (2) the effects of postural reflex mechanism on movement; (3) the ability to dissociate movements; and (4) the development of postural control in the three planes of space. These basic components provide the foundation for specific treatment techniques.

### Interplay between Stability and Mobility

The concepts of stability and mobility can be understood most effectively by defining dynamic movement. Dynamic movement refers to smooth, controlled, coordinated action based on a point of stability as its support. The part of the body in contact with the support surface can function as the point of stability. For example, the feet are the point of stability in a standing position.

Mobility is then achieved through a weight shift in any direction. Neurodevelopmental treatment assumes that normal movement requires the combination of stability and mobility. Each body part can perform both a stabilizing and mobilizing function, depending on the activity. For example, when the infant rocks in quadruped, the arms and legs provide stability for the trunk. When this same infant reaches for a toy in quadruped, the baby gets stability from his legs, trunk, and one arm so that the other upper extremity can reach for the toy in space.

**Effects of Postural Reflex Mechanism on Movement**

Neurodevelopmental treatment assumes that the postural reflex mechanism provides the foundation for the qualitative aspects of normal movement. The parts of the postural reflex mechanism (PRM) are postural tone, reciprocal innervation, and righting and equilibrium reactions.

For the purposes of this frame of reference, it is important to differentiate postural tone from muscle tone. Postural tone provides the background tone for normal movement and determines the muscle quality in overall patterns and distribution throughout the body rather than in specific muscles. Muscle tone is more often used to refer specifically to the internal state of muscle fiber tension within individual muscles and muscle groups. Normal postural tone must be low enough to allow movement against gravity (mobility) yet high enough to maintain a stable position against gravity (stability). Mature distribution of postural tone is reflected in greater tone proximally (for stability and postural alignment) and lower tone distally (for skilled refined movements).

Reciprocal innervation is the interplay between agonist and antagonist muscles during coordinated muscle activity. During graded movement, the agonist shortens and the antagonist lengthens, whereas in postural stabilization, the agonist and antagonist exert nearly equal force. The ability to control and grade movement depends on this interplay between muscle groups (Scherzer & Tscharnuter, 1990).

Righting and equilibrium reactions are two automatic movement patterns that occur during the first year of development and persist throughout life. Righting reactions restore and maintain the vertical position of the head in space, the alignment of the head and trunk, and the alignment of the trunk and limbs (Short-Degraff, 1988).

Postural alignment is a term often used to describe the presence of mature righting reactions. Equilibrium reactions build on already developing righting reactions, and they serve to maintain or regain balance during a shift in the center of gravity. This can be in response to a change within the person or to an external environmental change. Either the person moves, altering his center of gravity, or the support surface moves, requiring the person to make the necessary postural adjustment to maintain postural alignment.

**Ability to Dissociate Movements**

Dissociation, or the ability to differentiate movements between the various parts of the body, is indicative of maturation of the CNS. Dissociation of movement occurs in normal development within the first year of life and is characterized by separate movements between segments of the body (as well as within a given segment). Following the principles of normal development, dissociation proceeds from cephalo to caudal and from proximal to distal. Dissociation of head movements from movements of the shoulder girdle and trunk precedes dissociation of the trunk movements from pelvic movements. The ability to creep reciprocally demonstrates dissociation of the lower extremities from pelvic movements and from each other, as well as the movements of the upper extremities from the shoulder girdle and from each other. The ability to perform bilateral hand activities that involve stabilization of a toy with one hand and manipulation of its parts with the other hand demonstrates a higher level of dissociation.

### Development of Postural Control in the Three Planes of Space

Neurodevelopmental treatment assumes that motor control develops in a specific sequence in the three body planes. Developmentally, motor control occurs first in the sagittal plane, with extension and flexion against gravity. The next phase of development occurs in the frontal plane, with lateral righting. The final phase of development occurs in the transverse plane, adding the component of rotation (Scherzer & Tscharnuter, 1990). This progression is consistent in each developmental posture. In this frame of reference, the most significant developmental postures are prone, supine, sidelying, sitting, quadruped, kneeling, and standing. For example, the child is able to shift weight in the anterior-posterior plane in the prone position before shifting weight laterally. Control in the transverse plane, the last plane in which movement develops, is necessary for rotation (as in the transition from the prone position to sitting). This progression is then repeated in higher developmental positions such as sitting and standing.

## Sequences in Motor Development

Neurodevelopmental treatment assumes that motor development occurs sequentially with the sequences overlapping. It also assumes that previously developed skills prepare the child for later behaviors. While the baby is mastering a specific motor skill, he already is experimenting with the components in the subsequent stage. For example, infants perfect sitting balance at the same time as they begin to pull to stand. Movement sequences integrate righting and equilibrium reactions as well as previously attained motor abilities. This is reflected when children kneel and pull up on the furniture into a standing position. To perform this movement sequence, they have developed equilibrium reactions in quadruped to free the arms and pull into kneeling, balance between flexion and extension at the hips to elevate and extend the trunk, and the ability to weightshift laterally through the pelvis to half kneel and then to stand. The child may begin to experiment with lateral weightshifting in standing by taking a few cruising steps.

The NDT frame of reference assumes that the principles, components, and sequences that underlie normal movement also are essential to the development and performance of functional skills. This relates exclusively to the motor basis of functional skills and not to the sensory, perceptual, cognitive, and motivational bases of functional skills. Although infants and children who have abnormal patterns of movement certainly may attain some degree of independence in functional activities, their skill levels are compromised because of excessive reliance on compensatory patterns of movement. Compensatory patterns refer to those movements influenced by abnormal postural tone and habitual use. These are the abnormal movement patterns used repeatedly to achieve functional motor skills when normal movement patterns have not been established. For example, hyperextension of the head and neck is a compensatory movement pattern. The hypotonic child who has poor trunk stability may attempt to improve visual orientation in space through hyperextension of the head and neck.

Normal movement allows for the use of the most efficient patterns to accomplish functional tasks, such as playing on the floor, sitting at a table, freely moving in and out of positions to explore the environment, feeding, and dressing oneself.

## Variety of Movement

In normal development, infants show a variety of motor patterns when moving in and out of developmental positions and when interacting with objects. Infants rarely stay still. They move from one toy to another and are constantly changing their body positions.

## Abnormal Motor Development

A comprehensive understanding of abnormal motor development is equally important in the application of the NDT frame of reference. Knowledge of normal motor development provides a basis for identifying abnormal movement postures and patterns.

Abnormal development can be viewed in several ways. One way, proposed by Bly (1980), is that abnormal development occurs in "blocks" in the neck, shoulder girdle, pelvis, and hips, following the cephalocaudal progression of normal development. Another view, as stated by the Bobaths (1975, 1971a, 1971b) describes abnormal development as a lack of cortical inhibition that results from a damaged or immature nervous system. They emphasized the importance of abnormal postural tone combined with the gradual appearance of tonic reflex activity, as causing abnormal patterns of posture and movement.

Abnormal movements also may be seen from another perspective, as the persistence of primitive reflexes or as compensatory attempts to gain anti-gravity control. Both views are characterized by stereotypical patterns of movement. The cycle then moves from compensation to habit, resulting in changes in muscle length, that over time may cause orthopedic limitations in movement. Based on the specific type of tone of the child, varying clinical pictures of stereotypical patterns may be seen. Children with different types of neuromuscular disorders manifest different stereotypical patterns.

Although there are many ways of looking at the basis for abnormal movement, the subsequent problems that result from the abnormal development are the same. Clinically, the problems may be seen in the child's postural tone, reciprocal innervation, and development of righting and equilibrium reactions necessary for automatic movement. According to this frame of reference, there is a disruption in the normal sensory-motor-sensory feedback system as well as in the sequential development of postural control.

Problems in postural tone are assumed to have a significant impact on the development of abnormal movement patterns in this frame of reference. For example, in the development of the infant who has cerebral palsy, hypertonicity or hypotonicity initially may be the predominate characteristic. When this infant attempts to move against gravity, abnormal patterns of movement and posture become apparent. Patterns of extension tend to emerge first and appear to dominate the later motor patterns (Scherzer & Tscharnuter, 1990). As the infant matures, the tone may become increasingly hypertonic. Differences in tone may be observed in the trunk as opposed to the extremities. The extensor patterns for children with both types of tone are first seen as excessive cervical extension, that then proceeds down the spine. This extension is not counterbalanced with flexion and abdominal control in the high- and low-tone child. As the child continues to develop, differences in postural tone impact on the pelvis and hips, affecting sitting and the ability to pull to stand.

In abnormal development, abnormal movement also may result from a lack of dissociation. A lack of dissociation often is characterized by total patterns of movement, referred to as associated responses. For example, when movement of the head, shoulder girdle, trunk, and pelvis occurs in an associated pattern, there is a lack of rotation and normal righting reactions. This results in transitions from supine to prone or prone to supine positions being accomplished in a "log rolling" fashion, rather than rolling with segmental rotation. Another example can be seen in the lower extremities, where two primary patterns exist: complete extension of both legs or total flexion of both legs. Similar patterns also may be present in the upper extremities. These associated reactions limit the child's ability to perform independent functions, such as weightshifting to the side in the prone position or reaching forward with the other arm.

Another type of abnormal movement that results from a lack of dissociation is synergistic patterns. Synergistic patterns may be present within a leg or an arm. This occurs when distal movements are dominated by movements of the proximal joints. An example is when hand motions cannot be made independently but are completely controlled by movements made at the shoulder.

The identification of patterns of abnormal motor control used by a child helps to guide the therapist in selecting appropriate intervention techniques. It is assumed that the resultant compensatory patterns will become habitual ways of moving, without intervention. For example, the infant with excessive head hyperextension who lacks the counteracting flexion control may also elevate his shoulders to stabilize his head in an effort to maintain midline head control. This pattern of head hyperextension and shoulder elevation soon may become the preferred method of achieving and maintaining head control (Bly, 1980).

## Sensory Input as a Means of Bringing About Change

Central to NDT is the assumption that abnormal patterns of movement may be changed by altering sensory input to the CNS, thereby altering motor output. Furthermore, this may be done through the therapist's use of various techniques referred to as **handling**. Handling is when the therapist uses her hands on the child in a specified manner, using graded sensory input at key points of control. *Key points of control* are specific areas on the child's body selected for therapeutic handling. Key points may be proximal (such as the shoulder girdle, trunk, and pelvis) or distal (such as the hands and feet). Through handling, the therapist elicits and facilitates motor responses. Handling uses specific methods to decrease the frequency of abnormal patterns and to increase the occurrence of automatic normal movement reactions. Normal movement patterns facilitated by occupational therapists through handling must be goal directed and incorporated into functional activities. For handling to be effective, the therapist must grade touch and other sensory input that are finely tuned to the child's individual needs (Scherzer & Tscharnuter, 1990).

Another central assumption is that change must occur subcortically. Change results from the therapist's handling of the child to facilitate more normal tone and movement patterns. The development of movement in a child is achieved without skill and cognitive training methods.

# Function/Dysfunction Continua

Function/dysfunction continua provide therapists with descriptions of observable behaviors that are clinically relevant and that identify function and dysfunction in children.

## Postural Tone

Normal postural tone allows the person to move against gravity with mobility and ease. This amount of tone must be high enough to support the body against gravity and low enough to allow free movement. If postural tone is abnormal, then movement also will be abnormal or deficient. Postural tone can be abnormally high, resulting in excessive stability and difficulty moving against gravity, as in a child who has cerebral palsy with spastic quadriplegia, or postural tone can be abnormally low, resulting in excessive mobility and lack of control of movement, as in the child who has cerebral palsy with hypotonia (Fig. 5.1). Fluctuations in postural tone are also possible, as in the child who has cerebral palsy with athetosis, where tone can range from low to high, normal to high, or low to normal.

Dysfunction in postural tone also can be reflected in the pattern of distribution. Normal postural tone is lower distally. In dysfunction, as seen in the child who has cerebral palsy resulting in spastic quadriparesis, tone is higher distally than proximally. In addition, differences in the distribution of tone can be evident in the upper extremities, as in the child who has cerebral palsy that results in spastic diplegia. In these children, tone in the lower extremities is higher than in the upper extremities. Differences in tone also can be seen between the right and left sides of the body, as in the child who has hemiplegia.

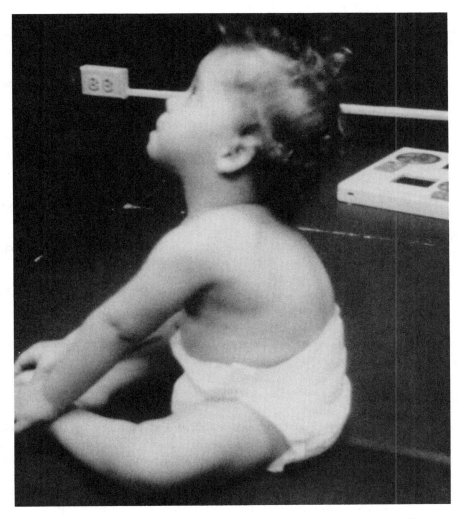

**Figure 5.1**   Hypotonic child in sitting position. Note the rounded spine and hyperextension of the neck.

| Normal Postural Tone | Abnormal Postural Tone |
| --- | --- |
| FUNCTION: Normal Postural Tone | DYSFUNCTION: Abnormal Postural Tone |
| BEHAVIORS INDICATIVE OF FUNCTION: | BEHAVIORS INDICATIVE OF DYS-FUNCTION: |
| Antigravity movement in and out of developmental positions with mature equilibrium reactions<br><br>Developmentally appropriate use of limbs for support, as well as finer adjustments during skilled activity | Hypotonicity<br>• Hypermobility and hyperextendability of joints<br>• Decreased degree of tension in muscles<br>• Limbs feel heavy on passive range of motion<br>• Limbs and body sink into any support surface<br><br>Fluctuating tone<br>• Presence of significant behaviors of hypertonicity, hypotonicity, and normal postural tone at varying times<br>• Presence of involuntary movements<br><br>Hypertonicity<br>• Increased muscle tone<br>• Resistance to passive range of motion<br>• Areas of the body with increased tone withdraw from contact with the support surface<br>• Presence of stretch reflex, clonus, or tremors |

## Stability/Mobility

The normal child combines stability and mobility on a foundation of normal postural tone when weightshifting and moving from one position to another. The functional end of the stability/mobility continuum is reflected in maturation of the righting and equilibrium reactions. This allows for dynamic stability and control over active movement. These concepts are illustrated by the normal child who is able to maintain sitting and then weightshift to the side to reach for a toy. The normal child has enough stability in the pelvis and trunk to allow mobility and free movement of the upper trunk, shoulder girdle, upper extremity, and head to obtain a toy out of reach. A child who lacks dynamic stability uses other mechanisms or compensations to achieve function. One such mechanism is the use of positional stability—that is, the use of the skeletal system rather than the neuromuscular system to achieve stability. The use of a posture with a broad base of support such as the hips in marked external rotation and abduction or **"W"** sitting (Fig. 5.2) are examples of a child's attempt to provide positional stability. Another example is the compensatory pattern of high guard posturing of the arms during sitting or ambulation, used in an attempt to achieve stability (Fig. 5.3). When high guard posturing is used to maintain balance, then the arms are not free to reach or grasp objects. Using an asymmetrical posture may also reflect the child's attempt to gain stability.

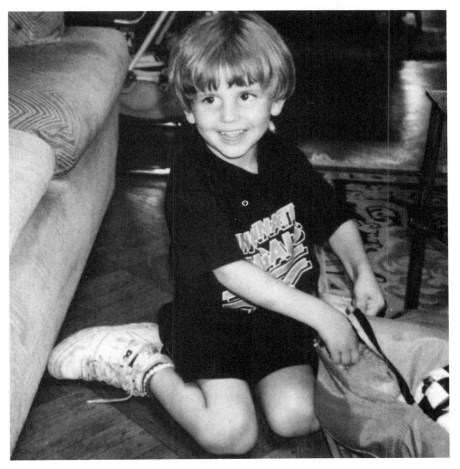

**Figure 5.2**    Child in a W-sitting posture to provide a wide base of support for sitting.

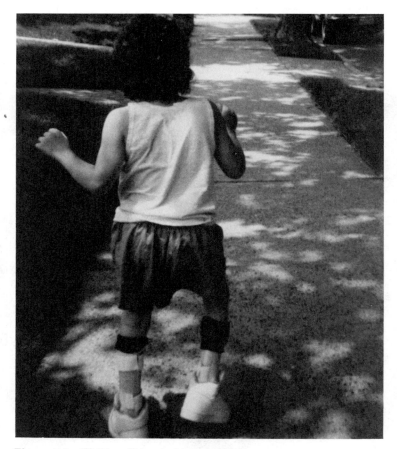

**Figure 5.3**   Child walking in high guard position.

| Dynamic Stability | Compensatory Stability |
|---|---|
| FUNCTION: Dynamic Stability | DYSFUNCTION: Compensatory Stability |
| BEHAVIORS INDICATIVE OF FUNCTION: | BEHAVIORS INDICATIVE OF DYSFUNCTION: |
| The ability to maintain and move in and out of developmental positions with mature righting and equilibrium reactions | Use of a wide base of support |
| | Use of upper extremities for stability beyond developmentally appropriate age |
| | Use of compensatory patterns such as persistence of the upper extremities in high guard position for maintaining or regaining balance during a weight shift; excessive reliance on protective reactions during weightshifting; persistence of asymmetrical patterns; variety of fixation patterns present (i.e. toe clawing, hand fisting) (Fig. 5.4) |
| | Exclusive use of "W" sitting position for sitting |

## Reciprocal Innervation as it Relates to Controlled Coordinated Movement

The child who develops normally has controlled coordinated movement throughout the full range of motion when moving. Reciprocal innervation allows this to occur through an interplay between agonist and antagonist muscle groups. In addition, controlled coordinated movement involves the timing, sequence, and rhythm of movement. In dysfunction, a lack of control is evident, along with an inability to coordinate movements, which is influenced by the child's postural tone. The child with low or fluctuating tone, characteristic of athetosis, uses the extremes of the ranges of motion and, therefore, has difficulty in controlling movement in the mid range. Conversely, the child who has high tone (spasticity) uses the mid range of motion and, therefore, has difficulty in achieving the full range of movement. The most skilled, controlled coordinated movements are evident in developmental hand manipulative skills.

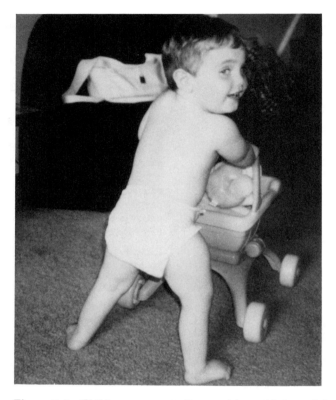

**Figure 5.4**   Child assumes standing position with legs abducted for a broad base of support. Note that toes are clawed for stability.

| Reciprocal Innervation | Lack of Reciprocal Innervation |
|---|---|
| FUNCTION: Controlled Coordinated Movement in Full Range of Motion | DYSFUNCTION: Mid-Range Control Only (Spasticity) |
| BEHAVIORS INDICATIVE OF FUNCTION: | BEHAVIORS INDICATIVE OF DYSFUNCTION: |
| Refined movement for skilled activities that reflect normal postural tone, dissociation, and various movement patterns | • Presence of synergistic stereotypic movement patterns influenced by increased postural tone<br>• Flexor patterns tend to predominate, especially under increased demands of gravity<br>• Full range of motion may be restricted |
| | DYSFUNCTION: End-Range Only (Athetosis and Low Tone) |
| | BEHAVIORS INDICATIVE OF DYSFUNCTION:<br>• Inability to grade movement transitions<br>• Excessive use of patterns of extension and flexion<br>• Difficulty in midline control |

## Righting and Equilibrium Reactions as They Relate to Postural Alignment

A lack of postural alignment in any or all of the body planes is considered dysfunctional. For example, in the sagittal plane, either a predominance of extensor patterns or an abnormal pull into flexion is considered dysfunctional. The development of righting reactions in the frontal plane also may be impaired, resulting in deficient active elongation on the weightbearing side and shortening on the nonweightbearing side. A third example demonstrates that postural alignment may be present in the sagittal and frontal planes but still can be deficient in the transverse plane, evidenced by a lack of rotation within the body axis. Children who demonstrate this type of dysfunction are not able to rotate their trunks freely to reach for a toy. These children instead would use lateral flexion—sidebending of the head and trunk—as a substitution. In addition, these children may need to rely on a broad base of support to maintain balance in various positions, or they may use their arms in compensatory fashion to protect against falling.

| Mature Righting/<br>Equilibrium Reactions | Immature/Absent Righting/<br>Equilibrium Reactions |
| --- | --- |
| FUNCTION: Postural Alignment | DYSFUNCTION: Lack of Postural Alignment |
| BEHAVIORS INDICATIVE OF FUNCTION:<br><br>Mature righting and equilibrium reactions in all positions | BEHAVIORS INDICATIVE OF DYSFUNCTION:<br><br>Excessive pull into flexion in upright positions<br><br>Predominance of head hyperextension<br><br>Inability to elongate muscles on weightbearing side of the body<br><br>Asymmetry |

## Dissociation

Dissociation is the ability to differentiate movements among various parts of the body. Movement patterns performed in an associated or synergistic way are indicative of dysfunction. These patterns frequently involve muscle contractions at various joints that tend to occur in a predictable pattern of movement, such as the upper extremity flexor synergy.

Persistence of these associated patterns also is dysfunctional. These associated reactions limit the child's ability to perform independent functions, such as weightshifting to the side in a prone position when reaching forward with one arm.

| Dissociated Movement Patterns Within and Between Body Parts | Associated or Synergistic Movement Patterns |
| --- | --- |
| FUNCTION: Dissociated/Differentiated Movement Within and Between Body Parts | DYSFUNCTION: Associated or Synergist Movement Patterns |
| BEHAVIORS INDICATIVE OF FUNCTION:<br><br>The ability to roll with rotation between shoulders and pelvis (Fig. 5.5)<br><br>The ability to use reciprocal leg movements in creeping and crawling (Fig. 5.7)<br><br>The ability to right head in all planes of space with shoulders maintained in proper alignment<br><br>When developmentally appropriate, to be able to hold a toy with one hand and manipulate its parts with the other | BEHAVIORS INDICATIVE OF DYSFUNCTION:<br><br>Log rolling (Fig. 5.6)<br><br>Bunny hopping<br><br>Pull to stand with lower extremities in extension, adduction, and internal rotation<br><br>Hand closing associated with flexion of the arm and hand opening with extension of the arm |

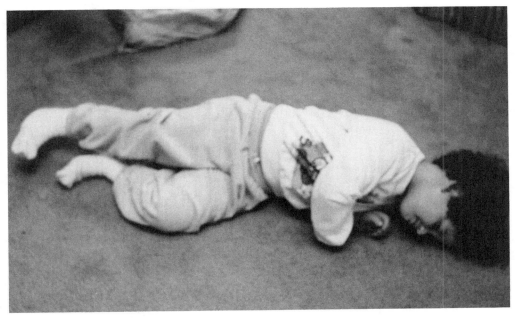

**Figure 5.5**    Normal segmental rolling.

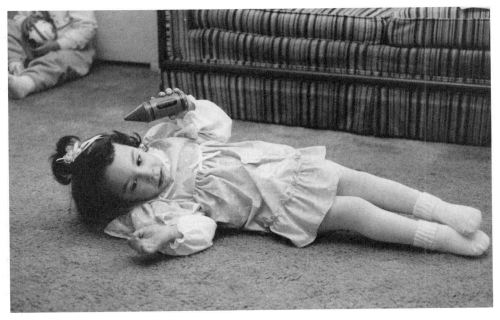

**Figure 5.6**    Log rolling.

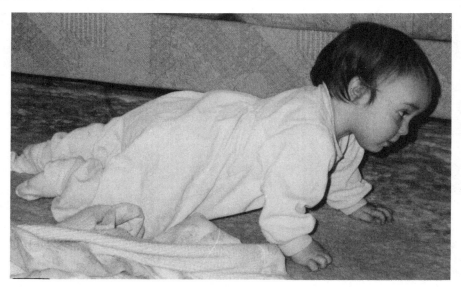

**Figure 5.7**  Normal child is able to dissociate movements of the upper and lower extremities in a reciprocal pattern.

## Variety of Movement

In normal development, infants show a variety of motor patterns when moving in and out of developmental positions and when interacting with objects. The presence of stereotypical movement patterns, such as persistence of primitive reflexes, is one indicator of dysfunction. Another stereotypical pattern may include posturing of the lower extremities with internal rotation and adduction. This would make it difficult to perform the external rotation and abduction necessary for sitting or standing activities. A stereotypical pattern of the upper extremities is shoulder elevation with scapular retraction. This pattern would impede functional skill development. A limitation of the variety of movement can interfere with the acquisition of independence as well as hamper the child's ability to interact with the environment.

In this continuum, the child who has full range of passive movement and no contractures or deformities is at the functional end of the continuum. Children restricted by abnormal tone and stereotypical movement patterns may develop contractures and deformities. Compensatory patterns of movement that are used repeatedly and become automatic also may contribute to the development of contractures and, ultimately, to deformities. The child who shows contractures or deformities with limitations in passive range of motion (PROM) is evidencing dysfunction. Intervention may prevent or correct deformities; however, the more consistently that these limited movements are used by the child, the more likely that dysfunction will occur.

| Variety of Movement Patterns | Stereotypical Movement Patterns<br>Reflexive Movement Patterns<br>Structural Deformities and Contractures |
|---|---|
| FUNCTION: Variety of Movement Patterns | DYSFUNCTION: Stereotypical Movement Patterns |
| BEHAVIORS INDICATIVE OF FUNCTION:<br><br>Uses varied repertoire of movement patterns based on the demands of the activity | BEHAVIORS INDICATIVE OF DYSFUNCTION:<br><br>Stereotypically, one or both lower extremities persist with extension, adduction, and internal rotation in all positions<br><br>Stereotypically, one or both upper extremities persist with shoulder elevation and retraction in all positions |
| BEHAVIORS INDICATIVE OF FUNCTION:<br><br><br>Uses varied repertoire of movement patterns based on the demands of the activity | BEHAVIORS INDICATIVE OF DYSFUNCTION:<br><br>Reflexive Movement Patterns<br>• Persistent asymmetrical tonic neck reflex that affects reaching and rolling<br>• Persistent symmetrical tonic neck reflex that affects crawling<br>• Persistent tonic labyrinthine reflex that affects sitting |

## Full Range of Motion Versus Structural Deformities and Contractures

| Full Passive Range of Motion | Contractures<br>Deformities |
|---|---|
| FUNCTION: Full Passive Range of Motion | DYSFUNCTION: Contractures, Deformities |
| BEHAVIORS INDICATIVE OF FUNCTION:<br>Full passive range of motion | BEHAVIORS INDICATIVE OF DYSFUNCTION:<br>Contractures<br>Deformities |

# Evaluation

Neurodevelopmental assessment is designed to identify and analyze characteristics of movement that may be associated with CNS dysfunction. It relies heavily on the therapist's ability to elicit responses to observe movement, categorize movement problems, and determine how these deficits interfere with the child's ability to acquire functional skills. When evaluating, the therapist needs to be able to adapt to the functional level of the child, including the child's age, specific needs, and severity of dysfunction. A complete occupational therapy assessment might include evaluation of oral-motor and feeding skills, gross and fine motor skills, sensory deficits, social-emotional factors, and cognitive skills. Not all of these areas, however, are addressed in this chapter.

Currently, no universally accepted format is available that uses the NDT frame of reference to evaluate a child who has CNS dysfunction. Numerous formats have been suggested for evaluation in this frame of reference (Bly, 1980; Bobath, 1975; Campbell, 1981). The evaluation delineated here is adapted from evaluations proposed by Scherzer and Tscharnuter (1990) and Boehme (1984). Although similarities exist in the observations and activities performed within a widely accepted format, when assessing a child who has CNS dysfunction, the therapist looks specifically for abnormal tone, tremors, and jerky, uncoordinated movement patterns that affect the quality of movement.

Traditional developmental evaluations used to assess children from birth to five years of age have several limitations. These standardized assessments have specific items or tasks to evaluate gross and fine motor skills, as well as other areas of development. The motor items, however, tend to measure only the acquisition of motor milestones, such as the ability to sit, stand, or grasp. These assessments do not analyze the specific factors that contribute to a child's inability to achieve a motor skill, nor do they address quality of movement issues.

For the most part, NDT assessments continue to rely on observation and on the therapist's sense when handling the child, as originally proposed by the Bobaths. Assessments are based almost exclusively on the observation of the child's spontaneous movements, as well as on selectively elicited movements brought about through handling by the therapist or caregiver. The challenge to the therapist is to summarize the common postural elements observed in all positions, based on the function/dysfunction continuum.

The NDT evaluation attempts to answer several key questions:

1. What is the influence of postural tone on the child's ability to move?
2. What normal postures are observed repeatedly at rest and during movement and when attempting to perform functional skills?
3. What abnormal postures are observed repeatedly at rest and during movement to perform functional skills?

**Table 5.1  NDT Evaluation Outline**

I. Overall Assessment of Functional Skills (What can the child do? At this point, the therapist is not concerned with the quality of movement but, rather, with the child's basic skills.)
   A. Gross Motor Abilities
   B. Upper Extremity Function
   C. Activities of Daily Living
II. Quality of Movement
   A. Postural Tone
   B. Developmental Postures and Transitions From One Position to Another Describe in terms of:
      1. Stability and Mobility
      2. Effects of Postural Reflex Mechanism on Movement
      3. Dissociation of Movement
      4. Postural Control in Three Planes of Space Stability and Mobility
      5. Variety of Movement Patterns
   C. Structural Limitations and Deformities

4. What may be the potential interference with the child's ability to achieve higher level motor and functional skills?

The entry-level therapist develops skills in this type of assessment by following a more structured evaluation approach, under the supervision of an experienced therapist. The outline presented in Table 5.1 provides some structured guidelines for NDT assessment.

## Overall Assessment of Functional Skills

Functional skills explore what the child can do without regard for the quality of movement. The therapist is concerned with the overall developmental picture of the child's functional skill performance with respect to the child's chronological age and his cognitive and sensory/perceptual levels. Another factor that should be considered, although it is not specific to this frame of reference, is the child's motivation. The therapist observes the child's ability (on a gross motor level) to achieve static balance in all developmental positions, the ability to make transitions from one position to another, and the ability to locomote.

The occupational therapist also is concerned with assessing upper extremity functional skills. These skills are described as they relate to the child's ability to use the arms for weightbearing, protective reactions, reaching and grasping, manipulating, and releasing objects in various positions.

Both gross motor and upper extremity functional performance skills contribute to the ability to perform activities of daily living (ADL). In this frame of reference, ADL is a discrete area of functional skills, an end result of gross motor and upper extremity function. Activities of daily living include participation in feeding, dressing, and self-care, as well as the ability to explore, to play, and then to learn from the environment. Again, this should be viewed in the context of the child's chronological age and cognitive level, as well as motivation as it relates to movement and interaction with the environment.

## *Quality of Movement*

Following a detailed description of the child's functional skills, therapists analyze the quality of movement used to accomplish these skills. As described in the theoretical base, quality of motor behavior also depends on the child's age and developmental level and may impact on the performance of functional skills. Certain behaviors considered age-appropriate for one child, may be immature or primitive for an older child. For example, the high guard posture in the sitting position at 5 or 6 months of age is normal, although it is abnormal for the twelve-month-old child. Simultaneously, other behaviors may be observed in both these children, irrespective of age, that are abnormal, pathological, or not generally seen at any time in normal development, such as the tonic reflexes.

Postural tone is very important in this frame of reference. It is examined with regard to three characteristics; the degree of stiffness, the distribution of tone, and the adaptability of tone in response to movement and handling. The child is evaluated in all developmental positions with respect to these characteristics. A detailed description is made of the child's posture at rest and the patterns used to achieve transitional movements, such as the progression of movement through space or changing of positions. This is done in each major position: supine, prone, quadruped, sitting, and standing. Observations follow the cephalo to caudal pattern from head, neck, shoulder girdle, trunk, pelvis, and then to the lower extremities. Consistent observations are then grouped together to develop summary statements about the child's quality of movement. These statements address postural alignment, dissociation of movement, stability, control and gradation of movement, and the variation of movement patterns.

Postural alignment is assessed in the three body planes (sagittal, frontal, and transverse) in which movement occurs, and in every developmental position as well. For example, a child with spasticity while sitting with his head hyperextended is out of alignment in the sagittal plane. A child with hemiplegia while standing asymmetrically with weight primarily on one lower extremity is out of alignment in the frontal plane. A child with spastic quadriplegia and who cannot roll with dissociation or rotation exhibits lack of alignment in the transverse plane.

Dissociation is the ability of the child to perform movement of one body part independent of another body part. An example is shoulder movement independent of pelvic movement, or movement of one leg in isolation to the rest of the body. Frequently the child with spastic diplegia is unable to pull into a standing position through the use of the half-kneel position. The child may achieve standing through use of symmetrical extension of both lower extremities and by pulling to stand with both upper extremities. Again, age is critical in the analysis of appropriate dissociation movement patterns.

Stability and mobility are described in the various positions in which the child functions. Specifically, the therapist is concerned with the postures or patterns used to maintain a position or to provide support for movement. For example, a child who does not have mature equilibrium reactions may use a broad base of support or a high guard posture to maintain balance.

Control and gradation of movement show the child's ability to coordinate movement smoothly and accurately through the reciprocal relationship between agonist and antagonist muscles. The ability to hold this transitional pattern demonstrates control and gradation of movement.

Variation of movement patterns constitute the repertoire that a child uses to perform functional tasks. Lack of variety may result in stereotypical patterns. This should be observed in the way that a child reaches for objects in various developmental postures, such as prone, sitting, and standing.

Of critical importance to occupational therapists is the impact of abnormal movement and posture on the child's use of his upper extremities for function and independence in self-care activities. Assessment of the upper extremities includes habitual postures and the influence of tone in weightbearing *and* nonweightbearing positions. This may be reflected in the child's ability to orient his limb in space and to use full range of reach in varied planes of movement. Specific observations of grasp, release, prehension, and in-hand as well as bilateral manipulation should be included.

## Standardized Evaluations

Recently, attempts have been made to standardize observations that address the quality of movement in young children. Standardized evaluations such as the Movement Assessment of Infants (MAI) (Campbell, 1981; Chandler, Andrews, & Swanson, 1980), the Posture and Fine Motor Assessment of Infants (PFMAI) (Case-Smith,1991) and the Tufts Assessment of Motor

Performance (Gans, Haley, Hallenberg, Main, Inacio & Fass, in press) attempt to assess the quality of movement. For example, the MAI addresses muscle tone, primitive reflexes, automatic reactions, and volitional movement. This is accomplished through observation. In these assessments, quality of movement is viewed separately from the developmental and functional behaviors of the child. These tests assess many of the concepts outlined in the previously identified function/dysfunction continua. It should be noted, however, that all areas are not fully addressed in these assessments. In addition, when using standardized tools, age limitations frequently interfere.

Neurodevelopmental treatment as a frame of reference is primarily concerned with motor behaviors. A thorough occupational therapy evaluation can supplement an NDT evaluation and should include sensory, oral-motor, perceptual, cognitive, and fine motor skills. Specialized assessments (Erhardt, 1982; Morris, 1990) beyond the format discussed in this chapter may provide more in-depth information on the development of fine motor and oral-motor skills. Sensory, perceptual, and cognitive functions also do not relate specifically to the NDT frame of reference and therefore were omitted here.

## Postulates Regarding Change

Postulates regarding change delineate the therapeutic environment that needs to be created, and they suggest the methods used by the therapist to facilitate change. For the NDT frame of reference, 16 postulates have been identified. When the results of evaluation indicate dysfunction, intervention focuses on the qualitative aspects of movement that interfere with the child's ability to develop skills or functional abilities. Different tonal abnormalities cause different problems that require different handling approaches. As previously described, the primary mode of intervention in NDT is handling by the therapist. Handling, which refers to techniques and methods to promote active movement in a child, assists the child in moving as independently as possible with "more normal" postural tone and movement patterns. Beyond hands-on interaction in individual treatment, handling also refers to lifting and positioning during other activities that occur throughout the child's day. Effective handling relies on the therapist's ability to understand and interpret the child's reactions and then to respond appropriately.

Four postulates are related to postural tone:

1. If the therapist is able to feel the child's muscle activation and the therapist can grade her touch accordingly, then the child will receive the optimum level of input to promote active participation in movement.

2. If the therapist is able to monitor the child's reactions to handling on input, then handling techniques may be modified easily.
3. If the child's movement is not automatic because of poor muscle control, then the therapist needs to provide graded therapeutic input. This would consist of various combinations of tactile and proprioceptive stimulation provided at different rates and speeds.

     Children with low tone frequently benefit from input at distal key points.

     Children with high tone frequently benefit from input at proximal key points.

     Children with low tone benefit from slow, controlled movements in limited ranges.

     Children with high tone benefit from the use of full range of movement and a variety of movement patterns with gradually increasing speed.
4. If therapeutic handling is used by all professionals and family members who have contact with the child, then the child has the most opportunities to move with "more normal" tone and patterns of movement.

Stability and mobility are the next general areas within the sequence of intervention, with two postulates:

5. To promote stability and mobility, the therapist must provide a sequence of intervention beginning with preparatory activities. These activities may include techniques that promote mobility in structures that indicate limitations in passive movement or techniques that promote stability through postural alignment of the body before active movement.

     Proximal stability may be facilitated through weightbearing, which requires cocontraction around a joint.

     Stability may be facilitated by applying intermittent compression directly to the muscles surrounding a joint.

     Mobility may be facilitated through activities that require wide ranges of movement.
6. If the therapist facilitates effective movement patterns and the child has ample opportunity to repeat these movement patterns, then these patterns will become integrated into his repertoire of motor behaviors.

The following two postulates relate to reciprocal innervation:

7. If the therapist provides inhibition and facilitation techniques in combination, controlled coordinated movements will be stimulated.

8. If the therapist uses handling techniques that inhibit abnormal patterns, then the child will develop greater stability and control over higher level movement sequences.

Two postulates relate to postural alignment. They are as follows:

9. If the therapist handles the child in a way that facilitates mature righting and equilibrium reactions in all developmental positions, then the child will have the potential to use these reactions to maintain normal postural alignment to engage in activities.
10. If the therapist facilitates reciprocal innervation leading to greater stability in the child and resulting in a smooth interplay between the agonist and antagonist muscles, then the child will be able to maintain and regain postural alignment.

There is one postulate that relates to dissociation:

11. If the therapist provides handling on either static or dynamic surfaces to facilitate differentiated motor responses, then dissociated movements will occur.

The development of a wide variety of movements is influenced by the child's environment, both human and nonhuman. The occupational therapist's use of objects and activities maximizes the child's motivation to engage in therapy and ultimately to improve motor abilities. The following four postulates relate to this area:

12. If movement achieved through handling is used in functional interaction within the environment, then the child has the greatest opportunity to develop functional skills.
13. If the therapist adapts the environment to take into account the child's developmental level, needs, and interests, then the maximum amount of stimulation will be provided to encourage motor skills.
14. If the therapist uses handling techniques when a child's attention is focused on a play activity, then it often is easier for the child to respond with an automatic movement pattern.
15. If the occupational therapist is responsive to the child's needs and encourages the child to initiate during treatment, then therapeutic handling will be an interactive and a meaningful process and the child will be more likely to initiate active movement to engage in purposeful activities.

To facilitate a full range of motion or to prevent contractures and deformities, adaptive equipment for positioning and orthotic devices are important to intervention. They can reinforce NDT therapeutic goals and aid in the prevention of abnormal patterns and deformities by providing consistent input. As the next postulate states

16. If preventative measures such as adaptive equipment and orthotic devices are provided, then the child will receive consistent input to prevent or reduce the occurrence of deformities and limitations.

# Application to Practice

The theoretical base and concepts of NDT as presented in this chapter constitute essential knowledge for entry-level occupational therapists who work with children who have neurological impairment. The application of these concepts requires skill and practice. Translating these concepts into treatment also may be learned effectively through supervision from an experienced therapist. Specialized training through continuing education workshops—ranging from two-day introductory courses to eight-week basic courses that lead to NDT certification—provide a comprehensive understanding and application of this frame of reference (Neurodevelopmental Treatment Association, Inc. P.O. Box 70, Oak Park, IL 60303).

Occupational therapists have a unique perspective on the quality of life of each child within the context of his family. This includes placing a high priority on functional ability. Within each intervention then, it is critical for the therapist to analyze the motor components of activities needed to accomplish the practical skills. This analysis assists the therapist in the development of functional and realistic goals for the child.

The ideal application of NDT uses a team approach that includes occupational therapy, physical therapy, speech therapy, special education, and the family. In each setting, such as school, home, clinic, or private practice, the occupational therapist must establish treatment priorities. The role and responsibilities of the occupational therapist may vary, depending on the other disciplines involved, as well as on the therapist's individual skills.

## Sequence of Intervention

A recommended sequence of intervention begins with preparatory activities. These activities may include techniques to promote mobility in structures that indicate limitations in passive movement[a] or techniques that facilitate alignment of the body before active movement. Then the therapist selects specific areas of the child's body for therapeutic handling. These key points may be proximal (such as the shoulder girdle, trunk, and pelvis) or distal (such as the hands and feet). The specific keys points used depend on the child's therapeutic needs. Following preparatory activities, active or automatic movement patterns should be facilitated, using continued therapeutic input at necessary key points of control. These active or automatic movement patterns are stimulated through graded input provided by the therapist handling the child. If movement is not automatic because of poor muscle control, graded therapeutic input consists of various combinations of tactile and proprioceptive stimulation provided at different rates and speeds. This sequence is completed when the desired response is incorporated into a functional interaction with the environment.

## Handling

Handling is graded sensory input provided by the therapist's hands at key points of control on the child's body. Handling includes any contact that the therapist's hands have with the child's body, resulting in active control or movement.

Handling is used to facilitate active or automatic movement patterns. The therapist's decision to facilitate at either proximal or distal key points of control often depends on the child's postural tone. For example, low-tone children frequently benefit from input at distal key points. This encourages active movement by the child while simultaneously preventing the child from depending on support from the therapist's hands and body. Handling at proximal key points often is used with the child with high tone. Abnormal patterns are prevented while providing the child with greater stability and control over higher level movement sequences. It is important to note that the therapist must maintain a constant awareness of her touch or degree of pressure to be responsive to the child's needs. When applying deep pressure, the therapist's hand is shaped to the child's body contour. During light or intermittent touch pressure, the therapist's hands follow the movement of the child and gently intervene to prevent abnormal responses.

The child with high tone (**spastic**) benefits from therapeutic handling that uses full range of movement and a variety of movement patterns with gradually increasing speed. Generally, handling of the child with spasticity

---

[a] Techniques that may be used to promote mobility include myofascial release and joint mobilization; however, it should be noted that these techniques are not part of the NDT frame of reference.

involves an interplay of techniques to reduce tightness and to facilitate active movement. The child with low tone (**hypotonic** or **athetoid**) benefits from slow, controlled movements in limited ranges. The hypotonic child frequently is treated in higher level antigravity positions (sitting and standing) to promote increased activation of proximal musculature.

One of the specific concerns of the occupational therapist is upper extremity movement and function. Specific handling techniques need to be used with children who have abnormal tone and movement patterns in the upper extremities and trunk. These tonal problems often manifest in difficulty with bilateral movements, reaching, grasping, releasing of objects, and in-hand manipulation skills (Exner, 1989). Another priority for the occupational therapist is to use handling techniques during self-care, including feeding, dressing, toileting, and personal hygiene.

Therapeutic handling also may require additional equipment, such as various sized balls, rolls, or benches. This equipment provides a static or dynamic surface, allowing the therapist to use her hands and body effectively to facilitate specific objectives, such as modulation of tone, weightshifting, and development of righting and equilibrium reactions.

## Inhibition and Facilitation

When handling, the therapist incorporates specific facilitation and inhibition techniques. Facilitation techniques involve direct input to stimulate muscle activity. The purpose is to produce a desired motor response. Conversely, inhibition involves decreasing abnormal muscular responses that interfere with movement. Another purpose of inhibition is to prevent increases in tone that may occur during movement and, thereby, to reduce the possibility of undesired muscle contractions.

Techniques such as tapping and intermittent compression facilitate normal muscle contraction and movement. The techniques provide proprioceptive and tactile stimulation (Boehme, 1988; Neurodevelopmental Association, 1990).

Tapping facilitates the large muscles of the trunk and increases postural tone. It also can be used to increase the contractile activity of specific muscle groups. The therapist taps over the belly of the muscle quickly, until the child responds with muscular contractions felt by the therapist. On observation, the child then begins to hold his trunk more independently or move his limbs actively. Tapping can be provided periodically, based on the child's ability to respond to this input. For example, the arches of the hands of a hypotonic child can be activated by tapping the child's palm repetitively with the therapist's finger pads (Boehme, 1988). Caution is urged when using this technique with spastic children because of the likelihood of eliciting abnormal motor responses.

Intermittent compression also is a form of tapping, sometimes referred to as *pressure tapping*. This technique is designed to facilitate cocontraction and usually is applied directly to the muscles that surround a joint that requires better stabilization. In working with a low-tone child to maintain an upright posture in sitting, the therapist's hands are placed on either side of the trunk. The hands apply a compressive force and remain in contact with the child's body with input toward the weightbearing surface. In this example, the therapist applies pressure to the child's torso in an inward and downward motion (Fig. 5.8).

Inhibition techniques can include traction or light joint compression, both of which decrease tone and undesirable movement patterns. These techniques are particularly effective in reducing flexor spasticity at the shoulder girdle and, even more so, tightness at the scapular humeral joint. When applying

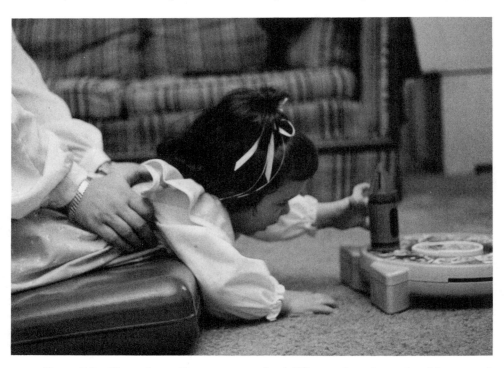

**Figure 5.8**    Therapist applies pressure to the child's torso in an inward and downward motion.

these inhibition techniques, the scapula should be stabilized on the rib cage by the palm of the therapist's hand placed at the inferior angle of the scapula. Simultaneously, the humerus is brought into external rotation and abduction by the therapist's other hand. The therapist maintains steady tension, elongating the muscles in this position. The stretch in this position, with gentle traction, inhibits the spastic muscles. Light joint compression can be used alternately, pushing the head of the humerus into the glenoid fossa before use of gentle traction.

Most often, inhibition and facilitation techniques are used in combination. As in the previous example that involved traction on the humerus, heavy compression also can be applied to the scapula in a downward rotated position to promote cocontraction of the scapula on the rib cage. In addition, techniques to inhibit tone may be used in conjunction with facilitatory techniques to obtain active movement. This may be evident when an occupational therapist places her hands over the scapula to prevent excessive elevation and abduction, while allowing increased range of reaching.

One end result of specific inhibition and facilitation techniques is the establishment of improved body alignment—such as righting reactions—that allows for more efficient movement and the emergence of mature equilibrium reactions. Alignment allows for the most efficient form of muscle cocontraction around a joint for stability. This stability then gives way to the greatest range and variability of active movement and control.

Facilitation and inhibition techniques are used repeatedly throughout the process of handling. They serve to prevent the reappearance of abnormal posturing or immobility, as well as to maintain the child's alignment and active participation.

## Weightshifting and Weightbearing

The therapist may use facilitation or inhibition handling techniques to encourage weightbearing and weightshifting. The goal of weightbearing and weightshifting is to promote postural alignment as well as to facilitate the child's ability to move in and out of positions and move through space.

All postural movements, whether gross or subtle, occur with a shift in weight. Shifts in weight, therefore, may occur in degrees of amplitude and in various planes (such as anterior-posterior, laterally, and diagonally). Children who have abnormal postural tone often have difficulty initiating, controlling, or grading a shift in weight. For example, the hypertonic child has difficulty initiating a weight shift, whereas the hypotonic child has difficulty grading a weight shift.

Weightbearing is when a child's body part or extremity maintains contact and exerts pressure against a surface such as the ground, therapy equipment, or, possibly, the therapist's body. Through weightbearing, cocontraction around a joint can be achieved, allowing for the development of greater proximal stability. This can be seen when children weight bear in quadruped and weight shift over extended arms as they move in and out of sitting. Weightshifting also occurs when children creep forward through space. This movement is important in the development of proximal to distal control; therefore, in a sequence of treatment, weightbearing may precede graded reaching or hand activities.

## Integration of Activities

For occupational therapists, activities that facilitate functional skills are essential. Play activities are especially important for children. Children who have motor impairments frequently have limited participation in play activities. The therapist who applies NDT therefore needs to be sensitive to the use of play activities during treatment (Anderson, Hinojosa & Stauch, 1988). Incorporating play fulfills a variety of therapeutic goals. Play (1) motivates or engages the child during therapy; (2) provides appropriate activity experiences as stimuli for normal movement patterns; and, (3) develops specific cognitive and perceptual skills.

It often is easier to elicit an automatic movement pattern through handling techniques when a child's attention is focused on a play activity. The therapist carefully selects the play activity to avoid the influence of excessive effort by the child, which may result in associated reactions.

Movements used during play often are similar to movements used in other aspects of life. The use of play activities during treatment, therefore, may encourage the use of the same movements in other activities such as ADL. An important element in this frame of reference is the development of appropriate movement patterns during treatment that can be generalized to ADL.

## Positioning and Adaptive Equipment

Positioning and equipment may be used as adjuncts to handling. They facilitate postural alignment and stability without hands-on contact by the therapist. The assumption is that this external stabilization allows more independent movement elsewhere. In addition, equipment reduces the likelihood of deformities and contractures that develop with habitual abnormal posturing and movement. Through the use of positioning and adaptive equipment designed specifically for the child's needs, the goals of therapy can be reinforced by parents and other professionals. This is discussed further in Chapter 8.

# Summary

The neurodevelopmental treatment frame of reference is based on the work of Berta and Karel Bobath in the 1940s. Other professionals in the field of pediatric rehabilitation have contributed extensively to this body of knowledge. This approach uses a "hands-on" method to facilitate movement patterns necessary for the acquisition of functional skills. Clinically, the approach is adapted and modified for use with children of varying ages and diagnoses.

The theoretical base of NDT is founded on a set of assumptions that provide the fundamental concepts for evaluation and intervention. The assumptions include concepts grounded in a knowledge about normal development, development of normal postural control, and understanding of components of movement. Normal development is subdivided further into four categories: principles of normal development, the sensory-motor-sensory feedback system, components of movement, and sequences of motor development. An understanding of abnormal motor control also provides essential guidance in the development of the frame of reference. Clinically, problems are seen in the quality of the child's postural tone, reciprocal innervation, and development of righting and equilibrium reactions necessary for automatic movement. Finally, the theoretical base assumes that treatment can be effective because "handling" alters the sensory input to the child's CNS and, thereby, changes the abnormal patterns of movement on a subcortical level. Handling allows for active participation within the context of functional activities so that learning can take place.

There are seven key function/dysfunction continua that provide therapists with descriptions of observable behaviors essential for the clinical assessment of most children. These continua provide the foundation for an NDT assessment, which is designed to identify and analyze dysfunction characteristics of movement associated with CNS dysfunction. The entry-level therapist is encouraged to follow a structured approach under the supervision of an experienced therapist to elicit the child's movement repertoire, categorize the movement problems, and determine how these deficits interfere with the child's ability to acquire functional skills.

Postulates regarding change delineate the environment that needs to be created and the techniques used by the therapist to facilitate change. These postulates emphasize the importance of consistent handling, active participation on the part of the child, responsibility of the therapist to the child's needs, creation of a motivating environment, use of ongoing assessment, incorporation of movement into functional activities, maximization of the therapist's sensory feedback through handling, and use of preventative strategies such as adaptive equipment and orthotic devices.

Application of the frame of reference requires practice, which is learned most effectively through supervision from an experienced therapist. Specialized training also is available through continuing education. Specific techniques used in this frame of reference include handling techniques that involve inhibition and facilitation of muscle activity. Combined with movement, this allows for functional interaction with the environment.

These techniques involve graded sensory input as well as incorporation of weightbearing and weightshifting to elicit automatic, active control. Play activities provide an essential component of motivation as well as a cognitive and perceptual stimulation. Adaptive equipment and positioning provide an adjunct to achieving the goals of therapy. The result is that the child acquires the movement components needed to achieve the greatest independence in developmentally appropriate areas of play, self-care, and school performance.

The NDT frame of reference provides the occupational therapist with a repertoire of handling techniques designed to improve a child's muscle tone and coordinated action. This allows for the emergence of stability and mobility necessary for mature postural reactions. The goal is to facilitate automatic movements used by the child in the acquisition of specific functional skills.

The NDT approach requires an ongoing process of problem solving to determine the movement components necessary for the performance of these functional skills (i.e., righting reactions, equilibrium reactions, active movements) as well as to analyze the child's responses to determine any interfering factors and missing components. It is a dynamic process in which the therapist may perform a range of activities, including elongating tight muscles, promoting mobility, and inhibiting spasticity and abnormal posturing within the context of goal-directed activity. The aim is for the child to achieve mastery in selected developmentally appropriate areas of play, self-care, and, ultimately, beginning school skills. Optimum achievement is possible when individual treatment is combined with activities at home and in school.

## OUTLINE OF NDT FRAME OF REFERENCE

I. History

II. Theoretical base
  A. Normal development
    1. Principles

a. Cephalocaudal
b. Proximal-distal
c. Gross to fine
2. Sensory-motor-sensory feedback
3. Components of normal development
   a. Interplay between stability and mobility
   b. Effects of postural reflex mechanism on movement
      1. Postural tone
      2. Muscle tone
      3. Reciprocal innervation
      4. Righting and equilibrium reactions
      5. Postural alignment
      6. Ability to dissociate movements
      7. Development of postural control in the three planes of space
4. Sequences of motor development
5. Variety of movement
B. Abnormal development
C. Sensory input as a means of bringing about change

III. Function/dysfunction continua
A. Postural tone
B. Stability-mobility
C. Reciprocal innervation
D. Postural alignment
E. Dissociation
F. Variety of movement
G. Full range of motion-structural deformities and contractures

IV. Evaluation
A. Overall assessment of functional skills
B. Availability of movement
C. Standardized evaluations

V. Postulates regarding change
A. Those that relate to postural tone
B. Those that relate to stability and mobility
C. Those that relate to reciprocal innervation
D. Those that relate to postural alignment
E. Those that relate to dissociation
F. Those that relate to maximizing the child's motivation to engage in therapy and, ultimately, to improve motor abilities
G. Those that relate to the use of adaptive equipment for positioning, or orthotic devices

VI. Application to practice
A. Sequence of intervention
B. Handling
C. Inhibition and facilitation
D. Weightshifting and weightbearing
E. Integration of activities
F. Positioning and adaptive equipment

## Acknowledgments

The photographs in Figures 5.5, 5.6, and 5.8 were taken by Steven A. Smith of New York.

## *References*

Anderson, J., Hinojosa, J., & Strauch, C. (1987). Integrating play in neurodevelopmental therapy (NDT). *American Journal of Occupational Therapy, 41*, 421–426.

Bly, L. (1980). Abnormal motor development. In D. Slaton, D. (ed.). *Development of movement in infancy.* University of North Carolina at Chapel Hill, Division of Physical Therapy, May 19–22, 1980.

Bobath, B. (1971a). *Abnormal postural reflex activity caused by brain lesions* (2nd Ed.). London: William Heineman Medical Books, Ltd.

Bobath, B. (1971b). Motor development, its effect on general development and application to the treatment of cerebral palsy. *Physiotherapy, 57*, 526–532.

Bobath, B. (1975, February). Sensorimotor development. *NDT Newsletters. 7*(1).

Boehme, R. (1984, May). Advanced NDT course in occupational therapy. New York: Long Island. Unpublished notes.

Boehme, R. (1988). *Improving upper body control.* Tucson, AZ: Therapy Skill Builders.

Campbell, P. (1981). Movement assessment of infants: An evaluation. *Physical and Occupational Therapy in Pediatrics, 1*(4), 53–57.

Campbell, P. (1986). Introduction to neurodevelopmental treatment. Pamphlet. Cuyahoga Falls, OH: Children's Hospital Medical Center of Akron.

Case-Smith, J. (1991). *Posture and fine motor assessment of infants* (research edition). Ohio State University.

Chandler, L. S., Andrews, M. S., & Swanson, M. W. (1980). *Movement Assessment of Infants: A manual*, Rolling Bay, WA.

Erhardt, R. P. (1982). *Developmental hand dysfunction: Theory, assessment, treatment.* Laurel, MD: Ramsco.

Exner, C. E. (1989). Development of hand functions. In P. N. Pratt & A. S. Allen (eds.) *Occupational therapy for children* (2nd ed.). St. Louis, MO: C. V. Mosby.

Gans, B. M., Haley, S. M., Hallenberg, S. C., Mann, N., Inacio, C. A., & Faas, R. M. (in press). Description and inter-observer reliability of the Tufts Assessment of Motor Performance. *American Journal of Physical Medicine and Rehabilitation.*

Kuypers, (1963). Organization of the motor systems, *International Journal of Neurology, 4*, 78–91.

Lawrence, & Hopkins, (1972). Developmental aspects of pyramidal motor control in Rhesus monkey. *Brain Research, 40*, 117–118.

Morris, S. E. (May, 1990). *The development of oral-motor skills in children receiving non-oral feedings,* (rev. ed.). Faber, VA: New Visions.

Neurodevelopmental treatment 8-week certification course manual. Oak Park, IL: Neurodevelopmental Association.

Scherzer, A. L., & Tscharnuter, I. (1990). *Early diagnosis and treatment in cerebral palsy,* (2nd Ed.). New York: Marcel Dekker.

Short-DeGraff, M. A. (1988). *Human development for occupational and physical therapists.* Baltimore, MD: Williams & Wilkins.

# 6

# Sensory Integrative Frame of Reference

JUDITH GIENCKE KIMBALL

Sensory integration is the process of organizing sensory information in the brain to make an adaptive response (Ayres, 1972a). An adaptive response occurs when a person successfully meets an environmental challenge. The sensory integrative frame of reference is applied when sensory system processing deficits make it difficult for a child to produce an appropriate adaptive response. In this chapter, the child's physical adaptive response and his reactions and behaviors, which include his emotional and ideational adaptive responses, are addressed. The primary consideration in sensory integration is that processing problems are related to subtle yet definable differences in neurological functioning, often called **soft signs** by physicians.

A. Jean Ayres, Ph.D., OTR, FAOTA, the originator of the theory of sensory integration, began actual work on the theory in the late 1950s. Dr. Ayres was an occupational therapist with a doctorate in educational psychology who did a postdoctoral fellowship at the Brain Research Institute of the University of California at Los Angeles. Her research is most commonly identified with learning disabled children; however, it has been extended to include many other forms of neurobehavioral development, including mental retardation, autism, sensory defensiveness, numerous behavioral disorders, and other neurosensory based problems.

Dr. Ayres made major contributions to the field of occupational therapy with the publication of the Southern California Sensory Integration Tests (SCSIT) in 1972 (1972b, 1980). The SCSIT was based on factor analytic studies that focused on the components of sensory integration, as well as other tests commonly used at the time with learning disabled children (Ayres, 1965, 1966a, 1966b, 1969, 1972a, 1972b, 1972c, 1972d, 1975b). Her 1977 study—using the Southern California Postrotary Nystagmus Test (1975a) (SCPNT)—supported the role of the vestibular system in sensory integrative dysfunction (Ayres, 1978). Earlier studies had already identified several deficit areas seen in children who had sensory integrative dysfunction, notably, problems with tactile discrimination, tactile defensiveness, perceptual difficulties, bilateral integration dysfunction, and dyspraxia (poor motor planning abilities). Later, factor analytic studies pinpointed left-hemisphere dysfunction, including auditory language disabilities, and right-hemisphere dysfunctions, such as deficits in perception and a lack of awareness of the left side of the body. Cumulatively, all the factor analytic studies resulted in a topology for identifying and treating sensory integrative problems. The topology included vestibular and bilateral integration problems, dyspraxia, left-hemisphere disorders, right-hemisphere disorders, and generalized sensory integrative dysfunction. These categories were used by occupational therapists until the late 1980s. (For a summary of Ayres' factor analytic studies and their contributions to the theory of sensory integration the reader is advised to see Clark, Mallioux, and Parham [1989]).

During the 1980s, Ayres developed and standardized the Sensory Integration and Praxis Tests (SIPT). These tests, published in 1989, were more specific to praxis and more in-depth than the SCSIT. Research using the SIPT indicates that the areas of dysfunction are similar to those already identified by the SCSIT. Because the SIPT tests are more complex and specific to praxis, their research findings expand our knowledge of the complexity and interrelationships in the central nervous system (CNS) (Kimball, 1990). According to Fisher, Murray, and Bundy (1991 p. 10), the patterns that were delineated by both cluster and factor analysis in the SIPT include

1. Somatosensory processing deficits
2. Poor bilateral integration and sequencing
3. Impaired somotopraxis
4. Poor praxis on verbal command
5. Visual praxis factor, more appropriately considered as poor visual perception and visuomotor coordination
   a. Poor form and space perception
   b. Visual construction deficits
   c. Visuomotor coordination deficits
6. Generalized sensory integrative dysfunction

The SIPT is scored by computer and generates a profile of the child's abilities compared against six patterns that emerged from SIPT standardization. These patterns include the following:

1. Low average bilateral integration and sequencing
2. Low average sensory integration and praxis
3. General sensory integrative dysfunction
4. Dyspraxia on verbal command
5. Visuo- and somatodyspraxia
6. High average sensory integration and praxis

Figure 6.1 is a chromagraph report that shows a child's scores on each of the SIPT tests, as well as the relationship to the six diagnostic clusters (SIPT, 1989).

# Theoretical Base of Sensory Integrative Frame of Reference

A knowledge of human development provides a starting point for understanding sensory integration. Sensory integration is far more complex, however, than the outward signs of function and skill development often associated with human development. The sensory integrative frame of reference focuses on the influences of the integration of the sensory systems that underlie the development of function and skills—that is, those sensory systems that organize the nervous system for actual acquisition of function (Fig. 6.2). This classic chart devised by Ayres is the starting point for understanding that function and skill are based on sensory system integration.

The sensory systems—or "senses" as they are labeled on Figure 6.2—that are important in the theoretical base of the sensory integrative frame of reference are the auditory, visual, vestibular, proprioceptive, and tactile systems. The vestibular, proprioceptive, and tactile systems are highlighted as the precursors to development of the auditory and visual systems. In fact, they are thought to be the precursors to the development of most end-product abilities. This perspective is different from the theoretical bases of other frames of reference, particularly those involved with cognitive development, which focus on the auditory and visual systems.

As Figure 6.2 is followed from left to right and the sensory systems integrate (i.e., "integration of their inputs'), the results are "end products" that reflect function and skills. The goal of occupational therapists who use a sensory integrative frame of reference is to facilitate the development of

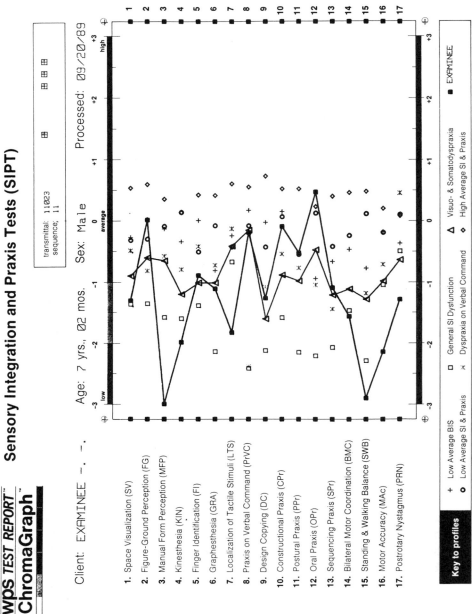

**Figure 6.1**   Sensory integration and praxis tests chromagraph Copyright © 1988 by Western Psychological Services. Reprinted by permission of the publisher, Western Psychological Services, 12031 Wilshire Boulevard, Los Angeles, California 90025.

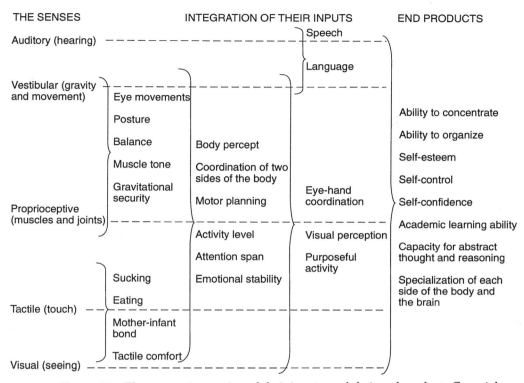

THE SENSES

Auditory (hearing)

Vestibular (gravity and movement)

Proprioceptive (muscles and joints)

Tactile (touch)

Visual (seeing)

INTEGRATION OF THEIR INPUTS

Speech

Language

Eye movements

Posture

Balance

Muscle tone

Gravitational security

Body percept

Coordination of two sides of the body

Motor planning

Eye-hand coordination

Activity level

Attention span

Emotional stability

Visual perception

Purposeful activity

Sucking

Eating

Mother-infant bond

Tactile comfort

END PRODUCTS

Ability to concentrate

Ability to organize

Self-esteem

Self-control

Self-confidence

Academic learning ability

Capacity for abstract thought and reasoning

Specialization of each side of the body and the brain

**Figure 6.2** The senses, integration of their inputs, and their end products Copyright © 1988 by Western Psychological Services. Reprinted by permission of the publisher, Western Psychological Services, 12031 Wilshire Boulevard, Los Angeles, California 90025.

these end products. The therapist is primarily concerned, however, with the integrity and integration of underlying sensory systems and the functional support capabilities that contribute to these end products. The occupational therapist directs the intervention at the sensory system and functional support capability levels (middle level of figure), in combination with facilitating an adaptive response, all of which result in the development of end-product abilities.

## Basic Concepts

The theoretical base of the sensory integrative frame of reference is unique in that it deals specifically with the contributions of the subcortical areas of the brain to human behavior. Dr. Ayres specifically stated that the brainstem was the primary area of integration and therefore played the greatest role in sensory integration. Structures of particular interest in the brainstem include the thalamus (master integrator of the brain), the vestibular nuclei and their interconnectors, and the reticular formation (particularly important in alerting and arousal). Dr. Ayres also postulated that the cerebellum plays a major role in sensory integration because of its processing of input related to gravity and movement. As this theoretical base evolved, the importance of other structures of the CNS were recognized. The limbic system has been identified because of its association with sympathetic arousal, which results in the survival (fight-or-flight) response often seen in people who exhibit sensory defensiveness (Ayres, 1979; Wilbarger & Wilbarger, 1991).

The cerebral cortex also is important to the theoretical base of sensory integration because of its contribution to praxis, particularly in the areas of ideation or a person's understanding of the need for movement. The entire CNS and the interplay or integration of all its systems are considered in sensory integration.

There are six basic assumptions that underlie CNS organization in sensory integration:

1) The central nervous system is hierarchically organized. Cortical processing relies on and depends on adequate organization of inputs supplied by the lower brain centers.
2) Meaningful registration of stimuli must occur before the CNS can make a response to it and, therefore, allow for higher functioning to occur.
3) The brain is innately organized to program a person to seek out stimulation that is organizing or beneficial in itself.
4) Input from one sensory system can facilitate or inhibit the state of the entire organism. Input from each system influences every other system, as well as the whole organism.
5) There is plasticity within the CNS.
6) Normal human development occurs sequentially.

*The central nervous system is hierarchically organized. Cortical processing relies on and depends on adequate organization of sensation supplied by the lower brain centers.* Phylogenetically, as the brain developed, newer and higher level structures, like the cerebral cortex, remained interconnected and depended on the adequate functioning of the older and lower level brain structures. The integration of sensory input provided by the lower brain centers allows the cortical or higher centers to process more complex and specialized information.

*Meaningful registration of the stimuli must occur before the brain can make a response to it and, therefore, allow higher functioning to occur, including adaptive responses.* The registration of sensory input must occur to signal a change in the environment, and this must be meaningful enough to alert the person. For example, if a child is not alerted to the possibility of falling when he starts to tip over, a balance response that is adaptive to the environmental situation cannot occur. In this example, the lack of registration may be caused by one of three things: (1) an inefficiency in the detecting mechanism—in this case, the vestibular system; (2) underarousal of the whole system; or, (3) a masking of the response by overarousal of many other systems.

*The brain is innately organized to program the person to seek out stimulation that is organizing or beneficial in itself.* To accomplish an adaptive response reinforces integration in sensory systems, but it also is based on input from those sensory systems. Children naturally seek out and engage in activities that optimally promote neural integration. This is referred to as the *inner drive for sensory integration.* For example, the jumping, climbing, and falling activities seen in most two-year-old children are related to the incipient understanding of gravity. At this age the child needs to experience his ability to move against gravity and needs to challenge gravity at all levels. Even adults seek out activities to give themselves a balanced "sensory diet." If we work at a desk, we might pick skiing, jogging, or aerobics to make us "feel better."

*Input from one sensory system can facilitate or inhibit the state of the entire organism. Input from each system influences every other system, as well as the whole organism.* In other words, facilitation and inhibition of a specific system do not have to occur within that system alone, but also can be achieved through the influence of inhibition and facilitation of other sensory systems. This powerful assumption provides the basis for the occupational therapist to treat dysfunction of one sensory system through intervention with another sensory system. It also demonstrates the vast interconnection between the function and structure of the CNS.

*There is plasticity within the central nervous system.* Brain processing and structure can be modified to bring about more optimal functioning. Using the sensory integrative frame of reference, intervention is directed at sensory systems and functional support levels to facilitate changes in the child's ability to produce an adaptive response. In many cases, this change is permanent and reflects a processing difference that cannot be attributed to learning alone. Although younger children are thought to have the most neural plasticity, experience has shown that change can occur throughout adulthood.

*Normal human development occurs sequentially.* The sensory integrative frame of reference is based on an understanding of the sequence of human development and on an understanding of the adaptive responses that children should be able to accomplish at each age level. If sensory system modulation and functional support capabilities are not integrated, then adaptive responses will not reach optimum levels. *Splinter skills* develop out of a need in specific situations, but their transferability to other situations is limited. The sensory integrative frame of reference focuses on developing integration, not on teaching splinter skills.

These assumptions, basic to CNS organization, are the foundation for the theoretical base of sensory integration.

## Sensory Systems

Particularly important to the theoretical base of sensory integration is an understanding of the vestibular, proprioceptive, and tactile systems. Although the neuroanatomy and neurophysiology of the systems are beyond the scope of this chapter, the chapter does assume a basic understanding of neuroscience. Functional connections will be emphasized, therefore with reference made only to the neuroscience that underlies these connections. (For a synopsis of neuroscience, the reader is referred to Moore in Gilfoyle, Grady, and Moore [1990]).

**Tactile System.**   This system has several different functions. Of particular interest is the ongoing interaction between the two major divisions of the body's tactile system: the dorsal column medial lemniscal and the anterolateral systems. (The head is served by the cranial nerves, particularly the trigeminal nerve).

The dorsal column medial lemniscal (DCML) system carries discriminative touch (specifically two-point discrimination), conscious proprioception, touch pressure, and vibration for the body. Of the two tactile systems, it is the newer phylogenetically. It plays a major role in the development of praxis. Wall (1970) identified an expanded role for the DCML system that is particularly pertinent to the development of praxis. He identified deficits in motor performance, especially voluntary exploratory movements, and deficits in attention, orientation, and anticipation with dorsal column lesion. (For a detailed discussion of this and related research the reader is referred to Cermak in Fisher et al. [1991, p. 151–154].)

The anterolateral system—composed of spinothalamic, spinoreticular, and spinotectal pathways—is a nonspecific, protective system that can produce sympathetic arousal. It also is a diffuse system that directs input into the reticular formation. It is responsible for the body sensations of pain, temperature, and crude touch (tickle and itch) and plays a major role in tactile defensive responses, such as an averse response to light touch that results from overarousal. Phylogenetically, this system is older than the DCML.

Adequate functioning of both major divisions of the tactile system is necessary for appropriate sensory integration. Problems in interpreting tactile input may result in difficulties in the end products, such as touch discrimination or praxis. (Praxis is the ability to motor plan a new, nonhabitual motor act.) In addition, the child may have difficulty in modulating tactile input. This can result in over- or underregistration of the tactile system. Overregistration is called *tactile defensiveness.*

**Proprioception.**    Proprioception is the understanding of where joints and muscles are in space. Proprioreceptors include the muscle spindles, the Golgi tendon organs, and mechanoreceptors of the skin. Proprioceptors work in conjunction with the vestibular system to give a sense of balance and position in space. All the muscles and joints are involved in this process; however, the neck joints and proximal limb joints, such as shoulders and hips, are of primary importance and give the most feedback to the CNS. Proprioception is a powerful system therapeutically.

**Vestibular System.**    The vestibular receptors, located in the inner ear, are composed of three semicircular canals at right angles to each other and the utricle and saccule. These structures are filled with endolymph and contain hair cells that send the signals concerning direction of movement when they are displaced within the endolymph because of head movement. The semicircular canals are responsible for detection of angular, fast, short bursts of motion, and results in phasic limb movements and momentary head righting. The utricle and saccule, which contain the otoliths (calcium carbonate crystals or the "rocks in your head") as well as endolymph and hair cells, are responsible for the detection of gravity (the "rocks" fall "down") and linear acceleration. Utricle stimulation results in tonic input to the limbs and maintained head righting.

According to Ayres (1979), the child's relationship to gravity is "more primal than the (child's) relationship to mother" (p. 40); or, Mother Earth's gravity is more important for security than a child's biological mother. Furthermore, Ayres described gravity as ". . . the most constant universal force in our lives" (Ayres, 1979, p. 40). She pointed out that all living things must relate to the earth's gravitational pull. Humans appear to be endowed with a strong drive to master gravity and to attain an upright position. This ability to move against gravity is one of the key movements a therapist looks for in a child, because it indicates a well-organized nervous system. Movement against gravity develops over time, as in (1) an infant's ability to raise its head off the mat at 1 month of age; (2) an infant's ability to raise his head, shoulders, and legs off the mat at 4 months of age; (3) a one-year-old child's ability to stand upright and walk; (4) a four-year-old child's ability to remain in a swing; and, (5) a school-aged child's love of movement activities that involve the challenge of gravity, such as jumping horses, skiing, or skateboarding.

The vestibular system makes connections through the vestibular nuclei in the brainstem and then sends information to higher levels in the brain. Dysfunction of the vestibular system, as seen in developmental problems, usually is caused by deficits in the integration of the vestibular input rather than by deficits in the vestibular receptors. Developmental vestibular problems can be functional, such as balance and coordination, or modulational (under- or overarousal), such as gravitational insecurity or intolerance to movement.

**Sensory Integrative Functions.**    The five systems previously discussed (auditory, visual, vestibular, proprioceptive, and tactile), provide the basis for development of the functional support capabilities that lead to the end-product abilities noted in Figure 6.2.

Table 6.1 shows the sensory integrative functions addressed in the sensory integrative frame of reference. To produce the desired adaptive response in an end-product ability, the person must have sensory system modulation within normal levels and reasonable functional support capabilities. Optimal functioning means that all systems and capabilities work integratively.

## Sensory System Modulation

The manner in which the sensory systems process input affects the quality of a child's ability to respond adaptively. Figure 6.3 shows the classic arousal curve commonly associated with the autonomic nervous system (ANS). Note that moderate arousal results in an optimal adaptive response, whereas high arousal results in behavioral disorganization and even anxiety or a negative emotional response. The key point often overlooked by health professionals is that arousal initiates a sympathetic, fight, flight, or freeze response. This reaction is the primary survival response of the organism. When arousal gets too high, the body responds as if to a serious survival threat. If it is not possible to fight or flee, then arousal does not dissipate easily, causing stress, anxiety, and difficulty in completing other adaptive responses. Persons who have sensory system modulation problems have more changeable arousal or

*Table 6.1*   Sensory Integrative Functions

Sensory System Modulation
  Tactile
  Auditory
  Relationship to gravity
  Movement level
  Oral arousal
  Olfactory arousal
  Visual arousal
  Attention level
  Postrotary nystagmus
  Sensitivity to movement
  Proprioceptive sensitivity
  Emotional level

Functional Support Capabilities
  Suck-swallow-breathe
  Tactile discrimination
  Other discriminative abilities
  Cocontraction
  Muscle tone
  Proprioception
  Balance and equilibrium
  Developmental reflexes
  Lateralization
  Bilateral integration

End-Product Abilities
  Praxis
  Form and space perception
  Behavior
  Academics
  Language and articulation
  Emotional tone
  Activity level
  Environment mastery

reaction levels than normal. This results in problems with adaptive response because their systems lack stability.

The sensory systems do not function independently. Arousal in several systems can combine, therefore, to increase arousal, and inhibition in several systems can combine to decrease arousal. The 12 sensory system responses that are considered to be contributors to modulation of arousal are listed under Sensory System Modulation in Table 6.1.

Sensory system modulation is influenced by the child's "sensory diet." Sensory diet is "related to the essential but changing need of all humans

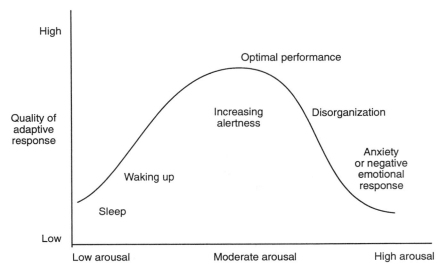

**Figure 6.3**  Classic Arousal Curve

to have an optimum amount of organizing and integrating sensation being registered by one's central nervous system at all times" (Wilbarger, 1984, p. 7). Sensory diet is the accumulation of the child's total sensory input and its effect. In normal children, the sensory diet acts as the only external modulating force that the nervous system needs under usual circumstances. Normally, a child seeks out varied sensory inputs to maintain normal modulation levels (see Fig. 6.3).

Usually, sensory system modulation fluctuates within a range of normal. Children who have sensory system modulation problems are much more variable than normal. Some children even react in a dangerous way and go from overarousal to physiological shutdown (Fig. 6.4). "Shutdown" appears to be an ANS response that can result in respiratory and cardiac irregularities and alterations in blood pressure that may produce decreased consciousness or shock. Shutdown results from severe overarousal that the nervous system cannot respond to in normal ways (Kimball, 1976; Kimball, 1977a). Other children may experience a dangerous possible variation in the pattern, which is also maladaptive, and go quickly from overarousal to underarousal but not to shutdown. This is thought to be a protective mechanism against severe sensory overload.

Severe physiological responses are infrequent but have been documented medically in at least two cases (Kimball, 1991). A more usual pattern is for a severely sensory overloaded person to shut off input and appear to be

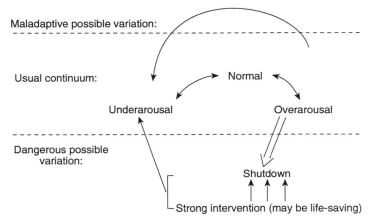

**Figure 6.4**   Sensory Systems Arousal Continuum

underaroused. When treatment is initiated with a child, he may quickly go to overarousal. Because treatment strategies are different for under- and overaroused children, this variation must be anticipated.

Each of the sensory systems also has an information processing component that discriminates appropriate aspects of the environment. Modulation problems mask the information components of the systems, often resulting in less than optimal ability to use the information processing systems. When sensory systems are well modulated, normal information processing is possible.

Normal tactile arousal/reactivity and integration allow children to differentiate among the types of tactile input that they experience. Ayres (1972a, 1975b) felt that the interplay between the two divisions of the body's tactile system gave the child a signal about being alert to a dangerous situation (anterolateral system) or differentiating what touch might imply (DCML). If this interplay is inaccurate, the anterolateral system may overarouse and cause the child to react as if in a survival situation when the stimulus warranted orientation only. When survival situations alert the nervous system, a fight-flight-freeze reaction might occur. Because most children react normally to touch, this overreaction could be interpreted as a behavior problem, when it actually is a variation in tactile system functioning called **tactile defensiveness**. We now know that much more than an interplay between the anterolateral and DCML systems is involved. Numerous ascending and descending controls exist on the two systems from many areas of the brain including the raphe spinal system, the reticular system, the limbic system, the hypothalamus, and the cortex (Chusid, 1979; DeGroot and Chusid, 1988;

Daube, Reagan, Sandok & Westmoreland, 1986; Fisher & Dunn 1983; Melzak & Wall, 1965; Pribram, 1975; Royeen, 1985; Routtenberg, 1968; Nieuwenhuys, Voogd, & van Huijzen, 1988; Kandel & Schwartz, 1985; Fisher et al., 1991). Important for treatment is the fact that all these functions in the head are served by cranial nerves, especially the trigeminal nerve, so that body input does not influence the head directly (Wilson-Panwels, Akesson, & Stewart, 1988). New research on neurotransmitters, particularly glutamate, and the finding that under extremely stressful conditions excess glutamate leads to cell death, certainly will contribute to a new understanding of sensory defensiveness in cases of abuse (Gold, Goodwin, & Chrousus, 1988a, 1988b; Fitzgerald, 1991; Dubner, 1991; Wilcox, 1991; Woolf, 1991).

Sounds, which are interpreted by the **auditory** system, alert children to changes in their environment that may or may not need attention and action. Usually, the only sounds that alert the child are those that need to be attended to. These differences may be caused by sound level, type, or novelty. Once the child has registered and has been aroused to the sound, he decides if action is necessary. If not, the sound can be ignored. When a normal hearing child is not alerted by sounds that may signify important changes in the environment, a state of underreactivity may exist. Because he has not been alerted, changes in the environment are not registered and, therefore, the child does not react adaptively.

In a state of overreactivity or defense, the child may be alerted to any environmental sounds, including those that do not require a response. Often the child is not able to habituate to a sound, therefore he continues to be alerted long after the sound is no longer novel. This state of overreactivity is called **auditory defensiveness**.

The gravity receptors in the vestibular mechanism, the otoliths in the utricle and saccule, normally alert children to changes in the relationship of their head position to **gravity** (Fig. 6.5). A change in head position that results in loss of equilibrium produces a compensatory response in the trunk and limbs to maintain balance. Children who are underreactive to gravity appear to be unaware of these changes in head position. They frequently will seek out strong movement input that even can be dangerous to them. Conversely, the child who is overreactive to changes in head position in relationship to gravity has a real fear or strong emotional response to situations that normally require only a balance reaction. This overreactivity is thought to be an otolithic response that is not being integrated appropriately. It is referred to as **gravitational insecurity**.

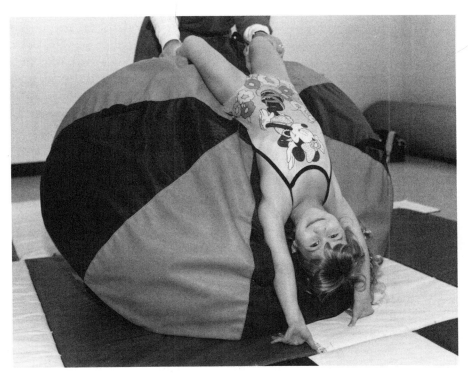

**Figure 6.5**   A gravitationally secure child; no fear responses noted.

**Movement** level refers to a child's need for nonpurposeful movement or much higher than normal levels of movement. Colloquially, this is described as "fidgeting" or being "motor driven." Normal children use movement to accomplish an end product, such as relocating from one place to another. The child who constantly needs to move to maintain a normal arousal level is referred to as **motor restless**. The child's need for movement probably is related to an overinhibition in the integration of vestibular input. This leads to his need to seek out more movement input to maintain a normal arousal/ reactivity level (Kimball, 1988). Sometimes it is difficult to differentiate between movement level and attention level. The child who has movement level modulation problem is motor restless and not necessarily distracted. He needs to move his body constantly and continually seeks out motor input. Conversely, the underreactive child may be slow moving, appearing to conserve movement.

Infants put objects in their mouths to learn about such things as texture, size, and shape and to fulfill the psychological need to mouthe. This is referred to as **oral arousal**. Some children are adverse to putting certain textures in their mouths. They refuse foods based on texture, not on taste. In severe cases, this can eliminate important foods from the child's diet, affecting nutrition. This overreactivity to textures is called **oral defensiveness**.

**Olfactory Arousal.** Odors can register powerfully because they go directly to the limbic system, referred to as the "smell brain," or the seat of emotions in the brain. Olfaction is the only sensory modality that does not have a synaptic connection in the thalamus before reaching higher centers. **Olfactory defensiveness** is the negative response to certain odors.

Children respond to **visual** stimuli by orienting to novel situations, checking them out, and then acting as required. The child who underregisters visual stimuli may not react appropriately in a situation that requires arousal and response. The child who is overreactive to visual stimuli might not be able to habituate; hence, he reacts to the visual stimulus as if it were constantly novel. An example of this is the fascination an autistic child may have with a revolving record.

If the child's **attention level** to all environmental input is either too high or too low, education will be difficult because his focus probably is not on academics. Attention level is modulated by the reticular system, and this system is influenced by all the other sensory systems. Moderate attention is required to interact effectively with the environment. Overreactivity to environmental input leaves the child deficient in his ability to screen out enough to attend to the "important" things, and underreactivity leaves the child with inadequate arousal for input to which he should respond. A child who has an overreactive attention level may be labeled as having an attention deficit disorder with or without hyperactivity. It is important to note that the label, **attention deficit disorder**, refers to the ability to attend cognitively, whereas the term **hyperactivity** often refers to motor restless behavior. These two terms sometimes are used interchangeably, but they really are distinctly different and should be defined separately.

**Postrotary nystagmus** is an ocular response attributed to the semicircular canals of the vestibular mechanism. It consists of rhythmic back and forth eye movement (nystagmus) following body rotation. This response is related to arousal/reactivity of the vestibular system (Ayres, 1976; Kimball, 1981; Kimball, 1986; Kimball, 1988). Underreactivity is thought to be related to excess inhibition in the lower brain centers. Conversely, overreactivity is thought to be caused by inadequate inhibition from the cerebral cortex. Underreactivity and overreactivity are both considered to be problematic.

**Sensitivity to movement** is thought to be mediated by the vestibular system. In sensitive persons, movement often triggers an autonomic reaction of nausea or vomiting. Sensitivity to movement may be caused by an intravestibular conflict, in which the semicircular canals and the otoliths send conflicting messages. Another possibility is a vestibular-ocular conflict, in which the vestibular mechanism and the eyes send conflicting messages. This may be the mechanism involved in carsickness and seasickness. For example, in carsickness, sitting in the front seat appears to lessen the sensitivity to movement because the person does not have to refocus the eyes constantly in relation to the moving environment. This is thought to reduce vestibular-ocular conflict.

**Proprioceptive sensitivity** refers to the child's response to joint or muscle movement, especially that initiated by someone else. When movements are not self-initiated, no feed-forward mechanisms are involved; only the less efficient feedback systems are used (see Praxis Section). Therefore no neurophysiological warning is given that the body is going to move. Movement by someone else could cause a negative response.

**Emotional** tone often is thought of as a purely psychological response; however, the sensory system antecedents of these behavioral responses need to be addressed. Children may have more or less than normal emotional variability because of their sensory systems, which are not interpreting input in a normal fashion. All the systems we have discussed contribute to emotional tone. Overreactivity may lead to hyperactivity, anxiety, or chronic stress. Underreactivity may mimic depression (Table 6.2).

## Functional Support Capabilities

These physical capabilities underlie and provide support for the end-product abilities. Functional support capabilities help integrate and modulate the input from the arousal/reactivity components of the sensory systems. They also integrate the information/discriminative components of these systems. The ten functional support capabilities are listed in Table 6.1.

**Suck-swallow-breathe** synchrony is a vital but often overlooked part of motor development. Appropriate muscle tone and stability need to develop in the tongue and jaw to allow nursing to occur with proper force, as well as synchronization of swallowing and breathing. This process proceeds to development of intercostal and diaphragm stability for good breath support for articulation. Neck and eye stability also are involved. All these things provide support for biting, chewing, phonation, vocal abilities, and postural control.

***Table 6.2*** Sensory System Arousal Continues

| Sensory System Arousal Levels | Functional Support Capabilities | | |
|---|---|---|---|
| | Low | Normal | High |
| High | Hyperactive Sensory defensive Poor end-product ability levels | Hyperactive Sensory defensive Behavior problems No motor problems | Hyperactive Sensory defensive Cortical signs |
| Normal | Normal sensory modulation Normal attention Few behavior problems Motor problems | Normal sensory modulation Normal attention Good end-product ability levels Good motor skills | Normal sensory modulation Cortically based attention problems |
| Low | Underaroused to pain, etc. Poor end-product ability levels Poor motor skills May be hyperactive | Normal motor skills Slow adaptation | Slow adaptation Cortical problems |

A child who does not develop these abilities may show a pattern of shallow, rapid breathing because of poor development of (low tone in) breathing musculature. This breathing pattern results in a sympathetic response. Other problems include drooling, poor eating (bite, chew, and swallow), poor stability in the neck and trunk, poor articulation, and misuse of the large proximal muscles that fixate (to help with breathing) rather than move freely to develop skilled motion. Remember that the head is controlled by the cranial nerves—different sensory pathways than the rest of the body—so, each of these problems must be evaluated and treated separately (Oetter, Richter, & Frick, 1992).

**Tactile discrimination** is the ability to perceive through touch and to define the spatial and temporal qualities of the environment by touch. As previously discussed, tactile discrimination is thought to be mediated largely by the DCML system (body) and trigeminal system (head). It helps to provide a basis for the normal development of praxis.

**Other Discriminative Abilities.**   All the sensory systems have an information processing component that provides discriminative information to the CNS. Constant discriminative input from all sensory systems orients the person to the environment and defines the way to modify or change behavior.

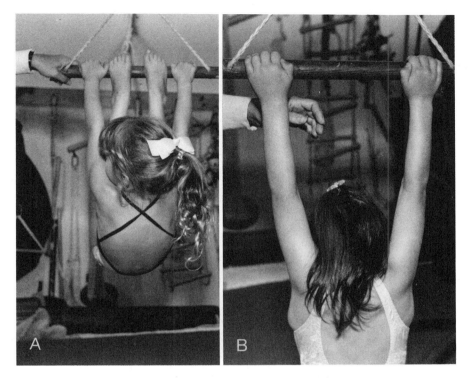

**Figure 6.6**  **A**. Mature response; note cocontraction throughout upper extremity and stable scapula; **B**, immature response; note holding on only with fingers and winging of scapular, indicating poor stability.

**Cocontraction**, the simultaneous contraction of agonist and antagonistic muscles, stabilizes joints for action and use. Cocontraction contributes to balance and also is believed to help form the basis for the development of movement patterns for praxis (Figs. 6.6A and 6.6B).

**Muscle tone** is the background level of muscle tension that is normal in everyone. Normal muscle tone also provides a basis for equilibrium, movement, and praxis.

**Proprioception** is the understanding of the body's position in space (consciously and unconsciously), based on feedback from joint, muscle, and skin receptors. Proprioception contributes to balance and equilibrium, muscle tone, and cocontraction.

**Balance and equilibrium**, as modulated by the vestibular system, is responsible for the ability to maintain posture and to move through the envi-

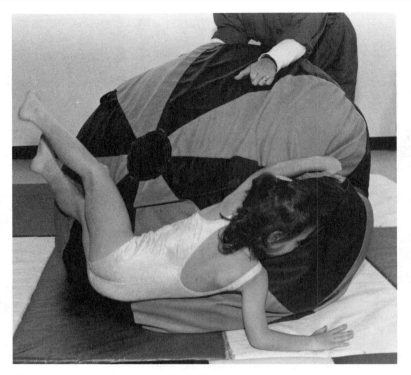

**Figure 6.7**   Less than optimal equilibrium response in prone position.

ronment. Balance and equilibrium contribute significantly to all the end-product abilities (Figs. 6.7, 6.8A, and 6.8B).

**Developmental reflexes** are species-dependent movement patterns evoked by sensory input. Some human examples are protective extension of the arms when falling and the asymmetrical tonic neck reflex. (Figs. 6.9A and 6.9B). Developmental reflexes can contribute to integration of movement by being present or absent, appropriately. They depend on age and developmental stage of the child and are influenced by arousal/registration level.

**Lateralization** involves the development of dominance in a hand, foot, and eye. The emergence of a dominant hand by the age of 5 or 6 years can signal that the brain has lateralized other functional abilities, for example, language to the left hemisphere, perceptual abilities to the right hemisphere. The lack of a dominant hand may signal lack of lateralization.

**Bilateral integration** is the ability to use both hands together in activities. One indicator of bilateral integration is the ability to cross midline efficiently.

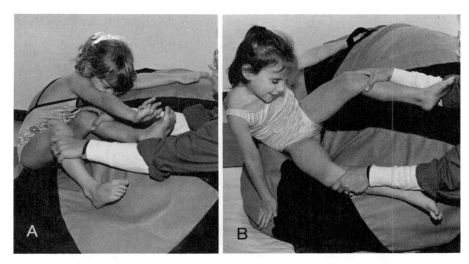

**Figure 6.8   A,** Mature response; balance reaction occurs in all parts of the body (even toes and trunk rotation) in response to balance challenge; **B,** Immature response; only head responds to balance challenge (note low tone in legs, winging of scapula, and holding on with upper hand).

All functional support levels are rated on a scale, from poor to good to excellent, with the exception of muscle tone and developmental reflexes. Muscle tone is rated low, normal, or high, with both low and high being abnormal. Developmental reflexes are rated hyporeflexive, normal, or hyper-reflexive, with both extremes being abnormal.

## End-Product Abilities

End-product abilities reflect integration of the sensory system modulation levels and functional support capabilities. The eight end-product abilities are listed on Table 6.1.

**Praxis** is often defined as motor planning, but it is much more. It is the ability to accomplish a nonhabitual motor act or the ability to coordinate the body through a complex movement that requires an adaptive response. According to Ayres (1985), "[P]raxis is a uniquely human skill that enables us to interact effectively with the physical world. It is one of the most critical links between brain and behavior. Praxis is to the physical world what speech is to the social world. Both enable interactions and transactions" (p. 1).

Praxis is complex and has been equated to motor intelligence. All aspects are detailed on the praxis figure (Fig. 6.10) and include ideation or conceptual-

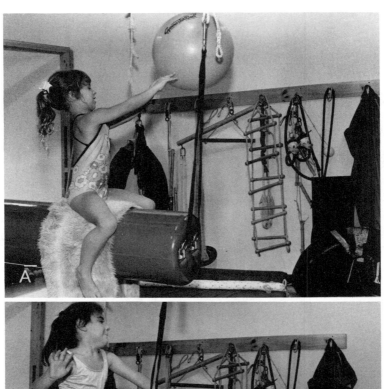

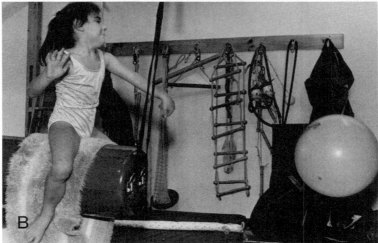

**Figure 6.9   A,** Mature response; child swinging on bolster swing can rotate trunk and use hands bilaterally and symmetrically to push large ball away; **B,** Immature response; child swinging on a bolster swing uses straight plane movement (less mature than rotation), and asymmetrical tonic neck is apparent in arms on attempting to push ball away.

ization; planning the course of action, including sequencing the actions; and, execution of adaptive responses.

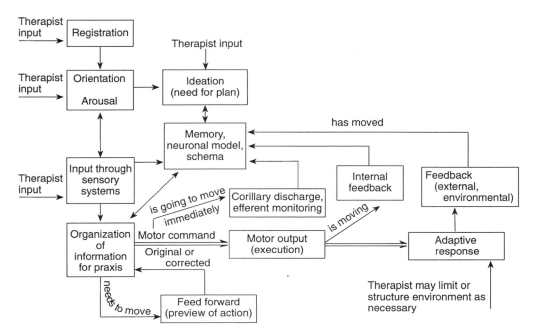

**Figure 6.10**   Neural Processes that Underlie Praxis: Sensory Integration Frame of Reference. Kimball, 1988.

This frame of reference assumes that praxis provides one basis for the development of academic abilities, behavior, articulation, emotional tone, and environmental mastery. Praxis probably is the most important organizational aspect of function that a person is able to accomplish. Children who have praxis problems are said to show "developmental dyspraxia" to distinguish that the problem is one of impairment of ability during development and not a loss of praxic ability like a stroke patient might experience (apraxia).

Dyspraxic children are "clumsy," and the problem is based on a complex interaction of less than optimal sensory processing, less than optimal functional support capabilities, and less than optimal ideation. Praxis is not a question of whether the child can accomplish the movement, but whether he can accomplish it with integration and quality.

**Form and space perception skills** are end-product skills that are thought to provide some basis for academic skills. Visual form and space perception can be broken down into various types, most of which are based on sensory motor processing deficits. Some children, however, show discrete visual spatial perception problems that are thought to be mediated by the right hemisphere.

**Behavior** as an end-product cannot be analyzed completely without the inclusion of the antecedent effects of sensory system modulation and functional support capabilities. Contrary to this perspective, psychologists view behavior mainly as an end-product of cognitive, social, and environmental interactions. In sensory integration, the sensory system antecedents must be evaluated for their own contributions before the psychosocial aspects are addressed.

**Academics**—scholastic abilities—usually are viewed in relation to difficulties in other end-product abilities, such as language, form and space perception, behavior, activity level, and emotional tone. Recently, academics have begun to be studied in terms of the antecedent effects of sensory system modulation, functional support system capabilities, and praxis.

**Language and articulation** abilities usually are evaluated by speech therapists. Occupational therapists also can contribute understanding of the underlying antecedents for difficulties in language and articulation, which sometimes can be traced to problems in sensory system modulation, functional support capabilities, and end-product abilities. The end-product component that is considered most important in this area is **praxis**. If the problem is one of articulation, the difficulty often lies in a praxis problem that can affect the speech musculature. This type of praxis problem includes difficulty in producing an appropriate adaptive response for sequencing. In addition, Ayres (1972a) has suggested that a pattern of language problems, particularly auditory language dysfunction, is related to left-hemisphere disorders.

**Emotional tone**, including stress level and self-esteem, is thought to be linked closely to sensory system modulation. If a number of components of sensory system modulation show overreactivity, then the person may be considered to be **sensory defensive** (Wilbarger & Royeen, 1987; Wilbarger & Wilbarger, 1991). Sensory defensiveness may result in behavioral and emotional problems, including anxiety. Often seen is the need to remain extremely organized, bordering on compulsion, to keep the environment under control, and to add no more arousal to the already overaroused sensory systems.

**Activity level**, including self-control, relates to the person's ability to stay cognitively and motorically focused. Although activity level often is thought to be related only to cognitive attention behaviors by other frames of reference, in this frame of reference it is assumed to be related to modulation in all sensory systems. A high activity level can be very functional and productive if it includes focus. A dysfunctional activity level includes motor restlessness and lack of focus, which may be mistaken for impaired attention span or cognitive deficits.

**Environmental mastery** involves the ability to produce a suitable adaptive response with appropriate praxis, emotional tone, activity level, behavior, and academic level. Environmental mastery involves a total repertoire of adaptive responses that reflect the integration of all sensory systems, the functional support capabilities, and, to some extent, all components of the end-product abilities. The child who has environmental mastery also has sensory integration at all levels.

Most components of the end-product abilities are rated from poor to good to excellent. The exceptions are behavior and activity level. Behavior usually is rated as poor to good. Activity level is rated as underactive to normal to overactive. Both over-and underactive activity levels are considered to be problematic.

## Praxis

In this frame of reference, dyspraxia is the major area of concern and is considered the most encompassing of all the problem areas. Specific knowledge of praxis, therefore, is important for understanding the client who has sensory integrative problems. Children who have dyspraxia have difficulty with the initial planning of a nonhabitual movement. They then have trouble internalizing the plan for the movement and, finally, have difficulty transferring the motor learning to a new situation and extracting the common components from previous learning so that they need only learn the differences or additions. A common example for adult readers would be learning to drive. Initially, attention must be given to all movements, then the process becomes internalized, and, finally, it transfers to the ability to drive any car (with modifications made only for differences among cars). Compare this to the dyspraxic child who learns to roller skate. The child works much harder than a normal child to learn the skill. Long after the other children have learned, the dyspraxic child is still not as fluent in his movements and has difficulty with unexpected situations that require a "new wrinkle" in the movement pattern—for example, a quick change in direction to avoid a child who has fallen in front of him while skating. And the transferability of this skill to a new, similar situation, like ice skating, is more limited than with the normal child.

The praxis process (see Fig. 6.10) starts with the child's registration of, or his attention to, some change in the environment. Once the child has registered a change in the environment, orientation and arousal must take place.

Orientation occurs after registration—a change in the environment—alerts the system to gather more information. This orientation is accompanied by a change in the arousal state and increased perceptual sensitivity. The child's system automatically makes a judgment about the significance of the stimuli being registered. This includes reallocation of attention and preparation for action.

Once the registration, orientation, and arousal have occurred, the situation is compared with established neuronal models by the CNS, allowing the child to move to ideation or to the realization of a need for a plan. At this point, the child begins organizing the information for movement—praxis—and may take in more input through the sensory systems to facilitate a better plan for action.

The first neuromechanism of the praxis sequence, that of **feed forward** or a preview for action, comes at the point of organizing for praxis. Feed forward is a neuromechanism that alerts the CNS to the need to move and compares the planned action with past models to ascertain the possibility of success. At this point, the CNS organizes a motor command and sends it forward. As the motor command is sent, afferent monitoring and corollary discharge occur. These signals alert the system that the child is going to move immediately. It is a preview monitoring of the command to move or an alerting of higher cortical centers that a command has been sent. Again there is a comparison with past experience, and a decision is made whether to continue with the motor command as sent or to correct it before the execution has begun. Once the motor execution has begun, **internal feedback** occurs. The CNS realizes that the body is moving, and, again, a comparison is made with past experience. Neural models of organization for praxis are rechecked, and, if necessary, the motor command can be corrected midstream. After the motor command is completed by accomplishing an adaptive response, feedback of an external or environmental nature occurs. The CNS realizes it has moved in a particular way and understands that it has or has not achieved the desired or adequate response. The whole process is then stored in the neural model or memory for future use. The above process is mostly nonconscious and may take only milliseconds.

The building up of neuronal models through this sequence is an active process. If the child does not organize himself for movement and does not originate and carry out the motor command and movement himself, then the only mechanisms that will be called into action are external and environmental feedback. Feedback is a very inefficient system and could be equated to learning how to ski with the learning occurring only from falling down.

Neuronal models are formed slowly and inefficiently with feedback only. This frame of reference assumes that if a child does not build neural models efficiently, then practicing a motor skill sometimes improves that motor skill but not the child's overall ability to coordinate or to extrapolate to other situations. In this frame of reference, the therapist's goal is to facilitate an active response from the child to build neuronal models. To achieve this, the therapist may add input at the following levels: registration, orientation, arousal, sensory systems, or ideation to facilitate a more appropriate adaptive response. The therapist also structures the environment to limit the complexity of the adaptive response to one within the child's developmental level.

The therapist must keep in mind at what level the problem occurs in the dyspraxic child. For example, if the problem is one of registration or arousal, the child may (1) not pay attention to the need to act on the environment, or (2) continually pay attention to the same stimulation so that no level of importance is assigned to it. This often is seen in autistic children who continually register an environmental stimulus (such as a moving object) without assigning significance.

Dyspraxia also may involve a problem in the ideation or understanding of the need for a plan. This may be seen in a child who attempts to accomplish an environmental action and accomplishes only a small piece of it. For example, a child swinging on a bolster swing has a ball thrown at him and allows the ball to hit him. The arousal may have occurred but the child did not understand that something needed to be done with the ball. Often, input through sensory systems, such as the vestibular, proprioceptive, and tactile systems, heightens the child's CNS ability to respond by summation over sensory systems. This assumption leads to one of the key treatment principles in sensory integration: Input from several sensory systems may be needed to achieve a registration or integration level sufficient for an adaptive response. For example, a child who has low muscle tone may not be able to balance himself on a moving surface, but after linear swinging on a bolster swing, jumping on a trampoline, and receiving heavy proprioceptive activity to proximal limb joints and neck, the child may be able not only to balance but also to catch a ball while balancing.

# Postulates of the Sensory Integration Theoretical Base

The evolving theoretical base of sensory integration presently includes 11 basic postulates. These postulates outline the elements that the occupational therapist must understand to apply this frame of reference. The postulates include the following:

1. Integration of sensory input is holistic—that is, all systems influence each other and the whole.
2. The child's behaviors are influenced by the state of the CNS. There is a relationship between certain behaviors and underlying CNS dysfunctions or inefficiencies. Some behaviors can be related to a specific sensory system but may be exhibited in many environments. Unless the basic problems are addressed or treated, the resultant behaviors will continue.
3. The functioning of the underlying sensory systems determines the quality of adaptive responses.
4. For integration to occur, meaningful registration of sensory input is required. Integration is reflected in an adaptive response.
5. When the child makes an appropriate adaptive response, this contributes further to the development of general sensory integrative abilities.
6. The child needs to be self-directed to act on the environment for the greatest potential change to occur in the underlying neurological organization and to result in an adaptive response.
7. Adaptive responses that are within the child's abilities should be used; therefore the child's developmental level must be assessed. These adaptive responses should be at the upper limits of the child's abilities to facilitate growth.
8. Sensory integration difficulties may arise from problems in two distinct areas: sensory system modulation levels and functional support capabilities. Either one or a combination of the two results in end-product ability problems.
9. Intervention is specific to the underlying deficits; it is not specific to behaviors. As adaptive responses become more organized, the child's behavior becomes more organized.
10. The child's behaviors can be modified through appropriate controlled sensory inputs that elicit or facilitate adaptive responses. Responses should be motor, emotional, and ideational ones.
11. Input from several sensory systems may be needed to achieve the registration level (arousal or inhibition) or integration level appropriate for an adaptive response.

## Function/Dysfunction Continua

Function/dysfunction continua in sensory integration help the therapist to determine the severity of the problem and to indicate the multiple systems that need to be addressed. Three continua are (1) sensory systems; (2) functional support capabilities; and, (3) end-product abilities (see Table 6.1).

## *Sensory System Modulation*

The way in which the sensory systems process input affects the quality of a child's ability to respond adaptively. Moderate reactivity results in an optimal adaptive response. Overreactivity/high arousal result in disorganization and even in anxiety or a negative emotional response. Underreactivity/low arousal result in partial or ineffective responses. When arousal gets too high, the child responds as if to a serious survival threat. If it is not possible to fight or flee, then the arousal does not dissipate easily, causing stress, anxiety, and difficulty in completing other adaptive responses. Persons who have sensory system modulation problems have more changeable reactivity/arousal levels than normal persons. The result can be problems with adaptive response because their systems lack stability. The sensory systems do not function independently. Arousal in each of several systems can combine, therefore, to produce high arousal, just as inhibition in several systems can combine to produce low arousal. The arousal or reactivity levels of each system need to be assessed, as do the information processing components of each system.

| Sensory System<br>Normal Response | Underregistration<br>Overregistration |
|---|---|
| *Tactile System:* | |
| FUNCTION: Normal tactile reactivity and integration | DYSFUNCTION: Difficulty differentiating tactile input |
| BEHAVIORS INDICATIVE OF FUNCTION: | BEHAVIORS INDICATIVE OF DYSFUNCTION: |
| Likes light touch<br>Differentiates types of touch<br>Discriminates and integrates touch from people, objects, animals, clothing | Underreactivity<br>  May not feel pain<br>  May not be aware of injury<br>  May not differentiate among<br>  types of touch |
| | Overreactivity<br>  Reacts negatively to light touch<br>  Perceives light touch as painful<br>  or irritating<br>  May not tolerate touch from<br>  certain types of clothing, objects,<br>  animals, or people |

*—continued*

*Auditory System*:

FUNCTION: Normal attention to sound

BEHAVIORS INDICATIVE OF FUNCTION:

Orients to noises, then reacts appropriately

DYSFUNCTION: Responds inappropriately to sound input

BEHAVIORS INDICATIVE OF DYSFUNCTION:

Underreactivity
May not orient to noises, no startle to loud sounds

Overreactivity
Overly distracted by noises
Startles easily to sounds
Upset at or appears annoyed by normal level sounds

*Relationship to Gravity*:

FUNCTION: Normal response to gravity

BEHAVIORS INDICATIVE OF FUNCTION:

Normal, respectful caution in dangerous-movement-related situations

DYSFUNCTION: Responds inappropriately to gravity

BEHAVIORS INDICATIVE OF DYSFUNCTION:

Underreactivity
No respect for heights, falling, or moving fast or moving in dangerous ways, even if caution is warranted

Overreactivity
Real fear, anxiety, or intense emotional reaction in response to movement situations that should only require alerting or changes in body/head position

*Movement Level*:

FUNCTION: Normal amount of movement

BEHAVIORS INDICATIVE OF FUNCTION:

Normal amount of movement

DYSFUNCTION: Atypical amount of movement

BEHAVIORS INDICATIVE OF DYSFUNCTION:

Underreactivity
Slow moving or appears to conserve movement
Overreactivity
Appears to be moving constantly

*Oral Arousal*:

FUNCTION: Normal oral response to food or objects

DYSFUNCTION: Inappropriate oral response to food or objects

BEHAVIORS INDICATIVE OF
FUNCTION:

Dislikes a few items because of
texture but normally will allow
food products to enter the mouth;
reacts because of taste

Discriminating with objects
not appropriate for mouthing

BEHAVIORS INDICATIVE OF
DYSFUNCTION:

Underreactivity

Will put anything into mouth
Does not seem to be bothered by
inappropriate items after the age
at which he should be aware of
inappropriateness

Overreactivity

Overly sensitive to texture of
items placed in mouth
Refuses many foods because of
texture, not taste
Dislikes objects in mouth (i.e.,
tooth brush, dentist's fingers or
drill)
Uses heavy chewing to calm self
Chews on inappropriate things
such as blankets

*Olfactory Arousal*:
FUNCTION: Normal level

BEHAVIORS INDICATIVE OF
FUNCTION:

Normal response to odors

DYSFUNCTION: Inappropriate
response to odors
BEHAVIORS INDICATIVE OF
DYSFUNCTION:

Underreactivity

Appears not to notice odors

Overreactivity

Very responsive to odors
Odors may make child upset or
nauseous
Odor may cause negative
"flashbacks"

*Visual System*:
FUNCTION: Normal orienting to
changes in the visual field

BEHAVIORS INDICATIVE OF
FUNCTION:

Normally orients to changes in the
visual field

DYSFUNCTION: Responds
inappropriately to changes in the
visual field
BEHAVIORS INDICATIVE OF
DYSFUNCTION:

Underreactivity

Underresponsive to changes in
the visual field
Underresponsive to objects that
enter the visual field
Underresponsive to changes in
movement, color and the like
even though visual acuity is
normal

—*continued*

Overreactivity
Orients persistently to objects
that are common (not unusual)
in the visual field
Difficulty habituating visually

*Attention Level:*

FUNCTION: Normal level of
attention

BEHAVIORS INDICATIVE OF
FUNCTION:

Normal level of attention

DYSFUNCTION: Inappropriate
attention levels

BEHAVIORS INDICATIVE OF
DYSFUNCTION:

Underreactivity
Appears to pay little or no
attention to environmental
changes that require an active
intervention or response

Overreactivity
Appears to be reacting constantly
to stimuli
Some reaction to stimuli may be
movement-related but also
includes all other sensory
systems

*Postrotary Nystagmus:*

FUNCTION: Normally dizzy after
rotary movement

BEHAVIORS INDICATIVE OF
FUNCTION:

Becomes dizzy normally after
rotary movement

DYSFUNCTION: Atypical response to
rotary movement

BEHAVIORS INDICATIVE OF
DYSFUNCTION:

Underreactivity
Does not show dizziness or
shows decreased dizziness after
rotary movement (referred to as
*depressed postrotary nystagmus*)

Overreactivity
Becomes overly dizzy after
rotary movement (referred to as
*prolonged postrotary nystagmus*)

*Sensitivity to Movement:*

FUNCTION: Normal response to
rotary or angular movement

BEHAVIORS INDICATIVE OF
FUNCTION:

Tolerates some rotary or angular
acceleration and then needs to stop
because of autonomic response

DYSFUNCTION: Atypical response to
rotary or angular movement

BEHAVIORS INDICATIVE OF
DYSFUNCTION:

Underreactivity
Tolerates excessive amounts of
rotary or angular acceleration
without an ANS response

Overreactivity
Tolerates very little or no rotary
or angular acceleration without
having an ANS response, usually
of nausea or "feeling funny"

*Proprioceptive Sensitivity*:

FUNCTION: Normal response to joint
or muscle movement

DYSFUNCTION: Negative response
to joint or muscle movement

BEHAVIORS INDICATIVE OF
FUNCTION:

BEHAVIORS INDICATIVE OF
DYSFUNCTION:

Normal registration and responses
to proprioceptive input provided
externally

Underreactivity
Does not appear to "feel" some
limb and muscle positions or
movements

Overreactivity
Overly sensitive to joint and
muscle movement provided
externally
Very aware of movements of
limbs

*Emotional Arousal*

FUNCTION: Normal expression of
emotions

DYSFUNCTION: Inappropriate
emotional response

BEHAVIORS INDICATIVE OF
FUNCTION:

BEHAVIORS INDICATIVE OF
DYSFUNCTION:

Normal expression of emotions

Underreactivity
Shows decreased levels of
emotions or the expression of
them

Overreactivity
Becomes upset by items that
might be considered trivial by
most other people

## Functional Support Capabilities

These physical capabilities underlie and provide support for the end-
product abilities. Functional support capabilities help integrate the input from
the sensory systems. Furthermore, they can be used to help modulate and
provide balance to the sensory systems.

| Specific Functional Capabilities | Poorly Developed Capabilities |
| --- | --- |
| *Suck-Swallow-Breathe:* | |
| FUNCTION: Normal response | DYSFUNCTION: Abnormal response |
| BEHAVIORS INDICATIVE OF FUNCTION: | BEHAVIORS INDICATIVE OF DYSFUNCTION: |
| Can synchronize suck-swallow-breathe patterns | Experiences difficulty with suck-swallow-breathe synchrony |
| Has good muscle tone stability and coordination in all suck, swallow breathe mechanisms | Muscle tone and stability are not developed enough to allow good coordination of suck-swallow-breathe mechanisms |
| *Tactile Discrimination:* | |
| FUNCTION: Good tactile discrimination | DYSFUNCTION: Poor tactile discrimination |
| BEHAVIORS INDICATIVE OF FUNCTION: | BEHAVIORS INDICATIVE OF DYSFUNCTION: |
| Ability to identify various shapes, textures, sizes by touch alone | Not able to differentiate objects haptically or cannot identify accurately by touch alone |
| Good two-point discrimination | Poor two-point discrimination |
| Good conscious proprioception (kinesthesia) | Poor conscious proprioception (kinesthesia) |
| Uses touch for information gathering | Poor differentiation of touch for information gathering |
| *Other Discriminative Abilities:* | |
| BEHAVIORS INDICATIVE OF FUNCTION: | BEHAVIORS INDICATIVE OF DYSFUNCTION: |
| Auditory Discrimination | |
| Ability to use auditory system for information gathering | Poor ability to use auditory system for information gathering in spite of normal hearing |
| Relationship to Gravity | |
| Normal balance response to change in head/body position in relation to gravity | Inefficient registration of change in head/body signaling; equilibrium/balance response needed |
| Postrotary Nystagmus | |
| Discriminates amount of dizziness | Difficulty in discriminating amount of dizziness |

Movement Level

| Movement goal-directed, focussed | Much non-goal-directed movement, unfocused |

Oral Discrimination

| Can discriminate taste and texture | Poor oral discrimination of taste and texture |

Olfactory Discrimination

| Can discriminate odors | Poor differentiation of odors |

Visual Discrimination

| Good visual discrimination | Poor acuity: uses glasses |
| Good visual acuity | Poor discrimination |

Proprioceptive Discrimination

| Uses proprioceptive abilities to discriminate force, velocity, and direction of movement | Is unable to judge force, velocity, or direction of movements accurately |

Attention Level

| Can attend well to take in more/ new information | Unable to attend well to take in new information |

Emotional Discrimination

| Discriminates meaning and expression of emotion in self and others | Difficulty in using emotional expression as a guide for action |

*Cocontraction:*

| FUNCTION: Good cocontraction | DYSFUNCTION: Poor cocontraction |
| BEHAVIORS INDICATIVE OF FUNCTION: | BEHAVIORS INDICATIVE OF DYSFUNCTION: |
| Ability to cocontract muscles around the joint so that the joint may be stabilized for action | Inability to cocontract muscles around the joints so that there is less than normal stabilization |

*Muscle Tone:*

| FUNCTION: Normal muscle tone | DYSFUNCTION: Atypical muscle tone |
| BEHAVIORS INDICATIVE OF FUNCTION: | BEHAVIORS INDICATIVE OF DYSFUNCTION: |
| Normal tone for stability of normal movement patterns | Low muscle tone; floppy tone Tone does not provide enough stability for some normal movement patterns |

*—continued*

High muscle tone
Too much tone for normal
movement patterns
Spasticity

*Balance and Equilibrium:*

FUNCTION: Good balance and
equilibrium

DYSFUNCTION: Poor balance and
equilibrium

BEHAVIORS INDICATIVE OF
FUNCTION:

BEHAVIORS INDICATIVE OF
DYSFUNCTION:

Good balance abilities

Usually exhibited in good overall
coordination

Difficulties in catching balance

*Developmental Reflexes:*

FUNCTION: Contribute to integration
of movement

DYSFUNCTION: Reflexes interfere
with movement

BEHAVIORS INDICATIVE OF
FUNCTION:

BEHAVIORS INDICATIVE OF
DYSFUNCTION:

Reflexes are "integrated" into
movement, are not obligatory

Difficulty moving against gravity
volitionally

May be obligatory movements in
postures, e.g., asymmetrical tonic
neck reflex with head turning

Certain positions or movements
may cause child to assume a
particular posture; example, back
arching in supine position

*Lateralization:*

FUNCTION: Lateralization of
function

DYSFUNCTION: Lack of or poor
lateralization

BEHAVIORS INDICATIVE OF
FUNCTION:

BEHAVIORS INDICATIVE OF
DYSFUNCTION:

Eye, hand, and foot dominance all
the same

No or mixed dominance

*Bilateral Integration:*

FUNCTION: Ability to use both
hands in bilateral activities

DYSFUNCTION: Difficulty in using
both hands in bilateral activities

BEHAVIORS INDICATIVE OF
FUNCTION:

BEHAVIORS INDICATIVE OF
DYSFUNCTION:

Smooth crossing of midline with
eyes and hands

Hands do not cross midline well

Eye blink, gaze shift, or eye jerk
when eyes cross midline

## End-Product Abilities

End-product abilities reflect integration of sensory system modulation and functional support levels. All these end-product ability levels can be scored on a poor to excellent continuum of function/dysfunction.

| End-Product Abilities | Poorly Developed End-Product Abilities |
|---|---|
| *Praxis:* | |
| FUNCTION: Ability to plan and coordinate complex nonhabitual movements that require an adaptive response | DYSFUNCTION: Difficulty motor planning and coordinating complex nonhabitual movements that require an adaptive response |
| BEHAVIORS INDICATIVE OF FUNCTION: | BEHAVIORS INDICATIVE OF DYSFUNCTION: |
| Ability to organize for nonhabitual movement to accomplish an appropriate adaptive response | Difficulty in organizing for movement or accomplishing an appropriate adaptive response |
| | Difficulty at any of the levels of integration may be seen in organization, sequencing, internalizing, or accomplishing the appropriate adaptive response |
| *Form and Space Perception:* | |
| FUNCTION: Good form and space perception | DYSFUNCTION: Poor form and space perception |
| BEHAVIORS INDICATIVE OF FUNCTION: | BEHAVIORS INDICATIVE OF DYSFUNCTION: |
| Able to use form and space perception effectively to produce adaptive responses | Difficulty in understanding and interpreting spatial relationships and figure-ground |
| | Contribution to difficulty with reading or math |
| *Behavior:* | |
| FUNCTION: Appropriate behavior | DYSFUNCTION: Inappropriate behavior |
| BEHAVIORS INDICATIVE OF FUNCTION: | BEHAVIORS INDICATIVE OF DYSFUNCTION: |
| Behaves appropriately in relationship to age, situation, and environment | Inappropriate behavior in relationship to age, situation, or environment |

—*continued*

*Academics:*

FUNCTION: Good academic performance

DYSFUNCTION: Poor academic performance

BEHAVIORS INDICATIVE OF FUNCTION:

BEHAVIORS INDICATIVE OF DYSFUNCTION:

Functioning at or above ability level

Functioning below ability level

*Language and Articulation:*

FUNCTION: Good language and articulation

DYSFUNCTION: Difficulty with language or articulation

BEHAVIORS INDICATIVE OF FUNCTION:

BEHAVIORS INDICATIVE OF DYSFUNCTION:

Language use is at age level

Language use is below age level

Articulation is at age-appropriate level

Articulation is worse than peers with no apparent structural cause

*Emotional Tone:*

FUNCTION: Balanced emotional tone, including good self-esteem

DYSFUNCTION: Inadequate emotional tone

BEHAVIORS INDICATIVE OF FUNCTION:

BEHAVIORS INDICATIVE OF DYSFUNCTION:

Emotional tone is balanced

Difficulty with emotional tone

Self-esteem is good and appropriate for age

Inadequate self-esteem
May be sensory defensive
May be compulsively organized

*Activity Level:*

FUNCTION: Normal activity level

DYSFUNCTION: Under or over activity level

BEHAVIORS INDICATIVE OF FUNCTION:

BEHAVIORS INDICATIVE OF DYSFUNCTION:

Normal activity for age level

Low activity level that may look like depression

Demonstrates appropriate self-control for age level

High activity level without focus, poor self-control

*Environmental Mastery:*

FUNCTION: Ability to function within the environment

DYSFUNCTION: Difficulty responding to environmental demands

| BEHAVIORS INDICATIVE OF FUNCTION: | BEHAVIORS INDICATIVE OF DYSFUNCTION: |
|---|---|
| Produces a suitable adaptive response with appropriate praxis emotional tone, activity level, behaviors, and academic performance | Demonstrates inappropriate adaptive responses; or poor response with inappropriate praxis, emotional tone, activity level, behavior, or academic performance |
| Understands and functions within the environment at an age-appropriate level | Difficulty in understanding and functioning within the environment at an age-appropriate level |

# Evaluation

Children referred to occupational therapy for suspected sensory integrative problems may present particular behaviors that often are interpreted as aberrant or as cortically based dysfunction. Such children are sometimes referred to physicians or psychologists before they are referred to an occupational therapist. (These behaviors are presented in Appendix 6A). It should be kept in mind that several symptoms together are indicative of sensory integrative dysfunction; one isolated symptom is not.

The evaluation of children for sensory integrative dysfunction is an intricate process. It requires that therapists be knowledgeable not only in this specific area but that they be well grounded in their understanding of development as well. Often children who are referred to an occupational therapist for evaluation already have been seen by several other professionals. The possible causes of the child's behaviors or motor deficits should be evaluated at all levels.

The following evaluation procedures are suggested for each of the function/dysfunction continua:

---

*Sensory System Modulation Levels*
*General (all systems):*

- Touch inventory for elementary school aged children (TIE) (Royeen, 1987; Royeen, 1990)
- Sensory motor history (Ayres Clinic, 1971)
- Sensory history (Wilbarger & Oetter, 1989; (Wilbarger & Wilbarger, 1991)
- Clinical observations
- Tactile defensiveness check list (Royeen, 1986)
- Overall sensory motor history
- Evaluation of sensory defensiveness (Wilbarger & Wilbarger, 1991)

*—continued*

*Specific:*

Relationship to Gravity

- Clinical observations, including equilibrium reactions in supine, sitting, and prone positions and reaction to moving equipment

Attention Level

- Observation
- Teacher report
- Parent report
- Physician report

Postrotary Nystagmus

- Southern California Postrotary Nystagmus Test (SCPNT) (Ayres, 1976; Kimball, 1981)

Sensitivity to Movement

- Clinical observations on the SCPNT
- Observations during other clinical observations
- Parent report

Emotional Arousal Level

- Psychological assessment

*Functional Support Capabilities:*

Suck-Swallow-Breathe

- Evaluation of oral mechanisms (Oetter & Richter, 1992)

Tactile Discrimination

- Sensory Integration and Praxis Test (SIPT) (Ayres, 1989)
- Teacher and parent reports

Cocontraction

- Clinical observations (Dunn, 1981; Fisher & Bundy, 1989)

Muscle Tone

- Clinical observations (Dunn, 1981)

Proprioception

- Clinical observations (Dunn, 1981)

Balance and Equilibrium

- Clinical observations (Dunn, 1981; Fisher & Bundy, 1989)
- Standing balance eyes open and closed, Sensory Integration and Praxis Tests (SIPT) (Ayres, 1989)
- Bruininks Oseretsky Test of Motor Proficiency (Bruininks, 1978)

Developmental Reflexes

- Clinical observations
- Parent report

Lateralization

- Clinical observations
- Parent report

Bilateral Integration

- Sensory Integration and Praxis Test (SIPT) (Ayres, 1989)

*End-Product Ability Levels*

Praxis

- SIPT
- Parent report
- Teacher report

Form and Space Perception

- SIPT
- Developmental Test of Visual-Motor Integration (DTVI) (Beery, 1989)
- Motor Free Visual Perception Test (MVPT) (Colarusso & Hammill, 1972)
- Parent report
- Teacher report
- Test of Visual-Perceptual Skills (non motor) (Gardner, 1988)

Behavior

- Clinical observations
- Parent report
- Teacher report
- Psychological evaluation

Academics

- School reports, including report cards
- Teacher report
- Educational assessment done by teacher and/or school psychologist (i.e., Wechsler Intelligence Scale for Children Revised, 1974); Kaufman Assessment Battery for Children (Kaufman & Kaufman, 1983)

Language and Articulation

- Evaluation is done by the speech pathologist
- Observations

Emotional Tone

- Observations
- Psychological report
- Social worker report
- Parent report
- Teacher report

*—continued*

Activity Level

- Observation
- Psychologist report
- Physician report
- Parent report
- Teacher report

Environmental Mastery

- Observation
- Child self-report
- Parent report
- Teacher report

---

The clinical observations suggested in this chapter should be conducted in a standardized way (Dunn, 1981). Clinical observations, histories, and checklists, and some standardized tests can be done by entry-level therapists. It is suggested that therapists should have some educational background in test administration before using standardized evaluations. The administration and interpretation of the SCSIT, SCPNT and SIPT require additional education. These are not considered entry-level occupational therapy skills and have been designed for therapists who have postprofessional degrees and clinical experience. There are extensive training programs, including certifications, that teach the administration and interpretation of these tests. Evaluation reports from other professionals may require interpretation by those specialized professionals. The occupational therapist is responsible, however, for interpreting the findings relative to this frame of reference.

When evaluating a child, the therapist may notice that problems in the sensory system modulation level often result in sensory defensiveness. Problems in functional support capabilities often result in decreased functional abilities. Both problems—those in sensory modulation level and functional support capabilities—influence the end-product ability levels. Although all end-product ability levels are important to the occupational therapist, one of primary concern is praxis, with the second concern being behavioral problems.

Dyspraxia is the key area of concern for the occupational therapist. It also is the most encompassing of the problem areas. Therefore, specific understanding of praxis is important in evaluating the child who demonstrates sensory integrative problems. The use of the praxis chart (see Fig. 6.10) and the clinical reasoning process (see Appendix 6D) helps the therapist to organize her thinking about the child's response. Furthermore, it helps the therapist to pinpoint where the problem occurs for the child. For example, using Figure 6.10, is the problem in registration, arousal, ideation, handling more or different sensory input, or responding to the limitation or structure of the environment?

Evaluation of sensory integrative problems involves a systematic appraisal of the child's functioning. Appendix 6B and Appendix 6C will help organize thinking during evaluation. The outline in Appendix B helps to organize results.

# Postulates Regarding Change

Postulates regarding change focus on the therapeutic environment needed to facilitate change. The occupational therapist does not create change in the child but facilitates optimum conditions in the environment so that change is most likely to occur. The interplay among the occupational therapist, the child, and the environment is complex and requires constant clinical reasoning. The clinical reasoning process is based on the therapist's observational abilities and on the organization of theoretical knowledge in the frame of reference.

In the sensory integrative frame of reference, 20 postulates have been identified. When the evaluation indicates dysfunction, intervention should be directed mainly at the sensory system modulation level or at the functional support capabilities level.

There are eight general postulates related to the use of the sensory integrative frame of reference:

1. If intervention involves several sensory systems and requires intersensory integration, then it will be more powerful and more likely to bring about an adaptive response.
2. If the therapist provides a situation in which the child can act on his environment, then the child will be more likely to produce adaptive responses. The child's self initiated actions also use the more efficient feed forward mechanisms rather than only feedback.
3. If the child is self-directed during therapy, then feed forward and corollary discharge will occur.
4. If the therapist provides a situation that requires an adaptive response that is developmentally appropriate, then the adaptive response is more likely to occur and more likely to promote growth.

5. If the activity presented to the child is challenging yet achievable, then it will facilitate an improved adaptive response.
6. If the therapist provides the child with a sense of emotional safety, then the child will be more likely to engage actively in the therapy process.
7. If the therapist provides the child with constant feedback during the therapy session, then the child will gain a greater understanding of what he is doing and what he has done.
8. If the therapist provides activities that involve controlled change and variety, then the child is more likely to make an adaptive response rather than develop a learned behavior.

If there are deficits in the sensory system modulation level, it is important to bring modulation within normal levels. There are six postulates regarding change related to sensory system modulation:

9. If sensory system modulation is within normal levels, then an adequate adaptive response is more likely to occur.
10. If a child is underreactive, then sensory system input may have to be of greater intensity or duration or more intentional for the child to be able to produce an adequate adaptive response. (Exception: those children who *look* underaroused but are really shut off because of severe overregistration.)
11. If a child is overreactive, then the usual adaptive response will reflect survival needs and not integration; therefore, the sensory system input will have to be modified for the child to produce an adequate adaptive response.
12. If modulating input is given to one system, then influence is seen in all systems because they are interdependent.
13. If the child's sensory diet is modified, then sensory system modulation is more likely to occur.
14. If the sensory system modulation level is normalized, then functional support capabilities and end-product abilities will be facilitated.

Functional support capabilities must be activated sufficiently to provide a base for organizing and supporting the adaptive responses. If perceptions, abilities, or feedback are faulty in these areas, they lead only to partially accurate adaptive responses. The partially accurate response is not even stable (always partially accurate in the same way) because of the inconsistent nature of the input from sensory systems and functional support capabilities; therefore, the client has inconsistent or inadequate information on which to base an adaptive response, leading to faulty motor patterns and learning. There are three postulates regarding change related to functional support capabilities:

15. If the therapist provides opportunity for input to the functional support areas at a level intentionally more intense or prolonged than that found in the environment, then functional support abilities are more likely to improve. (Remember that the body and head must be treated separately because of separate innervations.)

16. If the therapist provides opportunity for functional support reinforcement during active, child-initiated movement, then functional support capabilities are more likely to improve.

17. If the therapist provides opportunity for several functional support capabilities to be reinforced (integrated) simultaneously, then the capabilities are likely to improve.

There are three postulates regarding change related to end-product abilities:

18. If the therapist encourages the child to verbalize what he is doing during the therapy session, then he is more likely to build ideation.

19. If the child develops increased practic abilities and increased organization, then there will be a positive effect on other end-product abilities.

20. If the child is to build motor plans, then he must self-initiate the adaptive response process.

## Application to Practice

The specific techniques of the sensory integrative frame of reference differ from the techniques identified in the other frames of reference used by occupational therapists. Intervention in this frame of reference is mainly child-directed. That is, the child needs to act on his environment to produce the adaptive responses. This action by the child also produces the more efficient feed-forward mechanisms necessary for optimum adaptive response, rather than relying on the less-efficient feedback. In this frame of reference, the therapist is often nurturing and playful and is involved as an active participant in the treatment activities.

One goal of sensory integration is to achieve an effective adaptation to the environment through an improvement of CNS processing. The therapist encourages a large variety of activities and exploration, rarely repeating an

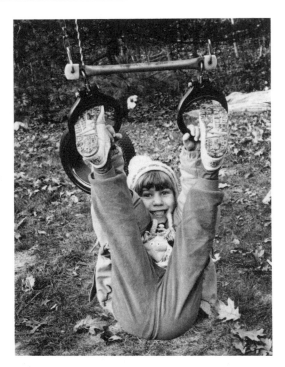

**Figure 6.11**
Sensory diet activity for home: trapeze and rings; provides proprioceptive and vestibular input.

activity. Activities should not be geared toward specific skill development through practice but should elicit an adaptive response.

In this frame of reference, intervention uses a treatment environment organized to help guide the therapy. Any activity in which the child wishes to engage can be used therapeutically if structured appropriately by the therapist. The child's spontaneous ability to produce an adaptive response and transfer it to other environments is one of the expected outcomes of a well-planned occupational therapy program.

Although direct intervention is done in a clinical setting, the child's activities may be orchestrated to contribute to a positive outcome through the "sensory diet." All the child's systems (including community, family, and school) are used. The community can offer modulating "sensory diet" activities such as gymnastics, dance, karate, or rollerskating. The family can carry out a home program to decrease sensory defensiveness as well as provide emotional support and monitoring of the sensory diet (Fig. 6.11). Also, the school can help contribute to increase success with end-product abilities, such as academics, once personnel understand the contribution of sensory systems functioning to the end products.

## Treatment Considerations

Occupational therapists who use a clinic-based sensory integrative approach need to be cognizant of three particular areas of treatment: the treatment environment, the child's responses, and the sequence of therapy.

### Treatment Environment

Occupational therapists who use this frame of reference need to be "environmental engineers." The safety of the child must be of primary importance. Some elements of physical safety in a treatment setting include the following:

- Sufficient space is needed to allow swinging movements, as well as running and jumping activities, and space for a scooter board ramp.
- Mats must provide sufficient padding for a fall from a height of up to 4 feet. Mats should be made of dense foam for the bottom 2 to 4 inches, topped by thick crash mats. Checking with the gymnastic association in the area will help determine the legal liability for numbers of inches of matting required for falls from particular heights.
- The floor of the clinic is also extremely important. If the clinic is built on a concrete floor, additional mats will be required. If possible, the clinic should have a wooden floor with a tile covering. Or, if wooden floors are not part of the structure, a wooden suspension floor can be built over the concrete floor to allow some give during falls. The tile on the clinic floor should be of a nondistracting color and pattern. This will reduce optokinetic nystagmus when the child is moving on the equipment.
- An overhead suspension system is necessary to allow safe suspension of swings such as net hammocks suspended by one point, trapezes, and bolsters and inner tubes suspended as swings. The overhead suspension must be capable of holding at least 500 pounds, (to hold an adult therapist and a large client at the same time on equipment). This 500-pound suspension needs to be safe during a swinging movement. There are many varieties of suspensions. Consult a professional engineer or an occupational therapy equipment supplier who also sells suspension equipment.

Clinical equipment includes materials with which children readily engage yet perceive as fun and challenging. Essential equipment includes scooter boards, a ramp, a trapeze, a net (pocket or sportsman's) hammock, assorted large therapy balls, a bolster swing, inner tube swings, a mini trampoline, an assortment of foam rubber pillows, cardboard stacking blocks, boxes, balls, bean bags, hula hoops, Theraband™, mouth toys, and sucking and chewing (oral motor) items, to name a few. Additional equipment may include a

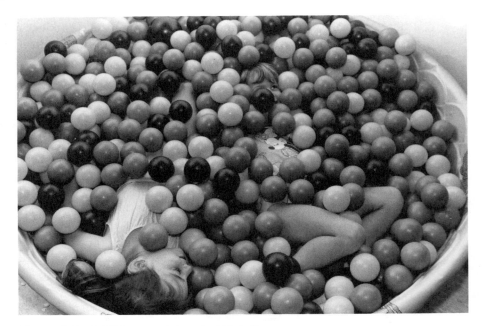

**Figure 6.12**   Inhibitory activity—bubbleballs.

waterbed mattress or air mattress on the floor of the clinic; a bubble ball bath or a large box filled with styrofoam packing material; a "Play all"™ roll; and, a Whizwheel™. Almost any active toy can be used in treatment. It is not the toy itself that is important, but the way in which the toy is used to obtain an optimal adaptive response (Figs. 6.12 & 6.13).

## General Considerations

In this frame of reference, therapy needs to be individually based, because the child's responses must be watched continually, and modifications must be made in treatment. Sometimes, small group activities may be used with several children. This limits the activities, however, to only those beneficial to all children and may limit the intensity of the therapy session.

The therapist must constantly observe the child's ANS responses during therapy so that overarousal and underarousal/registration do not occur. As discussed previously, severe overarousal/registration can lead to shutdown or even to shock. Some specific sensory integrative techniques have the potential to affect the nervous system positively. Conversely, they also have

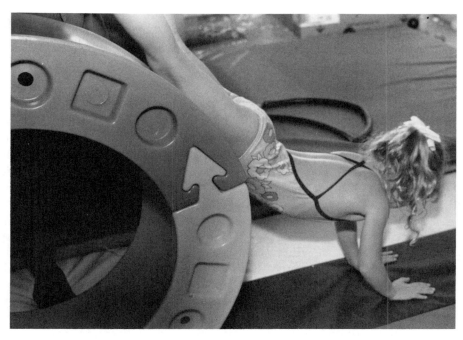

**Figure 6.13**  Maintaining extension in prone position while rolling off "Play-all." Note that therapist is holding feet for safety.

the possibility of having a strong negative effects if used incorrectly or carelessly.

During the therapy session, the therapist needs to give constant feedback to the child. Verbal feedback helps the child understand what he is doing and what has been done. Eliciting verbalization from the child about what he is doing is also helpful in building ideation. Any praise given to a child should be a real compliment, because children are attuned to fake praise. Consider positive comments on the process rather than on the end product. For example, use phrases such as "you really tried," "you must be proud of yourself for working so hard," or "that was the biggest jump you ever made."

The child needs to be self-directed or no feed forward or corollary discharge will occur. The role of the therapist is to **entice** the child to want to act on his environment. This can be done with organization of the environment to help the child choose the most beneficial activities. When the therapist cannot set up the environment to eliminate some distracting activities, the therapist should then guide the child's choices yet still allowing him to have some control. One method is to ask questions such as "Would you like to go ride on the bolster swing *or* on the scooter board?" This offers the child an opportunity to be involved in making choices and to build self-esteem.

An area of "default patterns" that therapists often fall into is the attempt to use particular pieces of equipment to get particular responses from the child and thereby insisting the child use those pieces of equipment. If the child comes into the room and immediately gravitates toward another activity or equipment, fast thinking on the part of the therapist can modify the activity to get the type of feedback and adaptive response the child needs. The occupational therapist needs to be always vigilant for creative possibilities to facilitate the adaptive responses while still using the child's desires and choices. Observing normal children on equipment can broaden the therapist's ideas about how equipment may be used.

Intervention that involves several sensory systems and requires intersensory integration is more powerful than intervention that uses just one system. For example, an activity that involves only swinging on a bolster swing is not nearly as integrative as an activity that involves swinging on a bolster swing and getting heavy proprioception by catching and throwing a three-foot ball. Tactile input can be added by putting a piece of fleece over the bolster and having the child sit on the bolster swing in shorts (see Fig. 6.9).

In the sensory integrative frame of reference, the aim is not to teach skills but to facilitate appropriate physical and emotional adaptive responses. The goal is to facilitate an adaptive response that can be used at any time in the child's life and can be adapted when the child needs it in other situations. The therapist should help build the child a motor and emotional repertoire.

In this frame of reference, intervention is based on the therapist's knowledge of the child's developmental level. Furthermore, activities are selected that require the adaptive responses within the upper levels of the child's capacity. To require only adaptive responses that are easy will not help the child to integrate new abilities. Conversely, to require a response that is too hard can cause disintegration, which could result in the child's loss of what he had gained previously in that particular therapy session.

The goal of intervention is to obtain a complex adaptive response that is integrated and results from multisensory input. What follows are some characteristics of an adaptive response in the sensory integrative frame of reference:

- An adaptive response is meaningful to the child, appropriate developmentally, socially, and psychologically, and specific to the situation.
- An adaptive response is not a taught skill or a rigid pattern of behavior but is elicited when needed.
- An adaptive response is reinforced by elicitation; therefore, adaptive responses are self-reinforcing, especially if they are integrated and work.

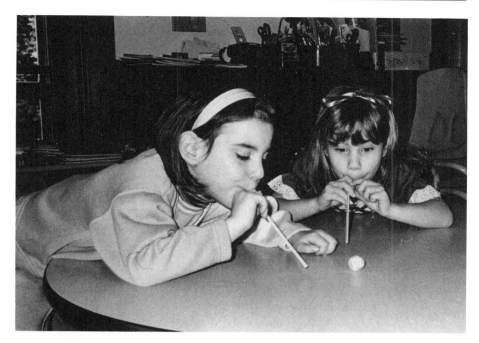

**Figure 6.14**  Oral-motor game: blowing ball with straws.

- An adaptive response requires active involvement of a child's central nervous system.
- An optimal adaptive response is achieved when the therapist interacts with the child, rather than instructing the child.
- An adaptive response should be within the child's developmental level. These adaptive responses should be at the upper limits of the child's abilities to promote growth. Care should be taken by the therapist not to push the limits of the child's abilities, because this may result in disorganization.
- Raw sensory stimulation (such as spinning a child for 10 minutes) is not sensory integration and will not elicit an integrated adaptive response.

Beyond the adaptive motor response, a therapist must address the adaptive emotional responses and the ideational responses. It is important that a child know what he is trying to do. Sometimes a therapist needs to initiate an activity by asking the child to verbalize what he is about to do. The therapist may need to provide the child with the first part of the sequence and then ask him to verbalize the next part. At other times, the therapist may need to demonstrate or actually help the child move through the activity before the child can take over for himself.

Remember that oral motor abilities must be facilitated separately from other motor abilities because of their separate neural systems (cranial nerves) (Fig. 6.14).

# Methods Used to Facilitate Adaptive Responses in Sensory Integration

Based on the identified needs of a child, the therapist selects appropriate activities and develops an actual plan for the sequence of the therapy session. The specific activities are not always planned; rather, the desired response is planned, such as flexion activities or two-step sequences. For example, a basic treatment sequence over time could include activities to (1) develop overall extension and flexion to achieve a balance in the use of the two patterns; (2) develop the ability to cross the midline of the body with the upper and lower extremities; (3) develop the ability to rotate the trunk during activities; and, (4) develop the ability to follow three-step directions. Before the activities are initiated, the therapist must prepare a child appropriately for success at each adaptive response. Listed below are some guidelines for facilitating an adaptive response:

- Address sensory system modulation problems first. If a child is on sympathetic arousal, the adaptive response will reflect survival needs, not integration.
- Avoid complex motor planning activities early in a session. Build up to complex motor planning activities through appropriate input and intermediary adaptive responses.
- Get the child involved actively in the activities and help him to succeed. Do not impose yourself, as a therapist, on the child (other than possibly in treating sensory defensiveness with brushing). Elicit the desired response through interaction.
- Intervention should be specific to the underlying sensory system deficits; it is not specific to behaviors. Practice may improve particular skills but does not improve the generalization of abilities.
- Balance the treatment session with structure and freedom. Neither free play nor total structure is therapeutic in the sensory integrative frame of reference. Some children come to therapy very self-directed—for instance, learning disabled children. Other children come to therapy not self-directed at all—for example, some autistic and mentally retarded children. For those who are not self-directed, the therapist might need to impose structure first and then work into more freedom.
- As a therapist, hypothesize about what the child understands and what is happening in his central nervous system. Answer the following questions: Does he know what he is going to be doing in the activity? Is he able to articulate it? Does he have the idea of what is required in the activity?

The therapist must capture the child's attention and motivation through her personality and through the activity. In this frame of reference, the occupational therapist is expected to have fun, act a little silly, and actually engage in play with the child. The best "problem" to have is that the child does not want to go home at the end of a therapy session and that the parent or care provider wonders why occupational therapy is so much fun for the child. Often, the therapist needs to explain to parents or care providers the importance of the child's having fun during therapy. Some parents or care provides may think that therapy should be hard work and that they are not getting their money's worth if it appears to be otherwise.

When selecting activities, the therapist must be sure that the activities are within the child's reach, but that they also extend that reach just a little, to the "achievable challenge." An activity that is too easy is not organizing; one that is too hard is disorganizing.

For children who are very dyspraxic or distractible, the therapist should avoid changing the whole activity. Instead, the therapist should change only part of the activity so that the required adaptive response is modified and neuronal models can be built. The therapy session should always end with the child's successful completion of an activity. (Go back to an activity that you know the child can execute successfully. If possible, give him a choice.)

The therapist must be infinitely flexible. In addition to changing adaptive responses quickly, she often must change her treatment plan because the child's sensory system modulation may be different from session to session. Activities that work at one time may not work at another. At all times, the therapist must keep in mind the child's treatment goals. In addition, she must realize that a specific activity is not essential to meet these goals, but that many activities will work. Flexibility will get the most positive results in a particular session.

It is critical that a therapist provide emotional safety for the child. The child must trust the therapist so that she can push him a little for better results. Part of the emotional adaptive response is laughter. Often music and singing can help integration. Some controlled fear also is appropriate. Young children, when learning about gravity and movement, often will challenge themselves by jumping off things (such as stairs) that are just a little higher than the ones they have tried before. This small element of fear can be arousing and exciting in therapy. The therapist must be careful, however, not to go overboard so that the fear becomes disintegrating.

Finally, it is important that a therapist recognize that improvement may not be linear, but stepwise with plateaus. Sometimes, especially in older children who have praxis problems, only small motor improvement occurs, but the children become much more organized. The child may retreat at times or refuse to do things previously done. He may be bored with the activity, have had a bad day, just not feel like doing the activity, or may hold back just before a large improvement. After significant change, children often need a chance to adjust or integrate the new level of learning. Demands from school or home, or a change in schedule also may intrude and could distract the child from a therapy session.

## Sequence of Treatment

As stated in the postulates regarding change, the sequence of treatment is (first) to modulate the sensory systems, (second) to work on the functional support capabilities within the adaptive responses, and (third) require adaptive responses necessary to build the end-product abilities. In the sensory integrative frame of reference, intervention follows the sequence of development. First, sensory modulation levels should be normalized to facilitate functional capabilities, bringing about adaptive responses.

## Sensory System Modulation

Sensory system modulation may be influenced in several ways. It is critical to keep in mind that arousal in one system can raise the set point (baseline) for the entire CNS. According to Wilbarger and Wilbarger (1991), a child who has sensory system modulation problems is called **sensory defensive** (SD). Sensory defensiveness can be rated as mild, moderate, or severe. Mild sensory defensive children are described as "picky," "overly sensitive," or "slightly controlling." They can be irritated by some sensations but not by others. They achieve at school and socially but need enormous control and effort to do so. When this control becomes too hard to maintain, they "fall apart."

The moderately SD child is affected in several areas of life (i.e., difficulty with social relations, self-care skills, or attention and behavior in school). The severely SD child is affected in every aspect of life. According to Wilbarger and Wilbarger (1991), these children usually have other diagnostic labels like severe developmental delay or emotionally disturbed. All SD children need treatment to deal with this primary problem and to enable other forms of treatment to be more effective. Treatment of sensory defensiveness can take several avenues: First, just diagnosing the problem can increase understanding of the child. Second, sensory systems can be influenced through a planned "sensory diet." And, third, direct intervention with a touch pressure brush may be needed. Sensory diet inputs can raise or lower the modulation level. What follows are some examples of excitatory and inhibitory activities:

*Excitatory Activities*
- Amusement park rides
- Fast driving
- Fast skiing
- Loud music
- Noisy parties
- Fast dancing
- Rock concerts
- Fast moving sports (i.e., basketball and soccer)
- A fast-paced job
- Worrying and anxiety
- Scary movies
- Riding on motorcycles

*Inhibitory Activities*
- Staying alone in a quiet room
- Dimming lights
- Soft music
- Heavy joint and muscle work (such as jogging, bike riding, slow weight lifting, karate, tap dancing, tackle football)
- Heavy touch pressure (such as massage)

Children who have sensory system modulation problems, also may need to have their sensory activities modified to help control modulation. More opportunity for activities that contribute to modulation may need to be provided. It seems apparent that some activities are calming and others are excitatory. Because of the type of dysfunction in some sensory systems, sometimes excitatory appearing activities have an inhibitory effect.

Children who have one type of hyperactivity, those who respond to stimulant medications (Ritalin®, Cylert®) to calm them, are considered to be experiencing underarousal to parts of the CNS (Kimball, 1986, 1988). Excitatory input, especially fast vestibular input, can override the underarousal and lead to modulation. In these children, the hyperactive behavior is seen as secondary to low arousal and serves to increase arousal rather than being caused by high arousal. Fast vestibular activities, particularly combined with proprioception, can normalize the sensory system functions in some children at least for short periods of time, and can reduce the "hyperactivity." There is mounting evidence that these changes may be more permanent.

Nonhyperactive children who have preferences for fast, intense movements (carnival rides, fast skiing, motorcycles, fast swinging, spinning) also have apparent underarousal or overinhibition in the lower brain centers, as discussed with depressed nystagmus. These fast movements actually modulate arousal to a more normal level.

Another way in which sensory systems are influenced for sensory defensive children is through direct intervention. The method of treatment involves direct input to decrease sensory defensiveness through the use of a specific type of nonscratching pressure brush followed by proprioceptive input to all joints (Wilbarger & Wilbarger, 1991). Only one particular surgical scrub brush (available through PDP products) has been found to provide the right input to effect the modulating response quickly (Wilbarger & Wilbarger, 1991). The fast, very firm, long-stroke brushing should be applied quickly on each extremity (hands, feet) and on the back but never on the stomach or face. This is then followed by 10 quick compressions of each joint. The joints can be compressed in groups by pushing the hands together, by jumping up and down, or by having another person push firmly (but not with too much pressure) on each set of joints 10 times. This treatment should take a total of about 1 minute and should be repeated 8 to 12 times per day for 1 to 2 weeks. The treatment should be monitored at all times by a specifically trained occupational therapist. If appropriate, maintenance treatment may need to continued. Because the mouth is controlled by a different part of the nervous system (the cranial nerves), oral defensiveness must be treated separately, with short, quick applications of firm pressure to the roof of the mouth (with the finger covered by a face cloth or by a plastic nipple) (Wilbarger & Wilbarger, 1991).

This pressure-proprioceptive treatment represents a departure from other treatments in this frame of reference in that it is "imposed lovingly" on the child (most children do love it). Some problems with sensory defensiveness are so resistant to change and have such a pervasive effect on a child's life that the imposition of input is the only way to "break through" and to begin normalizing the system. The true sensory defensive person rejects all therapeutic contact (Wilbarger & Wilbarger, 1991). In 1972, Ayres stated:

> Occasionally a therapist may be justified in applying stimuli in spite of discomfort for a few days in an effort to bring a sufficient shift in balance between the protective and discriminative response systems to enable development of tolerance to some stimuli. (p. 219)

The pressure brushing proprioceptive program can result in a decreased sensory defensiveness and more appropriate responses to sensory input. The

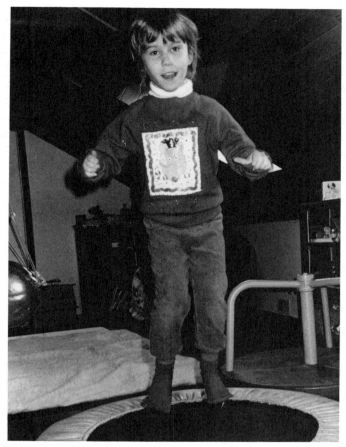

**Figure 6.15**   Sensory diet activity for home: minitrampoline.

parent or care provider may provide the program. This treatment must be closely monitored, however, by a therapist who has experience in sensory system dysfunction. For more information, the reader is directed to the videotape, *Occupational Therapy: Sensory Defensiveness* (Wilbarger, 1991).

Another method of sensory input, a "sensory diet," can be self-selected by the child (Fig. 6.15). Proprioception is important in sensory modulation and may be either joint compression or traction; thus, any heavy work, along with motor activity, that a child engages in will have a normalizing effect on the child's nervous system. Slow movement activities combined with proprioception are helpful for almost every child. Fast movement activities may have varying effects, depending on the child's nervous system. The neck joints and proximal limb joints, the shoulders and hips, are most responsive to proprioceptive input. A quick proprioceptive activity that can be used in a school classroom is 10 slow push-ups. Other easy proprioceptive activities that can be done at home are chin-ups with a chin-up bar, bouncing on a minitrampoline, doing push-ups against the wall, slow wrestling with others, jogging, bike riding, and roller-skating. One method of providing heavy proprioception to a child's neck joints is to lean couch cushions against the front of the couch and have the child kneel on all fours and push his head firmly, slowly, back and forth into the couch cushions. (Be careful not to injure the neck.) Once sensory system modulation is "normalized," or at least the arousal level is reduced, at the beginning of the treatment session, functional support capabilities and end-product abilities can be worked on. It is important to remember that different types of input can influence the nervous system for varying lengths of time. Tactile input can last up to 1 and $\frac{1}{2}$ hours, proprioceptive input up to 2 hours, and vestibular input up to 4 hours or more.

## Functional Support Capabilities

Activities to develop functional support capabilities are numerous and most activities incorporate more than one area. Cocontraction and muscle tone are best worked on with proprioception and balance equilibrium activities. The therapist needs to be reminded that in all interventions in which activity uses several sensory modalities, it is more likely that change will occur than when an activity is based on a single modality. Doing a proprioceptive activity while challenging equilibrium, therefore, can affect those two systems as well as cocontraction, muscle tone, and even the developmental reflexes and bilateral integration.

The more muscles and joints involved in the activity, the more input possible from the activity. The lower to the ground the activity (for example, non-standing), the more joints and muscles involved and the more elemental balance is required. Rather than the skill development approach of walking on a balance beam to enhance balance and equilibrium, a sensory integrative approach looks at the underlying integration inefficiency and treats it. Another example involves the use of a waterbed. If a therapist has a child kneel in the quadruped position on a waterbed so that his hands and knees both are touching the surface and are weightbearing, then the adaptive response may be to keep from falling over. If the therapist pushes on the waterbed and says "don't fall over," the adaptive response of the activity might be very elemental and be more of a learned rather than a developmental skill.

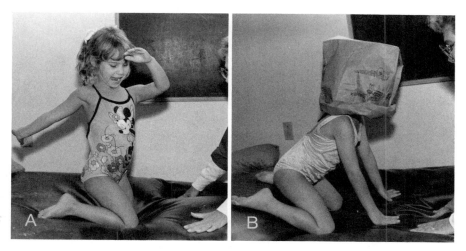

**Figure 6.16**  **A**, Mature response during equilibrium challenge (hurricane game) on waterbed; note rotation of trunk; **B**, challenge to equilibrium with vision occluded by bag (less upsetting than a blindfold).

Whereas, if the therapist states "you are a boat in the ocean and I am the hurricane and I am trying to sink you," and the therapist gets involved with making hurricane-type noises, blowing air at the child's face, and bouncing the waterbed around, then the child has an emotional as well as a physical adaptive response. Because the child concentrates on the **fun** of the game, the equilibrium reactions become more automatic and integrated (Fig. 6.16). The environment and activity have been set up for success and the most mature adaptive response possible. Involved in the activity, in addition to the equilibrium, are proprioception, cocontraction, and muscle tone. The activity can be changed if the therapist changes places with the child so that he becomes the hurricane and tries to sink the therapist. Another adaptation is to pretend that it is night—the child then has to "close his eyes" so that darkness ensues or a paper bag can be placed over his head so that his vision is occluded (Fig. 6.16). This makes the balance and equilibrium responses even more spontaneous because optical righting has been eliminated.

A common activity in an occupational therapy clinic—swinging on a bolster swing—can be used for balance, equilibrium, cocontraction, muscle tone, and proprioception at the same time. An adaptation of this activity consists of using a large three-foot ball thrown at the child (see Figs. 6.9A & 6.9B). This requires additional joint/muscle work to catch and to throw. The ball can be thrown from various angles as the bolster swing is moved. To change

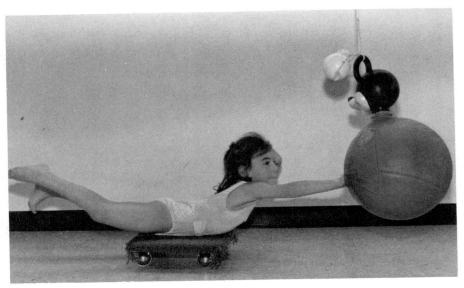

**Figure 6.17**   Prone extension position facilitated by ride down scooter ramp in prone position and reaching for suspended ball; note asymmetrical tonic neck reflex.

the activity, balls of different sizes and shapes or balloons can be thrown so that the child must make constant modifications and adaptations because of the different weights of the objects being caught or thrown. The constant change in this activity ensures an adaptive response and not a learned behavior. The swinging of the bolster swing also contributes greatly to making this an adaptive response that builds praxis rather than a learned behavior (as would be the case with practicing catching on a stationary surface).

The development of the ability to assume and maintain the prone extension posture is an indication of vestibular proprioceptive functioning. This position can be facilitated by placing a child prone on a scooter board and by doing many activities that require heavy proprioception and movement at the same time. Any activity down a scooter board ramp facilitated prone extension if a child is prone on the scooter board (Fig. 6.17). Another activity, scooter board basketball, which requires the prone child to throw the ball with two hands into a target a foot or two off the floor, also facilitates prone extension, whereas throwing with one hand does not. Activities done from a prone position in a net hammock are also appropriate (Figs. 6.18A & 6.18B).

For the inexperienced therapist, judging the quality of another antigravity response—the flexion response—is a difficult concept. It often appears that the child can do the response, but, if observed closely, the quality is not the

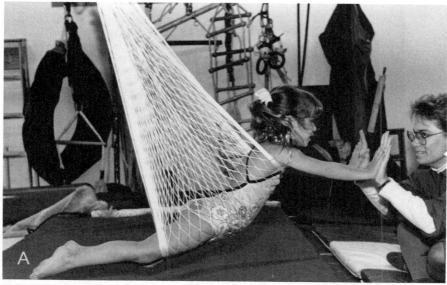

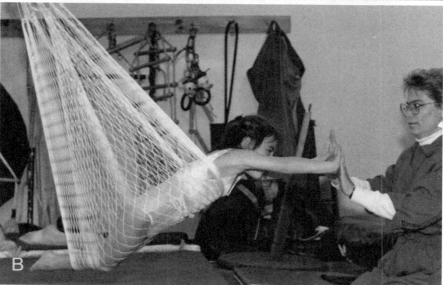

**Figure 6.18**   **A**, Mature response; 5-year-old child has symmetrical extension in prone position against gravity; **B**, Immature response; 6-year-old child has some asymmetry and flexion of hips in prone position, indicating difficulty moving against gravity. Pushing the therapist's hand with resistance adds proprioceptive reinforcement to this vestibular activity.

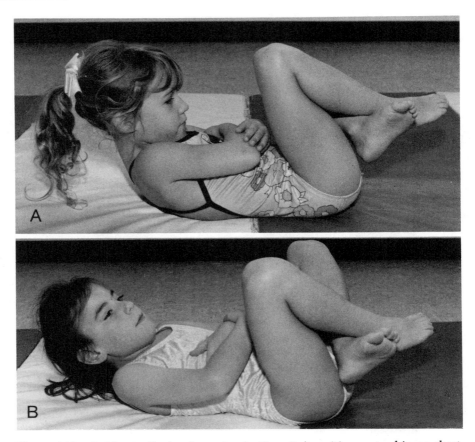

**Figure 6.19**   **A**, Mature flexion in supine (antigravity) position; note chin on chest, scapula off mat; **B**, Subtle immaturity in flexion in supine (antigravity) position; note chin not quite on chest and scapula on mat.

same as that of a normal child. Supine flexion is tested in the supine position on a mat where the child flexes his neck and knees off the floor at the same time. This often results in the knees being drawn up toward the stomach appropriately, but the neck is being lifted with a chin jut. In other words, extension occurs in place of flexion. This needs to be watched for and, if seen, indicates that the child is not producing a mature antigravity flexion response (Figs. 6.19A & 6.19B). The flexion response is extremely important not only in survival but also in articulation and swallowing. If the chin is jutted forward slightly in extension, this makes it difficult for the child to

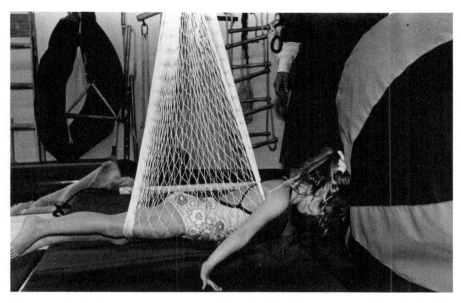

**Figure 6.20**   Neck proprioception; gentle pushing with head on mushroom ball while prone in net hammock.

articulate clearly, to chew, and to swallow effectively. Neck proprioception activities help greatly to reinforce the flexion response (Fig. 6.20).

Supine flexion is often a deficient response in children who are dyspraxic. The flexion pattern is extremely important to the child's development and is seen by Carl Sagan (1977) as being a primary survival pattern for mankind. Flexion follows a specific sequence of development that needs to be facilitated in a child who does not have a good flexion response. The first point is to maintain flexion, which can be facilitated in occupational therapy by placing a child on a flexion swing and having him maintain position as he swings. Holding flexion against gravity—for instance, holding onto the bottom side of a bolster swing—is the most difficult way to maintain flexion (Figs. 6.21A & 6.21B). Sitting in an inner tube and hugging it is also a way to facilitate flexion. The second level in developing flexion is to have a child assume the flexion position. In this case, a child can leave the flexion response momentarily by reaching for something while on the flexion swing and then can reassume the position (Figs. 6.22A & 6.22B; 6.23A & 6.23B). The third point in the development of flexion is being able to release flexion at the appropriate time. This can be seen in a child who can swing on a trapeze, lift his knees up over a barrier, and then jump into an inner tube or land on a desired space,

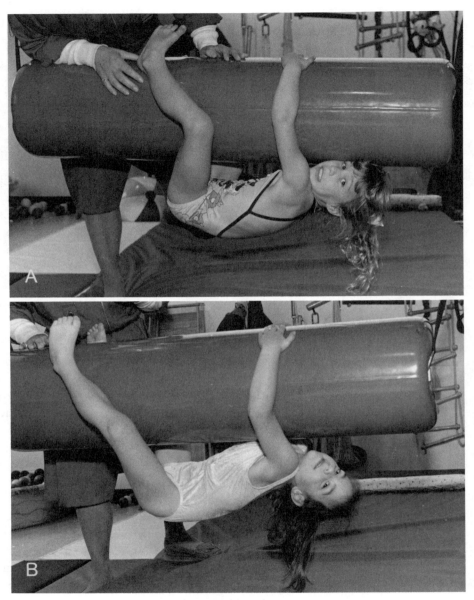

**Figure 6.21**   **A**, Mature response; 5-year-old child shows ability to hang on moving bolster swing in total flexion with good cocontraction (although expressing some fear); **B**, Immature response; extension in neck and back showing influence of gravity.

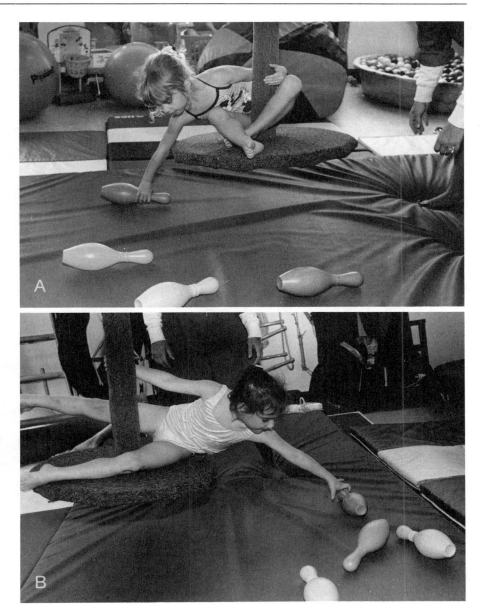

**Figure 6.22    A,** Mature response; 5-year-old child on moving flexion swing maintains flexion in lower body while extending arm to pick up bowling pin; **B,** Immature response; 6-year-old child on moving flexion swing extends whole body as arm extends to pick up pin.

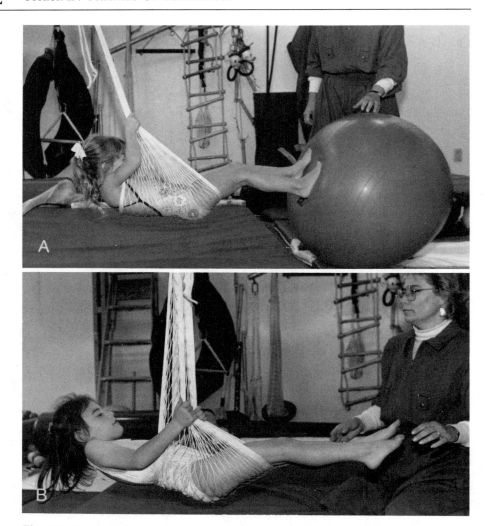

**Figure 6.23    A,** Mature response; ability to hold head (neck) in flexion against gravity and move legs into extension and flexion as needed to kick ball; **B,** Immature response; difficulty holding head (neck) and knees in flexion against gravity.

or swing on a trapeze and kick only the top box off from a pile (Fig. 6.24). This activity assumes that the child can initiate flexion, maintain it, and release it at appropriate times.

In a sensory integrative approach, the therapist needs to work through a normal motor developmental sequence of stability on which to build mobility. The particular sequence that can be followed is: (1) ability to assume the

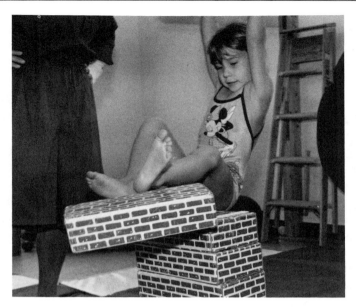

**Figure 6.24** Mature response; this 5-year-old child is able to flex selectively to kick the number of blocks desired off the pile, showing mature use of flexion abilities.

basic starting position; (2) develop stability in that position; (3) ability to move from the position in a straight plane movement; and, (4) integration of the movements and the addition of rotation.

An example of a normal motor developmental sequence is creeping in an infant. The child first gets up on all fours and generally falls down; then the child gets up on all fours and rocks back and forth, giving stability to the joints and strength to the muscles needed for the movement; after the rocking phase, the child begins a creeping movement, in a straight plane; and then, eventually, the child is able to add rotation, in that he can move around corners, pick up one hand, and turn to grab something all in the quadruped position. The same thing occurs in learning how to walk, where the child pulls up and sits down, then pulls up and cruises along the furniture in a straight plane motion, and then stands and walks in a somewhat controlled fall method with hands held up. Finally, as a more mature walker, the child adds some rotation in the upper body to the movement. (The same process can be seen in learning to ski).

Lateralization and bilateral integration also are addressed in functional support capabilities. Integrated movement in two planes is necessary for bilateral integration and in three planes for rotation (Oetter & Richter, 1992).

One method used to address this is the inclusion of rotation in an activity. Many children who have been identified as having sensory integrative dysfunction can be seen to be "straight plane" movers, that is, children who do not rotate their bodies but tend to move in straight, linear styles. Linear motion is indicative of earlier developmental organization. Beginning therapists need to be aware of the sequence, particularly rotation, because some children are able to accomplish a basic motor activity, but the quality is worse than normal because of the lack of integration of rotation. **Remember that treatment of praxis is not about whether the child can do an activity but about the quality of the movement** (see Figs. 6.9A, 6.9B; 6.16).

Getting children who have sensory integrative dysfunction to rotate can be a difficult task. The therapist must be creative in incorporating rotational movements into the adaptive responses. For instance, have a child catch a bean bag with his hands on one side of the bolster swing and then rotate around to throw the bag into a target placed far back on the child's other side. Often, the therapist observes that the child will switch hands to avoid crossing midline or rotating.

The development of the suck-swallow-breathe sequence is vital for the integration of good breathing and phonation, the development of muscle tone in the tongue and jaw, and stability and integrated movement of the head, neck, and trunk. The first place that midline stability and bilateral integration occur is in the eyes when a newborn sucks. Activities follow a sequence of suck-blow to bite-crunch to chew-lick (Oetter, Richter, & Frick, 1992). Examples of suck-blow would be to encourage the child to use a narrow straw for normal drinking but also to provide heavy things to suck through the straw such as pudding, sherbet, or fruit shakes. Strong flavors that stimulate the bitter and sour receptors at the back portion of the tongue help develop muscle tone in the back of tongue as well as jaw stability. Mouth toys such as fancy, unusual whistles and blowing games are encouraged (Fig. 6.25), and musical instruments are good for older children. Treatment of oral defensiveness also may need to be incorporated.

Biting and crunching activities include eating crunchy foods like carrots or popsicles (ice). Chew-lick activities include chewing bagels, gum, resistant candy (like caramel and licorice), and ice cream in a cone. Providing something for children to chew on between meals is indicated. Aquarium tubing can be tied in a knot and worn around the neck so that the child can reach it easily and put it into his mouth to chew on. Theratubing™ has better resistance to chewing but has a bad chemical taste; therefore, it needs to be soaked a long time before use (Oetter & Richter, 1992)

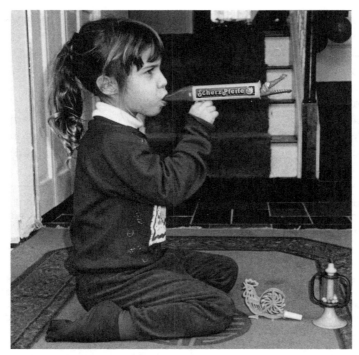

**Figure 6.25**   Mouth toys/whistles.

## *End-Product Abilities*

The end-product abilities are the combination of the child's sensory system modulation and functional support capabilities as well as his cognitive capabilities. Without the lower systems, the end-product abilities are difficult to develop at the highest level possible. It is often said of children who have sensory integration problems that they work so much harder than other children for inferior results.

**Praxis.**  The occupational therapist who uses the sensory integrative frame of reference is concerned primarily with praxis. The other end-product abilities may also be worked on directly in a treatment session but may be influenced indirectly in five major ways. First, the heightened organization gained by increasing practic abilities may affect other end-product abilities. Second, the increased feelings of mastery and self-esteem gained by producing and reinforcing appropriate adaptive motor responses may transfer to other end-product abilities. Third, the increased awareness of space and spatial perception gained by getting consistent internal feedback about the body in space impacts on the development of other end-product abilities. Fourth, articulation may be improved by incorporating head and neck movements in coordination activities. Fifth, increased motor sequencing abilities improve general sequencing abilities that then improve academics, because all academic activity involves a sequence.

The end-product abilities often are addressed in other frames of references, like those that focus on skill development and can be used as adjuncts to sensory integration, where the purpose is to change the child's nervous system responses. There are nine major guidelines for increasing a child's practic abilities:

- Therapists need to be sure that a child's sensory systems are modulated. A nervous system on overarousal/reactivity will produce any adaptive response focused mainly on survival (Fig. 6.26).

- Whenever possible, therapists should use functional support capabilities in activities (Figs. 6.27A & 6.27B).

- Therapists should organize the treatment session so that sensory system modulation occurs first, followed by functional support capabilities. Next, the therapist focuses on using functional support capabilities in conjunction with basic adaptive responses to achieve more integrated adaptive responses. For example, if the end-product practic response is to hit a ball with a bat while swinging on a bolster swing, then the preliminary activity might involve vestibular and proprioceptive input. These systems might be activated by having the child swing himself in the bolster by pushing and pulling on the bolster suspension rope (Fig. 6.28A, 6.28B, & 6.28C). Or, a therapist might select an activity that would require a more integrated adaptive response, such as having the child go down the ramp prone on a scooter board and pick up certain bowling pins whose colors are called out once the scooter has started, calling out "right hand blue, or left hand red." The preliminary activity might be to propel along prone on a scooter board by placing hands on the floor and pulling back hard, or by using both hands on a plunger to pull along. These preliminary activities activate the proprioceptor and vestibular systems so that they are more available to support the praxis activity. The probability of success is improved, and the nervous system has a better chance of using correct pathways to accomplish the activity, thereby building more accurate neuronal models for future use.

- Therapists need to have the equipment and space to provide appropriate sensory input, particularly vestibular input. Suspended equipment is necessary to give the child the opportunity to experience strong vestibular/proprioceptive input.

- Therapists should provide proprioceptive input whenever appropriate. Proprioception has been underused in treating sensory integrative dysfunction. Joint compression or traction, especially on the neck and proximal limb joints, the shoulders and hips, provides important input to help the child improve practic abilities. If a child is having difficulty with a praxis activity, the therapist might stop the activity and give 10 quick compressions to the child's joints involved in the activity, for example the arms, hands, and shoulders in a catching activity. Then the child should be asked to try the activity again. Often the therapist will observe significant changes in the child's ability to succeed at the activity.

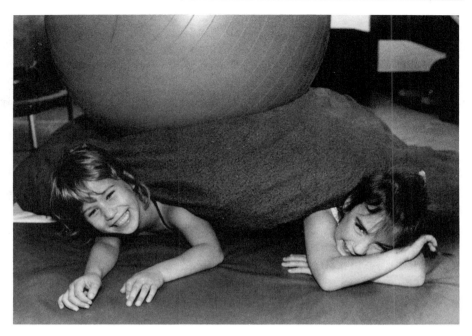

**Figure 6.26** Inhibitory activity: children pretending to be pizza dough are covered in sauce (mat pillow) and the cheese (ball) is rolled on with pressure.

- Therapists need to set up the treatment environment so the child can succeed. As stated previously, therapists should provide children with achievable challenges.

- When a child is inner directed and wants to do activities that a therapist had not anticipated, she should use quick clinical reasoning to use the child's activity to get an integrated adaptive response. For example, if a therapist has a bolster swing set up and the child arrives and wants to play on the large mushroom ball by throwing himself over it, rather than tell the child to get off the mushroom and get on the bolster, a therapist may make an adapted game out of being prone on the mushroom. The therapist could be King Kong, complete with roars, and try to knock the child off the mushroom. Or, bean bags or bowling pins could be scattered on the floor and the child could be asked to pick them up and throw them into a target while still prone over the mushroom.

- Neuronal models may be built by changing only a small portion of the required adaptive response. The whole activity does not have to change. This allows the adaptive response to remain adaptive and not become a learned activity. Furthermore, a small change gives a child a good chance to succeed because the activity is similar to a previous one and, therefore, does not require total reorganization. For example, if the activity is for a child to swing on a trapeze holding on with his hands, flexing his knees and hips so as not to knock down a pile of large blocks or boxes as he swings over, the activity could be graded by increasing the height of the boxes each time, or by having the child kick boxes off the pile (see Fig. 6.23). The activity of swinging on a trapeze to increase flexion abilities is being repeated, but it is not the same as practicing a skill because the adaptive response is changed each time, requiring the flexion pattern to be incorporated into a slightly different practic response.

*—continued*

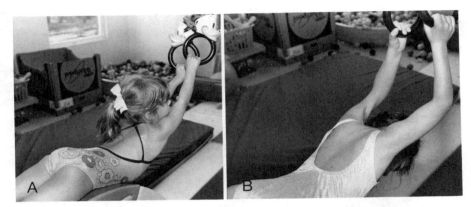

**Figure 6.27** **A,** Mature response; head up against gravity, good cocontraction in arms, strong proprioceptive input is used; **B,** Immature response; head down, influenced by gravity.

- Finally, therapists must be constantly inventive to change adaptive responses asked of the child. This poses a challenge for the therapist and also keeps things interesting for both the therapist and the child.

## Other End-Product Abilities

This frame of reference assumes that most other end-products, including academics (Ayres, 1976), are improved by addressing the child's sensory integrative problems. Other than praxis and incorporation of some form and space perception, the occupational therapist does not address other end-product abilities individually in her intervention. Instead, these abilities are gained through sensory integration, by combining sensory modulation, the development of functional support capabilities, and praxis. Environmental mastery becomes apparent for the child during occupational therapy using the sensory integrative frame of reference.

### Clinical Reasoning Process

Occupational therapy has long been considered an art as well as a science. Part of the art of occupational therapy is the clinical reasoning process that assists the therapist in developing and implementing the sequence of intervention. Appendix 6D explains this process. This table acts as a guide for the therapist to interpret the child's responses to evaluation or intervention and it is grounded in the therapist's knowledge base, careful evaluation of the

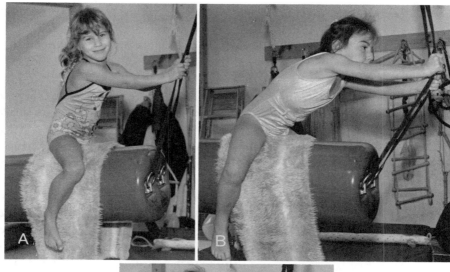

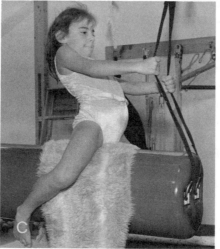

**Figure 6.28**  **A,** Mature response; ability to move bolster swing easily; **B,** Immature response; use of total body pattern to move bolster swing, note low tone in leg; **C,** immature response; use of total body pattern to move bolster swing; note lack of elbow flexion.

child, and ongoing evaluation of the intervention. What is best for the child today may be different tomorrow, based on new information about the child and his family or on additional theoretical information. One strength of the occupational therapist is her ability to change treatment as the situation shifts. Rarely does only one way exist to interact with a child.

The clinical reasoning chart (see Appendix 6D) can be used individually but is used best with another therapist. The critical thinking process (on the left side) is guided by the client-centered questions on the right. This involves the process of looking for causal explanations for behavior so that predictions can be made about clinical outcomes. The metacognitive portion is an exercise to reflect on the actual process that the therapist goes through— it is actually "thinking about our thinking." Its purpose is to extrapolate the critical thinking/clinical reasoning process in general ways to other clients or situations.

The clinical reasoning process may be used not only for evaluation but also for assessment of treatment outcomes. Steps 1 through 5 are used for evaluation and then are repeated, with the addition of steps 5A through 10 for assessment of treatment. Step 6—a critical one—often is overlooked by therapists. Therapists all have "default patterns" in their thinking, or areas that they ignore or do not pay as much attention to. If they can identify the type of default patterns that they have, then default patterns can be guarded against through consultation, peer review, case conferences, or just plain awareness. For example, the author discovered her default pattern to be an overconcern with safety that limited client activity choices. In one instance, the author's students produced a major improvement in one client by allowing an activity that the author had thought would be too dangerous but that was not. Becoming cognizant of her default pattern allowed the author to let clients experience the more intense activities they needed while still addressing safety issues.

## Summary

The occupational therapist who uses a sensory integrative approach may be called on to explain that approach in terms of its effect on the end-product abilities, especially in school systems. Many children who are referred to occupational therapy within a school setting have been identified as having handwriting problems, praxis problems, or behavior problems. When the therapist determines that the child has or may have a problem with sensory integration, the therapist can best serve the child by explaining sensory system modulation to his parents and teachers.

Some major behavior problems that become apparent in the school are related to sensory system modulation. For example, a child who has been identified as having sensory defensiveness might (1) hit out at another child who bumps him in the playground or in the lunch line; (2) refuse to use any sticky materials such as paste or fingerpaint; (3) become outraged if pushed off balance; (4) be fearful of walking down stairs; (5) cover his ears during public system announcements; (6) act out, mainly in the cafeteria; or, (7) become upset if the class schedule is changed for a special event. If the teacher understands these things as sensory defensiveness and not solely as behaviors, she could respond in a more effective way.

When the occupational therapist provides consultation about a child who has problems with sensory integration, she helps the teacher solve problems that affect her classroom. Poor handwriting could be related to poor praxis, poor muscle tone, or poor cocontraction. Poor attention span could be the result of sensory defensiveness. Poor perceptual skills contribute to problems in reading and mathematics. The most important contribution that the occupational therapist can make in the school environment is to explain to school personnel what these problems mean in terms of behavior, how changes in input to the child's nervous system can change behavior, and how the therapist and the school personnel can work together to help the child succeed.

As with school personnel, the occupational therapist can assist the families of children who have sensory integrative problems to understand the child and his behavior. At times, increased understanding may allow parents or other care providers to shed their blame for "causing" the child's problems. The understanding of sensory system modulation alone should produce a major difference in dealing with a child's behavior. The change in environment that a parent can influence can also result in beneficial changes well beyond the reach of a therapy session. It can also give parents the opportunity to interact optimally with their children, thereby increasing self-esteem for children and parents alike. This can also produce successful coping strategies. To explain sensory integration to parents or care providers can be one of the most empowering roles for a therapist.

## Outline for Sensory Integrative Frame of Reference

I. Theoretical base
  A. Basic concepts
    1. Contributions of the subcortical areas of the brain to human behavior
    2. Six basic assumptions that underlie nervous system organization
      a. Hierarchical organization
      b. Cortical processing
      c. Registration of stimuli
      d. Brain innate organization
      e. Input from sensory systems
      f. Plasticity

g. Sequential development
B. The sensory systems
  1. Tactile system
  2. Proprioception
  3. Vestibular system
C. Sensory integrative functions
  1. Sensory system modulation
    a. Tactile
    b. Auditory
    c. Relationship to gravity
    d. Movement level
    e. Oral arousal
    f. Olfactory arousal
    g. Visual arousal
    h. Attention level
    i. Postrotary nystagmus
    j. Sensitivity to movement
    k. Proprioceptive sensitivity
    l. Emotional level
  2. Functional support capabilities
    a. Suck-swallow-breathe
    b. Tactile discrimination
    c. Other discriminative abilities
    d. Cocontraction
    e. Muscle tone
    f. Proprioception
    g. Balance and equilibrium
    h. Developmental reflexes
    i. Lateralization
    j. Bilateral integration
  3. End-product abilities
    a. Praxis
    b. Form and space perception
    c. Behavior
    d. Academics
    e. Language and articulation
    f. Emotional tone
    g. Activity level
    h. Environment mastery
D. Praxis
  1. Organization of sensory information
  2. Neuromechanism of the praxis sequence
  3. Building neuronal models
  4. Dyspraxia
E. Postulates of the sensory integration theoretical base

II. Function/dysfunction continua
A. Sensory system modulation
B. Functional support capabilities
C. End-product abilities

III. Evaluation
   A. Presenting problems
   B. Specific evaluation procedures
   C. Clinical reasoning process

IV. Postulates regarding change
   A. Those that relate to the use of the sensory integrative frame of reference
   B. Those that relate to sensory system modulation
   C. Those that relate to functional support capabilities
   D. Those that relate to end-product abilities

V. Application to practice
   A. Treatment considerations
      1. Treatment environment
         a. Physical space
         b. Physical safety
         c. Clinical equipment
      2. General considerations
         a. Role of the therapist
            1. Monitoring
            2. Feedback to the child
         b. Child needs to be self-directed
         c. Activities that facilitate appropriate physical and emotional adaptive responses
         d. Characteristics of an adaptive response
            1. Meaningful to the child
            2. Elicited when needed
            3. Reinforced by elicitation
            4. Active involvement of a child's CNS
            5. Interaction between the child and therapist
            6. Within the child's developmental level
         e. Adaptive emotional responses and the ideational responses
   B. Methods to facilitate adaptive responses
      1. Adaptive responses
         a. Addressing sensory system modulation problems
         b. Build up to complex motor planning activities
         c. Get the child actively involved in the activities
         d. Intervention specific to the underlying sensory systems deficits
         e. Balance structure and freedom
      2. Therapist involvement
         a. Hypothesizing
         b. In activities
         c. Selection of activities the child can complete successfully
         d. Flexibility
         e. Emotional safety
   C. Sequence of treatment
      1. Modulate the sensory systems
         a. Inhibitory
         b. Excitatory
      2. Function support capabilities

3. End-product abilities
   a. Praxis abilities
   b. Other end-product abilities
D. Clinical reasoning process

### Acknowledgments

The author is grateful to Joanne Lavigne for her patient preparation of numerous drafts of this chapter; to Pat Wilbarger for her review of portions of the manuscript and her helpful suggestions for content revisions; to Patty Oetter and Pat Wilbarger for their insight into the newest sensory integrative theory; and to Emily Sarah Kimball, my daughter, who posed for the mature responses and to her friend who graciously posed for the contrast pictures so that therapists could learn.

All photographs in the chapter (with the exception of 6.11, 6.14, 6.15, 6.25) were taken by C.C. Church, Portland, ME. Other photographs were taken by J. Kimball.

### References

American Occupational Therapy Association (1989). Guidelines for occupational therapy services in school systems (2nd ed). Rockville, MD: Author.

Ayres, A. J. (1965). Patterns of perceptual-motor dysfunction in children: a factor analytic study. *Perceptual and Motor Skills, 20,* 335–368.

Ayres, A. J. (1966a). Interrelations among perceptual-motor abilities in a group of normal children. *American Journal of Occupational Therapy, 20,* 288–292.

Ayres, A. J. (1966b). Interrelations among perceptual-motor functions in children. *American Journal of Occupational Therapy, 20,* 68–71.

Ayres, A. J. (1969). Deficits in sensory integration in educationally handicapped children. *Journal of Learning Disabilities, 2,* 160–168.

Ayres, A. J. (1971). *Sensory motor history.* Torrance, CA: Ayres Clinic.

Ayres, A. J. (1972a). *Sensory integration and learning disorders.* Los Angeles: Western Psychological Services.

Ayres, A. J. (1972b). *Southern california sensory integration tests manual.* Los Angeles: Western Psychological Services.

Ayres, A. J. (1972c). Improving academic scores through sensory integration. *Journal of Learning Disabilities, 5,* 338–343.

Ayres, A. J. (1972d). Types of sensory integrative dysfunction among disabled learners. *American Journal of Occupational Therapy, 26,* 13–18.

Ayres, A. J. (1975a). *Southern california postrotary nystagmus test manual.* Los Angeles: Western Psychological Services.

Ayres, A. J. (1975b). Sensorimotor foundations of academic ability. In W. M. Cruickshank & D. P. Hallahan (Eds.). *Perceptual and learning disabilities in children* Vol. 2 (pp. 301–338). Syracuse, NY: Syracuse University Press.

Ayres, A. J. (1976). *The effect of sensory integrative therapy on learning disabled children: The final report of a research project.* Los Angeles: University of Southern California.

Ayres, A. J. (1978). Learning disabilities and the vestibular system. *Journal of Learning Disabilities, 11,* 18–29.

Ayres, A. J. (1979). *Sensory integration and the child.* Los Angeles: Western Psychological Services.

Ayres, A. J. (1980). *Southern california tests of sensory integration tests manual: (Rev. ed.).* Los Angeles: Western Psychological Services.

Ayres, A. J. (1985). *Developmental dyspraxia and adult-onset apraxia.* Torrance, CA: Sensory Integration International.

Ayres, A. J. (1989). *Sensory integration and praxis tests.* Los Angeles: Western Psychological Services.

Beery, E. (1989). *The developmental test of visual-motor integration* (3rd rev. ed.). Cleveland, OH: Modern Curriculum.

Bender, L. (1938). A visual-motor gestalt test and its clinical use (Res. Mon. No.3). New York: American Orthopsychiatric Association.

Bruininks, R. H. (1978). *Bruininks-Oseretsky test of motor proficiency examiner's manual.* Circle Pines, MN: American Guidance Service.

Chusid, J.G. (1979). *Correlative neuroanatomy and functional neurology* (17th ed.). Los Altos, CA: Lange Medical Publishers.

Clark, F. A., Mailloux, Z., & Parham, D. (1989). Sensory integration and children with learning disabilities. In P. N. Pratt & A. S. Allen (Eds.). *Occupational therapy for children* (2nd ed.) (pp. 457–507). St. Louis: C.V. Mosby.

Colarusso, R. P., & Hammill, D. D. (1972). *Motor free visual perception test.* Novato, CA: Academic Therapy.

Daube, J. R., Reagan, T. J., Sandok, B. A., and Westmoreland, B. F. (1986). *Medical neuroscience.* Boston: Little, Brown.

DeGangi, G., & Greenspan, S.I. (1989). *Test of sensory functions in infants.* Los Angeles, CA: Western Psychological Services.

DeGroot, J. & Chusid, J.G. (1988). *Correlative neuroanatomy* (12th ed.). Connecticut: Appleton and Lange.

DeQuiros, J.B., & Schrager, O. L. (1979). *Neuropsychological fundamentals in learning disabilities* (rev. ed.). Novato, CA: Academic Therapy.

Dubner, R. (1991). Neuronal plasticity and pain following peripheral tissue inflammation or nerve injury. *Proceedings of the VIth World Congress on Pain.* New York, NY: Elsevier Science Publishers BV

Dunn, W. (1981). *A guide to clinical observation in kindergartners.* Rockville, MD: American Occupational Therapy Association.

Farber, S. D. (1982). *Neurorehabilitation: A multisensory approach.* Philadelphia: W. B. Saunders.

Farber, S. D. (1989, May). Neuroscience and occupational therapy: Vital connections. Eleanor Clark Slagle Lectureship at the American Occupational Therapy Association Annual Conference, Baltimore, MD.

Fisher, A. G., & Dunn, W. (1983). Tactile defensiveness: Historical perspectives, new research: A theory grow. *Sensory Integration Special Interest Section Newsletter, 6*(2), 1–2.

Fisher, A. G., & Bundy, A.C. (1989). Vestibular stimulation in the treatment of postural and related disorders. In O. D. Payton, R. P. Fabio, S. V. Paris, E. J. Protas, & A. F. Van Sant (Eds.), *Manual of physical therapy techniques* (pp. 239–258). New York: Churchill-Livingstone.

Fisher, A. G., Murray, E. A., & Bundy, A. C. (1991). *Sensory integration theory and practice.* Philadelphia, PA: F. A. Davis.

Fitzgerald, M. (1991). The developmental neurobiology of pain. *Proceedings of the VIth World Congress on Pain.* New, NY: Elsevier Science Publishers BV.

Gardner, M. F. (1988). *Test of visual-perceptual skills* (non-motor). San Francisco, CA: Health Publishing Co., Children's Hospital.

Gilfoyle, E. M., Grady A. P., & Moore, J. C. (1990). *Children adapt.* Thorofare, NJ: Slack.

Gold, P. W., Goodwin, F. K., Chrousos, G. P. (August 11, 1988). Clinical and biochemical manifestations of depression: relations to the neurobiology of stress, (Pt I). *New England Journal of Medicine.*

Gold, P. W., Goodwin, F. K., Chrousos, G. P. (August 18, 1988). Clinical and biochemical manifestations of depression: relations to the neurobiology of stress, (Pt II). *New England Journal of Medicine.*

Kandel, E. R. & Schwartz, J. H. (1985). *Principles of neural science.* New York: Elsevier.

Kaufman A. S., & Kaufman, N. L. (1983). *Kaufman assessment battery for children.* Circle Pines: American Guidance Service.

Kimball, J. G. (1976). Vestibular stimulation and seizure activity. *Center for the Study of Sensory Integrative Dysfunction Newsletter* (now Sensory Integration International), July, Torrance, CA.

Kimball, J. G. (1977). Case History Follow Up Report, Center for *The Study of Sensory Integrative Dysfunction Newsletter* (now Sensory Integrative International), Torrance, CA.

Kimball, J. G. (1981). Normative comparison of the Southern California Postrotary Nystagmus Test: Los Angeles vs. Syracuse data. *American Journal of Occupational Therapy, 34,* 21–25.

Kimball, J. G. (1986). Prediction of methylphenidate (ritalin) responsiveness through sensory integrative testing. *American Journal of Occupational Therapy, 40,* 241–248.

Kimball J. G. (1988). Hypothesis for production of stimulant drug effectiveness utilizing sensory integrative diagnostic methods. *Journal of the American Osteopathic Association, 88,* 757–762.

Kimball, J. G. (1990). Using the sensory integration and praxis tests to measure change: a pilot study. *American Journal of Occupational Therapy, 44,* 603–608.

Kimball, J. G. (1991). *Personal case records,* Scarborough, ME.

Larson, K. A. (1982). The sensory history of developmentally delayed children with and without tactile defensiveness. *American Journal of Occupational Therapy, 36,* 590–596.

Melzack, R., & Wall P. D. (1965). Pain mechanisms: A new theory. *Science,* 150, 971–979.

Montagu, A. (1978). *Touching: The human significance of the skin.* New York: Harper & Row.

Nieuwenhuys, R., Voogd, J., & Van Huijzen, C. (1988). *The human central nervous system.* New York: Springer-Verlag.

Oetter, P., Richter, E., & Frick, S. (1992). *MORE integrating the mouth with sensory and postural function.* Hugo, MN: PDP Products.

Pribam, K. (1975). Arousal, activation and effort in the control of attention. *Psychological Review, 82,* 116–149.

Routtenberg, A. (1968). The two arousal hypothesis: reticular formation and limbic system. *Psychological Review, 75,* 1, 51–80.

Royeen, C. B. (1985). Domain specifications of the construct tactile defensiveness. *American Journal of Occupational Therapy, 39*(9), 596–599.

Royeen, C. B. (1986). Development of a scale measuring tactile defensiveness. *American Journal of Occupational Therapy, 46*, 414–419.

Royeen, C. B. (1987). Test-retest reliability of a touch scale for tactile defensiveness in children. *Physical and Occupational Therapy in Pediatrics, 7*(3), 45–52.

Royeen, C. B., & Fortune, J. C. (1990). TIE: Touch inventory for school aged children. *American Journal of Occupational Therapy, 44*, 155–160.

Sagan, C. (1977). *Dragons of eden.* New York: Random House.

Wall, P. D. (1970). Sensory of impulses traveling in the dorsal columns. *Brain, 93*, 505–524.

Wechsler, D. (1974). *Intelligence scale for children revised.* Psychological Corporation, NY.

Wilbarger, P. (1984). Planning an adequate "sensory diet"—application of sensory processing theory during the first year of life *Zero to three* Sept, 1991, 7–12.

Wilbarger, P. (1991). *Occupational therapy: sensory defensiveness,* 60-minute video, PDP Products, Hugo, MN.

Wilbarger, P., & Oetter, P. (October, 1989). Sensory processing disorders. Paper presented at the American Occupational Therapy Association Practice Symposium, St. Louis, MO.

Wilbarger, P., & Royeen, C. B. (May, 1987). Tactile defensiveness: Theory, applications and treatment. Annual Interdisciplinary Doctoral Conference, Sargent College, Boston University.

Wilbarger, P., & Wilbarger, J. (1991). *Sensory defensiveness in children 2–12.* Santa Barbara, CA: Avanti Education Programs.

Wilcox, G. L. (1991). Excitatory neurotransmitters and pain. In M. R. Bond, J. E. Charlton, & C. J. Woolf, W. (Eds). *Proceedings of the VIth World Congress on Pain.* New York, NY: Elsevier Science Publishers BV.

Wilson-Pauwels, L., Akesson, E., & Stewart, P. (1988). *Cranial nerves.* Philadelphia, PA: B.C. Becker, Inc.

Woolf, C. J. (1991). Central Mechanisms of acute Pain. In M. R. Bond, J. E. Charlton, & C. J. Woolf (Eds). *Proceedings of the VIth World Congress on Pain.* New York, NY: Elsevier Science Publishers BV

*Appendix 6A.*    Presenting Problems: Children with Suspected Sensory Integration Dysfunction

For the identification of sensory systems dysfunction, several symptoms must occur together.

INFANCY
>    Irritable baby
>    Low muscle tone
>    Poor sleep cycles
>    May dislike being held
>    May dislike being on back
>    May startle easily
>    Slow development—or less than normal quality of movement

TODDLER
>    Above may continue with addition of the following:
>    Short attention span
>    Clumsiness
>    Poor articulation
>    Overly upset by slight injury
>    Fear of walking on some surfaces
>    Fear of slides, other movements
>    Very messy eater
>    Slow language development
>    Rejects many foods because of texture

CHILDHOOD Pre K to 3rd grade
>    Above may continue with additon of the following:
>    Fine motor problems (i.e., hand writing, cutting, coloring)
>    Hyperactivity
>    Poor social skills
>    Impulsiveness
>    Cries easily
>    Dislikes textures (i.e., fingerpaint, food)
>    Difficulties in gross motor activities
>    Falls easily
>    Often accidently breaks toys during play
>    Strong dislike for certain types of clothing

MIDDLE CHILDHOOD 4th–6th grade
>    Above continues with additions of the following:
>    Increased academic problems/attention
>    Behavioral problems
>    Poorly organized or compulsively organized
>    Reversals in writing and reading
>    Trouble keeping up with peers in activities

## PRE-ADOLESCENCE

Above may continue with additions of the following:
Organization problems
Trouble finishing homework/attention
Immature in physical skills and social relationships
More pronounced behavioral problems (i.e., acts out, picks fights)
Loses or forgets things
Often socially isolated
Chooses individual sports (i.e., running, swimming)
Chooses heavy contact sports (i.e., football, soccer)
Avoids team sports (i.e., basketball, baseball)
May be overly emotional

**Appendix 6B.**    Occupational Therapy Evaluation of Sensory Integrative Abilities

Name _____    Referred by _____

Test Date _____

Date of Birth _____

Chronological Age _____

Presenting Problem _____

_____

_____

_____

_____

_____

_____

I. Sensory Systems Modulation/Sensory Defensiveness

| System | Indicators | Summary | Sensory Defensiveness Present |
|---|---|---|---|
| Tactile | | | |
| Auditory | | | |
| Vestibular | | | |
|    Relation to Gravity | | | |
|    Movement level | | | |
|    PRNT | | | |
|    Sensitivity to Movement | | | |
| Oral | | | |
| Olfactory | | | |
| Visual | | | |
| Attention | | | |
| Proprioception | | | |
| Emotion | | | |

II. Information/Discriminative System

| System | Indicators | Summary | Contribution to What End-Product Problem |
|---|---|---|---|
| Tactile | | | |
| Auditory | | | |
| Vestibular | | | |
|    Relation to Gravity | | | |
|    Movement level | | | |
|    PRNT | | | |
|    Sensitivity to | | | |
|      movement | | | |
| Oral | | | |
| Olfactory | | | |
| Visual | | | |
| Attention | | | |
| Proprioception | | | |
| Emotion | | | |

III. Functional Support Capabilities

| Area | Indicator | Summary | Contributions to What End-Product Problem |
|---|---|---|---|
| Suck-breath-swallow | | | |
| Cocontraction | | | |
| Muscle tone | | | |
| Proprioception | | | |
| Balance/equilibrium | | | |
| Integrated reflex | | | |
|    development | | | |
| Laterality | | | |
| Bilateral integration | | | |

IV. End-Product Abilities

| Praxis | Indicators | Tests Used | Summary |
|---|---|---|---|
| Behavior | | | |
| Academics | | | |
| Language/articulation | | | |
| Emotional tone | | | |
| Activity level | | | |
| Environmental | | | |
|    mastery | | | |

*Appendix 6C.*    Synthesis of Occupational Therapy Sensory Integrative Evaluation

1. Presenting problems:
   a. What are the presenting problems?
   b. Can they be grouped into clusters such as:
      — Sensory system modulation problems
      — Information/discrimination problems
      — Functional support capability problems
      — End-product problems
   c. What are the child's particular strengths?

2. Sensory systems modulation/sensory defensiveness
   a. What evidence of modulation problems do you have?
      — Sensory history
      — Presenting problems
      — Parent/teacher report
      — Your evaluations
   b. Is the child sensory defensive?
      — What sensory systems are involved?
      — How severe are the problems?
      — Would you rate them as mild, moderate or severe?
   c. What end-product abilities might be affected by these problems?

3. Information/discriminative systems
   a. What evidence of information/discriminative system problems do you have?
      — Presenting problems
      — Parent/teacher report
      — Reports from other professionals
      — Your evaluations
   b. What systems are involved?
      — Do modulation problems interefere with processing?
   c. What end-product abilities might be affected by these problems?
   d. What are the child's particular strengths?

4. Functional support capabilities
   a. What evidence of problems with functional support capabilities do you have?
      — Presenting problems
      — Parent/teacher report
      — Reports from other professionals
      — Your evaluations
   b. What capabilities are invovled?
   c. Do modulation or information system problems contribute to the problems?
   d. What end-product abilities might be affected by the functional support capability problems?

   e. What are the child's particular strengths?

5. End-product abilities

   a. What evidence of end-product ability problems do you have?
      — Presenting problems
      — Parent/teacher reports
      — Reports from other professionals
            — IQ assessments
            — Educational assessments
            — Psychological assessments
            — SIPT results (see explanation below)[a]
            — Your evaluations

   b. What end product abilities are involved?

   c. Do modulation, information system, or functional support problems contribute to the end-product problems?
      — How do they contribute?

   d. What are the child's particular strengths?

6. Summary

   a. What are the major end-product ability problems?

   b. Are they contributed to by modulation, information, or functional support problems?

   c. How does your evaluation relate to the presenting problems?

   d. Are the child's problem based in sensory integrative processing deficits of inefficiencies?

   e. What are the child's particular strengths?

   f. What treatment do you recommend?
      — Occupational therapy using a sensory integrative frame of reference
      — Occupational therapy using another frame of reference
      — Educational intervention (for cortically based problems)
      — Psychological referral (for non sensory defensive behavior problems)
      — Others

[a] The SIPT may be given only by therapists who have advanced training and certification in its administration. Most therapists who give the SIPT hold Masters degrees. The beginning therapist may use the SIPT evaluations done by other therapists in their evaluation process. Therapists may refer children to SIPT certified therapists for SIPT evaluation and then consult with them concerning treatment planning. For an in-depth analysis of the interpretation of the SIPT see Fisher et al. (1991).

***Appendix 6D.*** Clinical Reasoning: Causal Explanation and Prediction of Patient Treatment Outcomes

| CRITICAL THINKING PROCESS: | QUESTIONS TO BE CONSIDERED BY THE THERAPIST: |
| --- | --- |
| 1. Brainstorm causes for the unexpected | What are the possible causal explanations for the child's inability to produce an adaptive response? |
| 2. Focus | Based on brainstorming, identify general categories or multiple factors to focus on. |
| 3. Find evidence for and against each possible cause | What additional information is needed to identify which factors are more likely responsible to explain the child's inability to produce an adaptive response? |
| | At this point, what is inadequate in your knowledge base? Where can you get adequate information? |
| 4. Theoretical perspective | Based on the theoretical base of the frame of reference, consider which neural processes are most likely to produce deficits in the system. Consider the complexity of the central nervous system and limitation on knowledge. |
| 5. Evaluate evidence | Assess the child's and therapist's performance (on videotape if possible). |
| | What relevant evidence shows up? |
| | Which possible explanation does it support? |
| | "What is the best thing about my evaluation/treatment?" "What did I do well?" "What can I do differently to facilitate a better adaptive response in my client?" Develop treatment objectives. Return to number 1 and use process to evaluate treatment. |
| | Continue process during treatment. |
| 5a. Evaluate evidence continued | How do we know treatment is/is not working? |
| | What evidence has been overlooked or not fully understood? |
| 6. Look at possible default patterns | Can normal "blind spots" or default patterns be identified? How can they be guarded against? Who can help me in this area? |
| 7. Gather more evidence | Try other hypotheses. |

8. Make decision

Make judgement on most likely factor or set of factors responsible for client's behavior.

9. Prediction

Predict change that would occur if therapist changes input to client.

What should effect be on client if we are right; exactly what should happen?

10. Evaluation

How would you evaluate your treatment/ evaluation session?

METACOGNITION:

The metacognitive portion of the process involves discussion of the following questions:

1. Thinking about thinking

We will follow the clinical reasoning process in which you just engaged. You will examine your thinking and reasoning process.

2. Define steps

How did you actually make the prediction? Identify the steps in the process.

3. Evaluate process

What was the most important part of the process for you?

What was most valuable for you?

Do you feel that this all was necessary?

What was helpful in directing or stimulating your thinking?

What hindered your thinking?

4. Generalize

What parts of this process are applicable to other types of clinical populations?

What are the general concepts of clinical reasoning that you may extract from this proccess?

# 7

# Visual Perceptual Frame of Reference: An Information Processing Approach

VALORIE RICCIARDONE TODD

Occupational therapists have long been interested in visual perception and its contribution to task performance. In the search to formulate a sound theoretical basis for treatment strategies directed at modifying or overcoming visual perceptual problems in children, occupational therapists have been influenced by cognitive and developmental psychology (Gibson, J.J., 1966; Gibson, E.J., 1969; Piaget, 1953), neurology (Luria, 1980), education (Frostig, 1973; Kephart, 1971), and optometry (Getman, 1965). In addition, occupational therapists, including Ayres (1972), Abreu (1984), Bouska (1985), Toglia (1989), and Warren (1990), have developed their own guidelines for intervention related to visual perceptual dysfunction.

Visual perception is the ability to interpret and use what is seen. Interpretation is a mental process involving cognition, which gives meaning to the visual stimulus. It is the continuous combined impact of visual experience, intersensory communication, and cognitive growth that serves the development of visual perceptual abilities. In this frame of reference perception is viewed as a cognitive process that "changes as a function of learning, labelling, and experience" (Mussen, Conger, & Kagan, 1969, p. 287).

Many children who have physical, developmental, or learning disabilities demonstrate difficulty interpreting and using visual information effectively from their environments. These children are described as having visual perceptual problems because they have not acquired adequate visual perceptual skills in spite of normal vision.

Visual acuity and ocular motor skills greatly influence visual perceptual performance. Researchers (Chedru, Leblanc, & Lhermitte, 1973; Gianutsos, 1987) and occupational therapists (Bouska, 1985; Warren, 1990) describe specific information about the direct influence that basic visual skills have on visual perceptual performance. They have proposed that visual perceptual deficits often may be misdiagnosed. They claim that what sometimes appear to be visual perceptual deficits actually are visual problems or ocular motor disturbances. Accordingly, it is essential that occupational therapists acquire information on vision and ocular motor skills to assist in assessing and analyzing their influence on visual perception and functional performance.

## Theoretical Base

The visual system has neural interconnections with all the other sensory systems (Ayres, 1972). During the processing of visual information, input received through the visual system is integrated with information from the other sensory systems. The importance of this intersensory integration cannot be undervalued; however, it will not be addressed in this chapter (see Chapter 6). This frame of reference addresses only those children who have adequate visual and ocular motor skills but who are unable to process and use visual input efficiently. It assumes that intersensory integration is adequate.

Visual perception is an interactive product that involves the reception of input through the visual system, intersensory integration of that visual input, and cognitive analysis. Each of these components does not function independently, but, rather, each influences the other and depends on one another to function optimally. As a child matures, visual perception depends on the function of the central nervous system (CNS), especially on cortical structures. Maturational improvements are seen through the increased speed, amount, and complexity of visual information that a child can process. Visual perception is not based on passive reception but occurs through an active process between the child and his environment. The child learns to perceive visually as he attends to, sorts out, and organizes visual information selectively based on previous experiences.

This theoretical base is divided into three major sections. The first section summarizes the information processing model and its relationship to visual perception. The second section defines and describes three cognitive processing skills integral to this frame of reference: visual attention, visual memory, and visual discrimination. The third section discusses the influence that learning has on the development of visual perceptual skills.

## Information Processing Approach

The information processing model explains the flow of information through the human cognitive system. It focuses on how the learner attends to, recognizes, transforms, stores, and retrieves information for later use (Miller, 1983). The information processing model also specifies the cognitive skills necessary to perform a visual perceptual task. It stipulates how important it is to understand the underlying reasons for failure or the conditions that influence performance (Toglia, 1989). The insert that follows summarizes the basic components of the model:

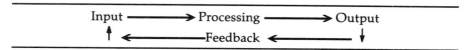

The flow of information begins with sensory input that is then processed. Processing requires that the sensory input be attended to, compared with previously stored information, transformed into some mental representation, and assigned meaning or acted on (Miller, 1983). All, or any of these operations, may be simultaneous or sequential.

Learning occurs from an interaction between the learner and his environment. Characteristics of the person that influence learning include prior knowledge, attitudes, motives, and cognitive style. Important characteristics of the task are whether it is visual or verbal, concrete or abstract, and so forth (Biehler & Snowman, 1990). Output can be observable behavior that reflects whether or not learning has occurred, or it can be mental information that is stored (Miller, 1983). Outputs that depend on visual perception include gross motor skills, fine motor skills, self-care, play, speech, and certain academic tasks. It is assumed in this model that learning has taken place when there is change in the child's observable behavior.

Feedback to the system comes from output, reinforcing observable behavior, and providing new input. It can be internal or external. Internal feedback comes from within the child. It consists of sensory and cognitive responses to the input that serve either to reinforce the output or to provide information that helps the child modify the output. External feedback is new input provided from another source that is separate from the child. It may come from another person or from the environment. For example, the therapist may point out that one triangle looks different from the others. An example of feedback from the environment would be when a child trips off a curb and has not seen the curb as a step. Feedback—both internal and external—is critical to learning and to the adaption of new experiences.

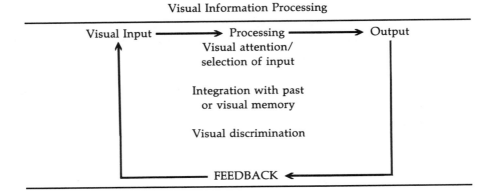

Visual Information Processing

From sensory **input** received through the visual system (visual input), children obtain information about their external environment. Visual input is received through the structures of the eye and is transmitted to the visual cortex, where it then is processed. The external presentation of visual input may be simple or complex, occur in small or great amounts, be in high or low contrast, or be organized or scattered. The presentation of visual input places varying demands on the ability to process effectively.

In using the information processing model to explain aspects of visual perception, three fundamental components are: **visual attention,** which involves the selection of visual input; **visual memory,** which involves the integration of visual information with previous experiences; and, **visual discrimination,** which is the ability to detect features of stimuli for perceptual differentiation, matching, and sorting.

## Processing Skills for Visual Perception

It is assumed that the cognitive processing skills of visual attention, visual memory, and visual discrimination depend on each other to function optimally. These skills are thought to overlap. It is believed that a deficit in any one of these skills can interfere with visual perceptual processing.

## Visual Attention

Visual attention is the ability to concentrate visually on some part or parts of the tangible environment. It is subject to the child's learning, experience, and developmental/cognitive level. As the child's ability to conceptualize and think about what he sees expands, so does his visual attention. Stimuli that attract attention are "objects, people, events and tasks that provide novelty, complexity, conflict, surprise and uncertainty . . . and that are presented for moderate or intermediate duration" (DeGangi & Porges, 1990). Three components of visual attention that affect learning are alertness, selective attention, and vigilance (DeGangi & Porges, 1990; Posner & Rafal, 1987).

Arousal is the transition from sleep to a waking state; **alerting,** however, is the transition from waking to attentive and alert state needed for active learning and adaptive behavior (Meldman, 1970). Children and adults alike usually adjust to any change or novelty in their environments. They habituate, or stop attending, however, when the stimuli are familiar and recognized or after repeated presentations. Characteristics that elicit orienting behavior are light, movement, and stimuli of high contrast and contour.

Because people have a limited capacity to attend, it is necessary to screen out irrelevant information. **Selective attention** is the ability to choose relevant visual information while ignoring the less relevant information. Selective attention often depends on the child's ability to attach some meaning to the visual array or to his reason for attending to a particular task (Levine, 1987). As familiarity and meaning increase, selective attention changes so that the child can habituate and screen out the familiar or unnecessary stimuli. In this way, he is free to attend to novel stimuli or to change the focus of his attention. Selective attention also is affected by the structure of the environment. It is easier to attend to and remember environmental features that are visually simple, organized, and nondistracting. An environment that is cluttered, disorganized, and highly stimulating often increases alerting behaviors and does not encourage a child to attend selectively to any one feature. If the child becomes overwhelmed by disorganization or distracting features, he will withdraw or become over active.

**Vigilance** is the conscious mental effort to concentrate and persist at a visual task. The quantitative aspect of attention determines the length of time a child spends on a visual task. This is affected by the child's understanding of the task requirements, motivation, problem solving skills, and reasoning capabilities, all of which determine his ability to sustain mental effort. Vigilance allows for deeper cognitive analysis.

### Visual Memory

The availability of stored information is essential to visual perception and learning. As visual information is received by a child, it is compared to and contrasted with previously experienced information that has been stored. Visual memory is defined as the ability to retain and recall past visual experiences.

Visual information needs to be coded for storage. This occurs through "control processes" that determine how the information is encoded. The initial control processes include attention, recognition, and rehearsal (Biehler & Snowman, 1990).

As previously stated, a child must be able to attend to information to remember it. Visual attention varies according to the task and the child's previous experiences. Visual recognition builds on attention and memory in that information is directed toward the meaning attached to or encoding the new information for future use. The way in which data are stored is not understood completely (Levine, 1987). Visual memory is classified according to its duration (i.e., short-term memory or long-term memory).

Visual short-term memory or "working memory" can hold a limited number of unrelated bits of information (seven, as in a telephone number) for approximately 30 seconds (Short-DeGraff, 1988). It has limited capacity and the information disappears if it is not processed further. Visual long-term memory is the permanent storehouse that has expansive capacity.

For information to be used later, it first must be coded and then stored in long-term memory. Coding of information depends on the child's ability to understand and structure data. He needs to associate new data with information already stored in his memory. If he has nothing to use for comparison, he may use rehearsal strategies. Maintenance rehearsal or pure repetition is used to hold information for immediate use. It has no effect on long-term storage. Elaborate rehearsal relates new information to information already stored in long-term memory and facilitates the transfer of this combined information to long-term memory. Coding in long-term memory may occur through semantic or linguistic associations or through imagery, categorization, and seriation. Imagery involves the relation of incoming data to meaningful images. Categorization involves the grouping of data into classes and subclasses, such as fruits and apples. Seriation requires the organization of data in a particular sequence.

Visual memory expands, allowing the child to deal with increased amounts of information, increased amounts of detail, and then, eventually, with visual sequences. A child must be able to remember increasing amounts of visual detail to allow him to compare and contrast complex designs; otherwise, speed and accuracy are sacrificed by constant rechecking (Banus, 1971). Children develop and learn how to use various techniques to remember data. Precision, speed of recall, and ease with which children can retrieve information all are indispensable learning skills (Levine, 1987).

Retrieval of information depends on registration and storage abilities. Recovery of information may be facilitated by association skills that link units of information together, and by recognition skills which rely on cues to elicit memory of a previously encountered stimulus. As a child becomes more capable of associating new information with a larger knowledge base, his memory improves. Simultaneously, as cognitive skills are refined, the child's capacity to store more information in long-term memory increases. The rate of retrieval expands, resulting in a more rapid ability to recognize and name visual information. By the age of seven years, the child is better able to use mnemonic strategies that involve rehearsal and imaging (Levine, 1987).

### Visual Discrimination

The learning of visual perceptual skills is believed to be similar to the learning of other skills. Part of this frame of reference draws from E. J. Gibson's theory of perceptual learning or perceptual differentiation learning (1963). Gibson (1963) proposed that a child must learn to deal with the vast amount of information that comes from his environment. The child learns to do this by responding to certain distinctive features in a specialized way. Consistent with this perspective, specific principles are fundamental to the cognitive analysis of visual information as it is transformed into visual discrimination.

Visual discrimination is the ability to detect distinctive features of a stimulus so that it can be recognized or identified as being the same as or different from a similar visual stimulus. This skill area is commonly thought to be synonymous with the label **visual perception.** Visual discrimination changes with age and is characterized by an increasing ability to recognize objects and to differentiate stimuli by attending to an increasing number of distinctive features. Distinctive features are the unique, identifiable, and distinguishable characteristics of a stimulus (Gibson, 1963). As the child develops, greater differentiation and precision occur in recognizing similarities and differences in visual stimuli. In this frame of reference, the development of visual discrimination is assumed to proceed from general to specific; from the whole to its parts; from concrete to abstract; and, from the familiar to the novel. These postulates about the formation of visual discrimination serve as the basis for the acquisition of specific visual discrimination skills.

**General to Specific.**    Initially, a child learns to recognize and discriminate objects based on attention to global structure and not by specific characteristics or details. Recognition of objects often is learned within the context of a familiar activity, for instance, through the child's repeated sensory motor play and functional use of an item. As experiences with objects increase, the child begins to group visually similar objects into what Piaget called **classes** (Richmond, 1970). Classes signify groups of objects with shared characteristics. To classify similar objects, the child must be able to extract the features that make the object part of a class. For example, a child may see a variety of cups and learn that they are cups because they hold liquid and have handles. Simultaneously, he may notice differences among cups and is able then to identify one specific cup as his own.

Labeling plays an important role in the process of visual discrimination. When objects are given distinctive names, it is easier for the child to perceive them as separate and different from each other (Mussen, Conger, & Kagan, 1969). Although children do not need to have language skills to develop visual discrimination skills, it is beneficial and facilitates the process.

As objects become more recognizable and classifiable, attention is paid not only to the overall shape or configuration but also to an item's specific characteristics. Gradually, the child is able to analyze more than one property at a time. Simultaneously, the ability develops to analyze the whole against the parts.

**Whole to Parts.**    To understand the relationship of the whole to its parts in visual discrimination requires not only the ability to recognize whole forms but also to become more aware of spatial organization and the relationship between components. The details of forms may be important, but so is the relationship between the details, which makes the process of differentiation more complicated (Kephart, 1971).

The development of discrimination of the whole to its parts is sequential. First, the child tends to be global in his observations. He perceives and reacts to an entire stimulus rather than to its parts, particularly if the stimulus is strange or not meaningful (Mussen, Conger, & Kagan, 1969). Then, he is able to attend to specific parts or to the whole, depending on his ability to understand the parts. If the parts are not understandable, he will attend to and categorize the stimulus by its global configuration. At this time, between the ages of four to seven years, some children can attend to the component parts but may have difficulty in relating these data back to the whole. Finally, children are able to attend to the whole and its parts simultaneously.

**Concrete to Abstract.** Another dimension in the acquisition of visual discrimination skills is the ability to go from concrete to abstract. Recognition skills begin with interactions between real objects that can be seen, felt, and manipulated. Then a child develops the ability to relate to and recognize familiar objects in two dimensions, in pictures. This is an example of symbolic or representational abilities that begin to emerge at this time. Young children develop the ability to see a picture as a representation of an object, just as later, when words become symbolic labels for objects. The progression in visual discrimination from concrete to abstract then moves from the concrete object to more representative forms (photographs, realistic colored drawings, line drawings, and, finally, abstract representations).

**Familiar to Novel.** Discrimination also progresses from familiar to unfamiliar or novel. As a child learns and has more experiences, he becomes familiar with more stimuli. Consequently, processing demands change. In looking at new visual stimuli, many children first may try to extract some familiar component to assist in recognizing or matching things to past experiences. Then, they may identify the different properties of the object so that they can see it as a new and distinct item.

## *Learning Visual Perceptual Skills*

This frame of reference is based on the belief that the development of visual perceptual skills is learned. According to this assumption, visual perception requires that the child make sense out of what he sees based on visual stimuli as he interacts with his environment. Learning provides the means to achieve this understanding. It is assumed that for visual stimuli to be understood and used, information from the visual system must be processed mentally and learning must take place. This mental processing involves more than conscious awareness and knowledge of objects through attention; it involves the integration of visual information through the cognitive realm of understanding. This includes the mental processes of thinking, understanding, knowing, and judging. The development of visual perceptual skills, therefore, is affected by learning and can be influenced directly by the teaching-learning process. More advanced learning results in abilities to sequence, categorize, form concepts, perform intellectual operations in space, problem solve, and generalize.

Research indicates that at birth a child has rudimentary visual skills (Anderson, 1986). As a child matures and interacts with his environment—which requires the use of the visual system—he refines his visual perceptual abilities. The development of specific visual perceptual skills is learned and influenced by the child's capabilities and the opportunities provided by his environment. Through this learning process, vision becomes seeing and the child acquires the essential skills that permit him to deal effectively with the spatial world.

## Specific Visual Discrimination Abilities

As visual attention and visual memory develop, specific visual discrimination abilities begin to emerge. They can be delineated in terms of recognition, matching, and sorting. Each requires the ability to note similarities and differences with increasing complexity and then relates these data back to previously stored information. This process is called **differentiation,** which is the cognitive aspect of noting similarities and differences and which results in the skills of recognition, matching, and sorting.

### Recognition

Recognition is the ability to note key features of a stimulus and relate them to memory (Biehler & Snowman, 1990). Memory is important to recognition because the identification of a familiar object requires comparison against stored information. Recognition is the first step in the development of visual differentiation. It requires the child to note and remember features that make an object identifiable. As the child matures, more sophisticated visual discrimination abilities allow the child to recognize more subtle similarities and differences among objects and then label them. Gradually, he is able to recognize immediately a wide variety of stimuli. As these recognition skills expand, they allow for quicker, more accurate, and more refined interpretations of the visual world. An example of this occurs in reading when words become recognizable immediately as opposed to sounding out each letter to read the word. Thus, reading becomes quicker and easier.

### Matching

Another visual discrimination skill is matching. Matching is the ability to note the similarities among visual stimuli. In matching tasks, a specific object or quality is identified (Fig. 7.1). Then all other stimuli are compared to that object or quality, to identify whether it is the same or different. Toddlers and preschoolers spend a lot of time examining things to see whether or not they match. During these stages of development, when children are involved in a single matching task, they may switch the attribute that they are matching because they have not developed "rule-bound" behavior.

Matching skills tend to develop sequentially. Children initially match things based on similarities rather than on differences. In young children, this leads to overgeneralization. As the child's range of skills expands, the child sees and attends to new and different aspects of objects, even those that are familiar to him (Ruff, 1980). The distinctive features of an object's attributes, such as size, color, and shape, become increasingly more relevant. This provides the child with the ability to match along these parameters. Then the child is able to sort and categorize objects in various ways based on one or more distinctive features.

Matching according to the attributes of size, color, and shape seems to precede the ability to differentiate spatial changes. Younger children often do not pay attention to changes in position (Gibson, 1963). For example, a child views his teddy bear as his teddy bear no matter what position it is in or from what position he views it. Such perception is based on the child's ability to see objects as having invariant properties; this is known as **perceptual constancy.** This early skill may explain why younger children relate to an "M" in the same way that they relate to a "W" and a "b" in the same way as a "d" because the letters apparently look alike, no matter what their position may be.

Children begin to detect the positional difference of upside-down and right-side-up (inversions) before left and right (reversals) or before other spatial orientations (angles or tilt). As children get older, about the age of seven years, spatial orientations seem to become more relevant. Children become more able to detect and react to such things as reversals and angle tilt. This may be one reason why reversals by children are common until the age of seven.

### Sorting

Another visual discrimination skill is sorting. Sorting does not rely only on noting visual similarities and differences; it actually is a higher level of cognitive skill. When sorting, the child is asked to look at a group of items and determine which one is different (Fig. 7.2). This sorting or categorizing task does not usually provide a concrete sample or stimulus for comparison.

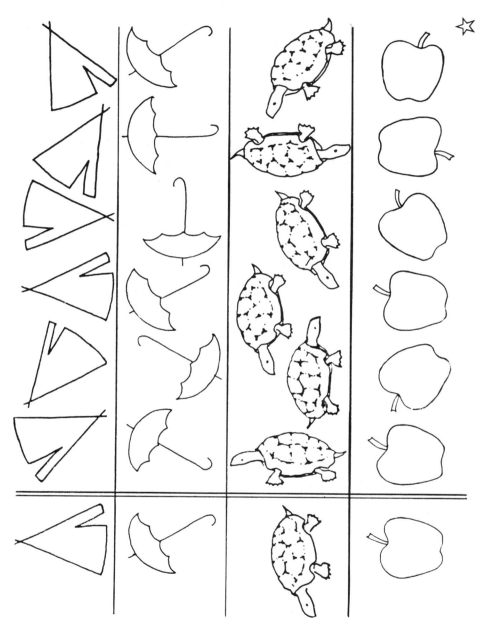

Figure 7.1.   A matching task

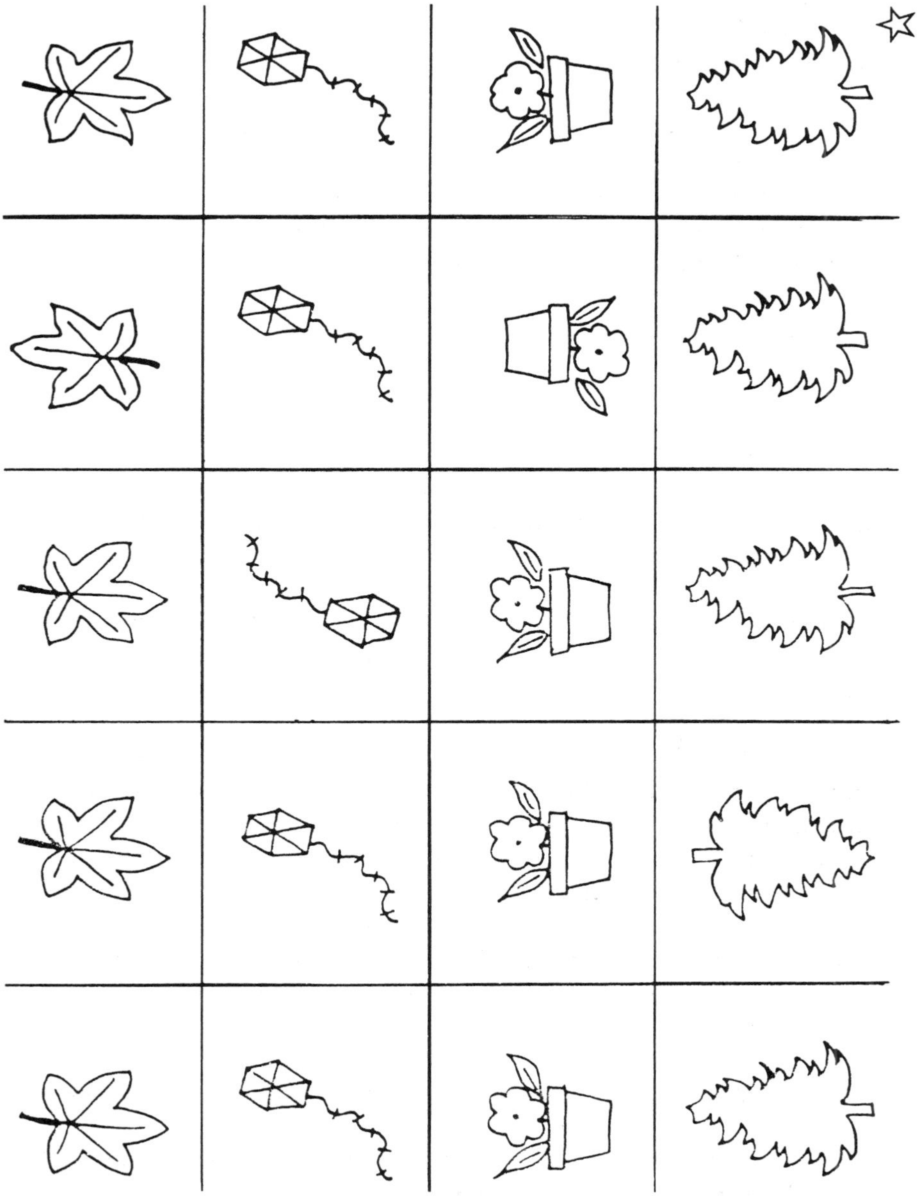

Figure 7.2   A sorting task

Instead, it requires the child to determine mentally a quality or category on which similarities or differences can be noted. It is more abstract because it requires mental manipulation and visual comparison of each item to others in some organized fashion. A similar cognitive ability, seriation, must be used in size sequencing tasks, such as nesting cups and graduated pegs. The child must be able to determine size relationships among a group of objects and then be able to organize them in a graduated series. This requires simultaneous comparisons of each item to the others in the group. The greater the number of items, the more complex the task. Story sequence cards are even more abstract because interpretations about the actions in each picture must be made and then organized into a logical sequence.

## Summary

Visual perception is an interactive result of sensory input received through the visual system, intersensory integration, and cognitive analysis. The information processing model provides a means for understanding how sensory input, such as visual information, is processed. Combined with cognitive analysis, it provides a useful model for explaining the process of turning sensory input received through the visual system into visual perception.

Three cognitive processing skills fundamental to visual perception are visual attention, visual memory, and visual discrimination. Important aspects of visual attention that affect learning are alertness, selective attention, and vigilance. Visual memory involves the coding and storage of information into long-term and short-term memory. Visual discrimination is assumed to proceed from general to specific; from the whole to its parts; from the concrete to the abstract; and, from the familiar to the novel. Discrimination skills depend on visual attention and visual memory.

Specific visual discrimination skills include the cognitive process of noting similarities and differences, which results in the skills of recognition, matching, and sorting. Three major theoretical postulates form the basis of this frame of reference:

1. Visual perception is learned through interaction with the human and nonhuman environments.
2. The acquisition of visual perceptual skills is a complex process affected by learning and moves from general to specific, whole to parts, concrete to abstract, and familiar to novel.
3. Although each visual perceptual skill develops in its own sequence, the acquisition of each skill affects the acquisition of other skills.

# Function/Dysfunction Continua

Function/dysfunction continua provide therapists with descriptions of observable behaviors that are clinically relevant and that identify function as well as dysfunction in children.

## *Visual Attention*

Visual attention provides a child with information about the physical environment and his relationship in it. It informs him of the presence and physical characteristics of objects and people. It assists him in knowing where he is in space and about his relationship to objects in the environment.

The child must be in a balanced state of arousal, ready to receive visual information. Selective attention assists in choosing which of the available stimuli is most likely to be useful. This is refined even more through learning, where the child understands the relationship of the whole to its parts. Vigilance to visual stimuli allows for greater precision in the discrimination of subtle differences among stimuli.

If a child has difficulty in visual attention, then visual perception may be affected. The child may be overaroused or underaroused by sensory input received through the visual system. He may not be able to select the features that require more attention or analysis. In addition, he may miss the relationships between objects needed for further recognition, discrimination or storage. If he is unable to persist in an activity because of short attention span, he may miss important details or relationships between stimuli. He may not attend long enough to store information in his memory.

**Alertness**

| Normal visual attention | Overattentive<br>Underattentive<br>Poorly sustained |
|---|---|
| FUNCTION: Normal state of arousal | DYSFUNCTION: Poorly maintained level of arousal |
| BEHAVIORS INDICATIVE OF FUNCTION: | BEHAVIORS INDICATIVE OF DYSFUNCTION: |
| Alert, attentive to visual stimuli | Overattentive:<br>Overly distracted by visual stimuli |

*—continued*

Orients to visual stimuli
comfortably and easily

Demonstrates adequate amount
and length of wakefulness

Sleeps restfully and for adequate
amount of time

Normal activity level

Continual visual searching
behaviors, rarely maintains
attention

Underattentive:
Difficult to arouse or alert to
visual stimuli

"Habituates" quickly to stimuli
that are too simple or too
complex

Fatigues easily after attempts to
attend; sleeps or "tunes out";
looks away, shuts eyes, moves
away

Erratic sleep/wake cycles; restless
sleep patterns; tired during
daytime

Poorly sustained attention:
General high activity level;
constant need to move and
interact with the environment

Easily distracted by objects,
persons, and things in the
environment

## Selective Attention

| Selectively Attends to Visual Stimuli | Reduced Ability to Selectively Attend to Visual Stimuli |
|---|---|
| FUNCTION: Ability to attend to relevant visual information while inhibiting irrelevant information | DYSFUNCTION: Difficulty in selecting and attending to relevant visual information |
| BEHAVIORS INDICATIVE OF FUNCTION: | BEHAVIORS INDICATIVE OF DYSFUNCTION: |
| Able to orient to and visually attend to relevant stimuli | Difficulty screening out unimportant information |
| Screens out unimportant visual information | Tends to focus on irrelevant or unimportant stimuli |
| Attends to an object in an array, such as a detail in a picture or a word in a sentence | Easily confused or distracted by unimportant stimuli, details, or extraneous stimuli |
| | Difficulty attending visually to information that would be helpful to a task |

**Vigilance**

| Concentrate on and Persist at a Visual Task | Reduced Persistence on a Visual Task |
| --- | --- |
| FUNCTION: Ability to concentrate on and persist at a visual task | DYSFUNCTION: Unable to concentrate or persist on a visual task |
| BEHAVIORS INDICATIVE OF FUNCTION: | BEHAVIORS INDICATIVE OF DYSFUNCTION: |
| Visually attends to task for appropriate length of time for adequate performance | Cursory examination of visual stimuli; is not vigilant enough to allow for identifying visual details |
| | Cannot maintain visual attention for an appropriate length of time to allow for adequate performance |

## *Memory*

Children who exhibit functional memory skills can recognize familiar people, objects, and symbols. Adequate visual attention is a prerequisite for the development of functional short-term and long-term memory skills. Short-term memory is particularly susceptible to distraction. Some children who have long-term memory deficits may have a tendency to remember unusual, nonsalient data that are not pertinent to the task. They often have a good selective memory for specific information, but this ability is not generalized. These children may rely too heavily on rote. They are less likely to relate new information to prior knowledge (Levine, 1987).

**Visual Memory**

| Adequate Visual Memory | Poor Short-Term Memory; Poor Long-Term Memory |
| --- | --- |
| FUNCTION: Ability to adequately recall visual information | DYSFUNCTION: Poor or reduced ability to recall visual information to store & retrieve visual information in short- or long-term memory |
| BEHAVIORS INDICATIVE OF FUNCTION: | BEHAVIORS INDICATIVE OF DYSFUNCTION: |
| Visually attends well enough to remember visual stimuli | Fails to attend to visual input adequately enough for storage |
| Identifies visual stimuli that were presented, even briefly | Inability to recognize or match visual stimuli presented previously |

*—continued*

| | |
|---|---|
| Remembers sound-symbol relationships for reading | May have good memory for life experiences but not for factual material |
| Remembers sequences needed for writing words | Poor ability to use mnemonic strategies for storage and relies on rote; fails to relate information to prior knowledge |
| Able to use mnemonic strategies to improve memory stores | Response time may be prolonged as memory is explored |
| | Inconsistent recall abilities |

## Specific Visual Discrimination Abilities

As a child develops the ability to detect various features that make objects unique, he develops a complementary ability to recognize and discriminate objects. When he begins to notice the similarities and differences among many objects, he can match and sort by shape, size, color, number, position, and detail.

Children who have problems with perceptual differentiation are unable to identify objects from their features. These children also have difficulty in recognizing similarities and differences between similar stimuli. Because of these deficits, such children usually are unable to make quick, accurate, and refined interpretations of visual information.

Some children demonstrate poor visual discrimination through difficulty in matching tasks. They may continue to match along a more general feature and not attend to other distinguishing characteristics or details. Some children have difficulty in distinguishing similar shapes or size and color differences. Such deficits in school-aged children may be noticed on worksheets that require the child to find a match to a stimulus figure. The child may perform adequately when the choices are highly disparate from the stimulus, but errors tend to increase when many details or differences are subtle. These children may go on to have difficulties in recognizing letters and numbers, which may affect their abilities to write and read.

Some children demonstrate poor visual discrimination in their difficulty to perform sorting tasks. Their task performance is much like that of children who have difficulties with matching. For example, the child who has problems with sorting may be unable to pick out like figures from a row of stimuli.

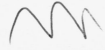

**Specific Visual Disc**

| **Adequate Sp** | **equate Visual** |
| **Discriminat** | **mination Skills** |

FUNCTION: Ability to recognize, match, and sort based on visual stimuli

DYSFUNCTION: Inadequate ability to recognize, match, and sort

BEHAVIORS INDICATIVE OF FUNCTION:

BEHAVIORS INDICATIVE OF DYSFUNCTION:

Recognizes previously experienced objects and symbols

Matches objects, shapes, and symbols based on color, size, shape, and position

Sorts objects, shapes, and symbols based on color, size, shape, and position

Responds appropriately to component parts (details) within a complex visual design while maintaining relationship to the whole

Attends to spatial orientation of letters, numbers, words, and so forth

Able to distinguish proper spatial orientation and identify reversed letters, numbers, and so forth.

Poor recognition skills of familiar objects or symbols

Poor matching skills

Difficulty in matching objects, shapes, colors, and symbols

Difficulty in matching same shape presented in a different spatial orientation

Confuses similar shapes, such as square/rectangle, and letters, such as b/d, u/n, m/w, K/X , E/ F, A/H, M/W, O/Q, P/R, g/p/q

Poor sorting skills

Requires a stimulus to match; unable to formulate mental set

Unable to determine which object, shape, or symbol is different in an array

Difficulty in recognizing form within a complex field (embedded or overlapping)

Overlooks details and misses the important information

Overattends to details and misses the big picture

Reverses letters, numbers, and words

Poor organizational abilities; confuses where to start and how to proceed

# Evaluation

Before assessing visual perceptual skills, it is important for occupational therapists to screen for visual difficulties. Although occupational therapists are not expected to perform vision evaluations, they may screen children for visual input disorders, to make appropriate referrals to other professionals. Included in Appendix 7.A is an appropriate tool for clinical vision screening. In addition to this tool, Appendix 7.A also includes a checklist that may be useful in documenting behaviors that might warrant a complete ophthalmic evaluation.

When assessing a child's visual perception, a therapist should use age-appropriate visual input. If the task is too complex for the child to perform, the therapist should simplify it to a level of presentation where the child is successful. In this way, a therapist presents tasks at the child's functional level and can determine what modifications are needed to elicit the child's best performance.

## *Visual Attention Skills*

Visual attention skills often are related to a child's general attention abilities. To observe a child who performs various tasks and activities provides the therapist with a good indication of that child's overall attention skills, including visual attention. When possible, the therapist should assess a child's attention span in a variety of environments and under various conditions. For example, a child may perform optimally in a one-to-one situation over a relatively short period of time but may be unable to attend in the classroom. He may perform his best for a new person but does not perform consistently for familiar people, like his parents or teachers. Both parents and teachers are important sources of information about the setting in which a child might be having difficulty attending or concentrating. When it is not possible to interview a parent or teacher and additional information is needed, a therapist may find that a questionnaire is helpful.

When assessing a child, it is important to realize that even some age-appropriate tasks can provoke inattention and distraction because of the child's inability to perform the task. Assessment of a child's visual attention skills can be guided by answering the following questions:

What types of visual stimuli attract and hold his attention?
Are additional sensory cues necessary, such as auditory or tactile cues to gain his attention?

Does he become annoyed by attempts to engage his attention?
How much structure is necessary to gain his attention?
How long can he attend to age-appropriate visual tasks?
Is he "overly active" or "hyperactive" and truly unable to sit still?
Is he lethargic and difficult to arouse?
What types of stimuli (auditory, visual, olfactory, movement) distract him from the task?
Does he demonstrate incessant visual searching?
Does he tend to "tune out" visually?
Does he become fatigued during tasks that require sustained visual attention?
Does his performance deteriorate or improve with certain types of tasks?
Can he be redirected to the task?
Can his distraction level be decreased by restructuring the environment?
Are manipulative, three-dimensional objects more alluring than pictures?
Are colored pictures more interesting than black and white pictures?

## Evaluation of Visual Memory

Again, reports from parents and teachers regarding a child's memory may be helpful. These reports are especially valuable in gaining data about a child's long-term memory. Some questions to guide assessment in this area are:

Is the child better at remembering experiences that are multisensory and autobiographical than remembering isolated bits of semantic information (school work)?
Is he consistent in his ability to recognize and name objects or symbols (letters or numbers)?
Does he remember old, familiar stimuli but have difficulty with new, unfamiliar stimuli?
Does information have to be repeated for him to remember it?
Is his memory erratic? That is, does he sometimes remember information one day and forget it the next?

Several standardized assessments exist to test short-term visual memory for children over four years of age. Two standardized tests that have sections specifically related to visual memory are the Motor Free Visual Perceptual Test (MVPT) (Collarusso & Hammill, 1972) and the Test of Visual Perceptual Skills (TVPS) (Gardner, 1982).

To gain information about how a child codes his visual information for storage, a therapist can question the child about how he remembers the figure. Did he name the figure (semantic memory)? Did he rely on immediate revisualization (eidetic memory)? Did he look at one part or another, or did he take in the gestalt? During the assessment, the therapist needs to consider how effective the child's strategies are. To collect additional information, a therapist may suggest an alternative strategy to assess whether the child is able to use it.

Error analysis of the task performance and the individual items of the standardized assessments may reveal that a child is having difficulty in "remembering" visual stimuli when he must choose from an array of figures. Selection of a matching figure from an array of figures requires that a child be able to attend to internal details or to spatial rotations. Memory may be influenced by poor discrimination abilities.

If a child is having difficulty with a standardized test and it appears that the problem lies with sustaining visual attention, the therapist may want to adapt the testing procedures. Before each item the therapist may want to cue the child to keep his eyes on the page until the page is turned. Then, the therapist should not turn the page until the child makes eye contact with the stimulus. In this case, the standardized scores cannot be used.

## Evaluation of Specific Visual Discrimination Skills

Before the age of four, a child has basic visual discrimination skills acquired through the use of matching tasks with three-dimensional objects. Matching identical objects precedes matching pictures and symbols such as shapes, letters, and numbers. Matching progresses along the parameters of size, shape, color, texture, and, eventually, position and increasing amount of detail.

Formboards and single-piece puzzles are ways to evaluate early discrimination of shape. Nesting blocks and graduated cylinders—types of sorting tasks—indicate how a child is beginning to perceive size relationships among a group of same-shaped items. Does the child use a lot of trial and error or does he "see" some relationships before touching the item? Does he use trial and error after it is no longer age-appropriate? Does the child appear to have a plan or does he work at random? For some skills, norms can be found in many developmental checklists.

Many tests for visual perception also assess visual discrimination in two dimensions after the age of four. Most of these tests separate visual discrimination into different subtests, such as form constancy, form discrimination, figure-ground, and spatial relationships. These tests often overlap, however, and do not test one parameter exclusive of the others. Form constancy is one such example. The child must be able to identify a given form (usually located as a detail in one figure) in an array of several figures. This item can require figure-ground skills, selective attention, or the ability to discriminate a whole form from its parts. For our purposes, these motor-free matching tests of visual perception assess visual discrimination capabilities across the parameters of general to specific, whole to parts, simple to complex, few to many, concrete to abstract, and familiar to novel. Like their counterparts in language evaluation, these tests can be considered to delineate the child's "receptive" visual perceptual capabilities. Other visual motor tasks can be considered to show the "expressive" visual perceptual capabilities. When a child is doing poorly in this type of matching task—for instance, of identifying one stimulus in an array of four or five—the therapist must often do her own task analysis to determine where the breakdown in visual analysis may be. She needs to look at the items along the parameters of total to parts, simple to complex, and few to many, as well as to changes in spatial orientations.

Some children begin to have difficulty when the amount of detail within a figure begins to increase, when a number of the choices closely resemble the stimulus, or when the stimulus is abstract or unfamiliar. They also may have a problem when the differentiating characteristic is a change in position. It may be easy to determine whether a figure is upside down (inverted) but not whether it is tilted or reversed (left/right confusion).

Because of specific deficits, a child may be unable to respond to a standardized test. Sometimes, modifications of the test yield more useful information. It is important to note that this invalidates the test score but it may provide information that helps the therapist in the intervention process. For example, children who have scanning or attention problems may perform better on discrimination tasks if each item in the array is presented in isolation by covering all others (Fig. 7.3). In this way a therapist can see discrimination abilities at a simple level and recognize the interference when multiple stimuli are present.

Many tests of visual perception include a section in which the child is asked to identify which stimulus is different. Young children especially have a difficult time with this, possibly because of poor language comprehension of the concept "different." Sometimes it is because of a poor ability to sort— that is, the ability to establish a class by which all but one of the stimuli match. The therapist must determine which factor may be interfering in this task. Possible factors are (1) difficulty with language concept; (2) inability to sort cognitively; or (3) poor visual discrimination of the items in the set.

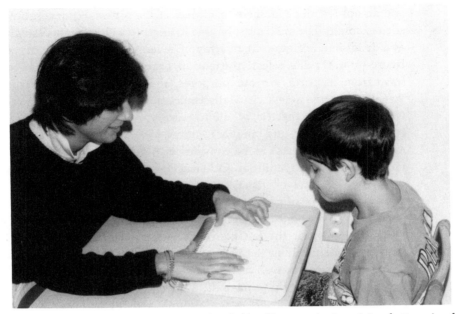

**Figure 7.3**    Eliminating extraneous visual stimuli can assist in gaining better visual attention.

Tests commonly used to evaluate visual perception include motor tasks that rely heavily on visual discrimination skills, particularly parts-to-whole relationships. These "expressive" tasks may include the copying of three-dimensional block designs and two-dimensional graphic designs. Block designs are included in many developmental assessments such as the Miller Assessment for Preschooler (Miller 1982) and the Peabody Developmental Motor Scales (Folio & Fewell, 1983), and usually are located in the fine motor or adaptive skills sections of these tests.

These tasks are not used to assess the quality of motor output but, rather, the ability to process a complex form, break it down into its components and reorganize the parts into an accurate copy (Fig. 7.4). The child's motor control must be looked at separately. If a child has a motor deficit, these tests may not be appropriate.

When a therapist presents three-dimensional tasks, she can gain a great deal of information about a child's specific visual discrimination skills. A therapist should observe the following:

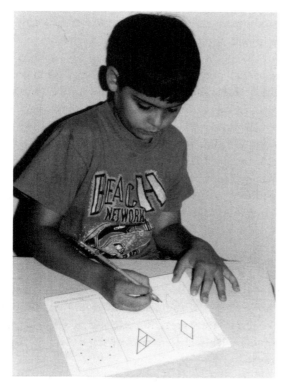

**Figure 7.4**   Copying two-dimensional designs

- The child's ability to orient vertical, horizontal, diagonal, and circular spatial coordinates.
- The child's ability to use "null space" in designs.
- The child's ability to combine lines and planes to make a shape or design.
- The child's attention to details. For example, are all the parts present? If some parts are missing, which are they? If there are extras, what has been added?
- The child's ability to orient the parts in relation to one another.
- The child's errors in rotation, inversion, and reversal.

Another technique for assessing specific visual discrimination skills involves design copy or reproduction of a presented design. Motor control influence sometimes can be reduced when a child is given larger objects from which to copy designs, or when vertical building is not required and designs lie flat on a surface. In addition, larger spaces on which to copy graphic designs sometimes can improve perceptual performance and decrease motor demands.

Beyond analyzing the visual perceptual errors that a child makes when performing a motor task, a therapist can find out additional information about how a child processes information by talking with him. Specifically, a therapist can ask a child if he thinks his reproduction matches the stimulus. If he can identify his errors in duplication and attributes them to the fact that his hand did not do what he wanted it to, then the problem may be in motor control rather than in visual perception. Whenever a therapist asks a child to describe what he is doing or why, she should be sensitive to the child's ability to admit his own errors and then take this factor into consideration.

## *Summary*

A child usually is referred for occupational therapy evaluation because of an observable performance deficit. In this frame of reference, problems of concern are caused by inadequate interpretation and use of visual input. This determination has to be made within the context of the overall occupational therapy evaluation findings.

When the evaluation is completed, all information must be analyzed and interpreted within a broader context of the child's other capabilities, which may include visual receptor skills; sensory motor processing, fine motor control, and skill development; and, other cognitively based processes such as language, reasoning, and problem-solving. The complete occupational therapy evaluation could include many of these areas. Additional information may be obtained by reviewing other records, such as psychological, speech, and language reports. When analyzing visual perceptual performance, it must be viewed within the context of other cortical skills. Often, visual perceptual problems are seen in conjunction with other cortically based problems, such as language, reasoning, and problem-solving difficulties. When visual perceptual problems are identified in conjunction with other cortically based problems, it is important not to isolate the visual perceptual deficits from other problems. Analysis of evaluation findings determines whether the poor performance on the visual perceptual part of the evaluation is primarily caused by deficiencies in visual perceptual skill areas or whether it is a reflection of global cognitive difficulties, inadequate visual reception, or poor motor abilities.

# Postulates Regarding Change

When the evaluation results indicate a perceptual dysfunction, the therapist must address the components that interfere with function. The postulates regarding change can be used to formulate treatment strategies for the perceptually impaired child.

Five general postulates are related to the use of learning within this frame of reference:

1. If a child is provided with an environment that includes appropriate visual stimulation, then the child will likely respond to the stimulation and learn from interaction with his environment.
2. If a child is provided appropriate visual learning experiences, then he will learn to direct his attention, memory, and discrimination abilities cognitively.
3. Learning is increased when it begins at the child's current level and proceeds at a rate that is comfortable for the child.
4. Learning is facilitated if a child is provided challenging activities at or slightly beyond his current functional level.
5. Learning is enhanced when a child understands what is to be learned and the reason for learning.

It is important that a child develop visual attention to gain visual information about his physical environment. Four postulates regarding change are related to visual attention:

6. Visual attention is facilitated when the child is in an appropriate state of physical and mental preparedness.
7. Visual attention is facilitated by novelty, complexity, conflict, surprise, and uncertainty.
8. Selective visual attention is enhanced when less relevant stimuli are at a minimum.
9. Concentration and persistence in visual tasks increase if motivation, comprehension, and intrinsic interest are present.

Adequate visual attention is a prerequisite for the development of functional short-term and long-term memory skills. Four postulates regarding change are related to visual memory:

10. Visual memory is enhanced when visual attention, motivation, and comprehension are present.
11. Visual memory is enhanced when a visual stimulus is combined with additional sensory input such as tactile, proprioceptive, or auditory input.
12. Visual memory is enhanced through repetition. Repetition can be exact or varied.
13. Visual memory is enhanced by seriation, imagery, and mnemonic strategies.

Six postulates regarding changes are related to visual discrimination:

14. If visual stimuli are presented in a clearly organized manner then visual attention, memory, and discrimination are enhanced.
15. Visual discrimination is enhanced when the visual arrangement is presented clearly, organized simply, and properly positioned in relationship to the child, in a well lit environment.
16. Visual discrimination is enhanced by drawing specific attention to the distinctive features of the object, recognition, and verbal labeling.
17. Object recognition is enhanced by sensory motor play and functional use of objects.
18. Visual discrimination is enhanced when the visual stimuli are presented along the continua of general to specific, whole to parts, familiar to unfamiliar, and concrete to abstract.
19. Visual discrimination is enhanced when relationships among stimuli or internal parts of the visual stimulus are recognized.

# Application to Practice

Intervention related to visual perception difficulties requires that a child learn to attend to visual information and to use cognitive analysis to process that sensory input.

## *Teaching/Learning*

This frame of reference is based on the belief that the development of visual perceptual skills is a learned process. The occupational therapist who uses this frame of reference is concerned with how a child **learns** to make sense out of what he sees. An essential aspect of occupational therapy intervention is to facilitate the child's learning through the teaching/learning process. Teaching principles are used by a therapist to help a child process visual stimuli in a meaningful way. Learning requires a child to change his attitudes about specific stimuli based on repeated experiences. A therapist assists in this learning process by creating an environment that encourages a positive change in the child's behavior.

Based on the work of Mosey (1986), the following principles of learning have been accepted as fundamental for this frame of reference:

---

- To foster learning, a therapist selects activities and creates an environment that reflects a child's aptitude, age, sex, and interests.

- A child's learning is affected by his motivation to engage in or complete a specific activity. His learning is increased if he is actively involved in the activity.

- A child is more likely to learn from an experience if he initiates and engages in the activity himself.

- For a child to learn from an experience, it must begin at the child's current level of functioning and proceed at a rate that is comfortable for him.

- Learning is enhanced if the child receives positive reinforcement and feedback as the consequence of his action.

- Trial and error, shaping, and imitation of models all are important learning techniques.

- Repetition and practice are important aspects of learning.

- For a child's learning to be optimized, the learning environment needs to be supportive and appropriate for the activity.

- When planning a learning experience, a therapist must be prepared to deal with the child's conflicts and the frustrations inherent in the learning process.

---

These general teaching/learning principles apply to all aspects of intervention within this frame of reference.

## Visual Attention

Visual attention is facilitated when the child is appropriately prepared, both physically and mentally. When a child has difficulty with any aspect of visual attention, the therapist must be concerned with creating an environment that improves his attention and task performance.

Knowledge about a child's overall alertness and emotional state is important to know so that therapy sessions and activities can be organized properly. General sensory stimulation or inhibition may need to be performed during or before visually oriented activities. At times, the sensory integrative frame of reference (see Chapter 6) may be effective before the visual perceptual frame of reference is used. If a child is overaroused, sensory and motor

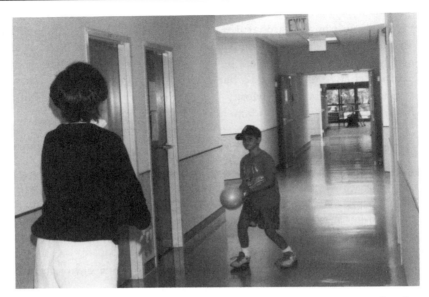

**Figure 7.5**  Visual attention can be encouraged through various eye-hand coordination activities.

activities may be used to calm him. If a child is underaroused, motor activities can be used to alert him. Movement activities can be used alternately throughout a session, either to release tensions or to provide stimulation that is organizing and actually assists in refocusing the child's attention to more demanding visual tasks. Motor activities that require eye-hand coordination, such as pointing, throwing, placing, and stacking, can encourage a child to attend visually to what his body and hands are doing or need to do (Fig. 7.5). At other times, movement may need to be restricted when attention to tabletop activities, such as paper and pencil tasks, is desired (Fig. 7.6). A child may need to be positioned in a chair at a table in such a way that provides clear boundaries and limits his ability to leave the activity on impulse.

Intervention specific for visual attention involves structuring, activity selection, activity modification, and therapist verbalization and cuing.

### Visual Attention—Structuring

The structure of a treatment session can help the child's visual attention. When organizing the treatment session, a therapist needs to decide how long a child is able to attend given the activities selected. One way to organize a treatment session is for the therapist to select one major activity that involves several different tasks. In this way, the child's visual attention is assisted in

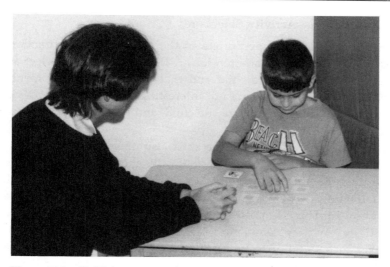

**Figure 7.6** Child is positioned to maintain attention to task and limit impulsivity. Visual distractions have been minimized.

small segments of increasing lengths with several different tasks. One method of structuring such a treatment session is to alternate activities in a circular fashion—that is, a therapist selects an activity that involves four tasks for a 30-minute treatment session. The activity may include familiar, previously successful tasks or new tasks, which may require attention of different lengths to complete. The child chooses the first activity from the group, and when it is completed or when attention wanes, the task is changed. During the treatment session, the child alternates only among the four tasks, elaborating or repeating as needed.

For the child who has a longer attention span, the goal may be to increase the cumulative length of time he attends to one task or activity. In this case, a therapist might organize the treatment session around one major activity.

If a child is involved in planning the treatment session with the therapist, he may be more motivated to attend and participate. A child often attends better when he knows what is coming next, when he knows what constitutes task completion, when he has had some choices in the tasks or materials, and when he knows when the activity is going to end. Listing the activities together, by picture or words, can give a predictable structure to the session. It is important to include "clean up time" within the structure of the treatment session because it helps a child attend to a designated structure, to know the end of the activity, and to develop good work habits.

### Visual Attention—Activity Selection

Almost any activity appropriate to the child's level of functioning can be used to stimulate visual attention. A therapist needs to select activities, however, that interest the child and that are at his developmental level. Activities that are too easy are not interesting or motivating. Activities that are too difficult may discourage the child, and he may not be motivated to participate.

When selecting activities, a therapist also must consider the amount of time needed for completion. The various tasks should be able to be completed within the time frame that the child can attend, because task completion is self-motivating. An activity needs to last slightly longer than the visual attention span. This is important because the child then will want to complete the activity. Activity completion is motivating and reinforcing. As a child improves in his ability to be alert visually and attentive, the duration of activities can be increased. As the child's attention for familiar activities increases, a therapist can sustain that activity for a longer time through repetition or addition of new tasks or components. As visual attention improves even more complex visual activities can be introduced and repeated.

Depending on the child, familiar or novel activities may stimulate prolonged interest. A therapist should use a combination of the familiar and novel, because familiar activities allow a child to recapitulate positive learning experiences and to learn by experiencing the activities in new and varying ways in different situations. Novel activities encourage a child to engage in new and different things, and they also encourage the generalization of learned skills.

Activities selected to gain or maintain a child's visual attention should use tasks or materials that are interesting. Young children may like brightly colored toys that move and make sounds. Older children may enjoy objects that can be manipulated or that depict a theme, such as dinosaurs, dolls or cartoon characters (Fig. 7.7).

### Visual Attention—Activity Modification

How an activity is presented to a child who has poor visual attention affects performance. If the treatment goal is to increase a child's attention within a unfamiliar single activity, then a therapist needs to know the child's capability and adapt the tasks in ways that were previously successful. Challenging the child in a positive way to complete more repetitions of a task can motivate some children. For example, a therapist may say, "See if you can beat your record and do two cards instead of one," or "I bet you can!" For

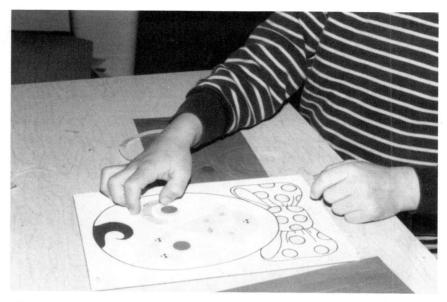

**Figure 7.7** This activity is selected because of the child's interest in stickers. This task requires shape and size matching as well as color coding.

another child, the use of a timer can be beneficial in keeping the child on the task. In this case, a therapist may say, "Let's see if you can finish this design in 2 minutes instead of 5"; or "You worked for 10 whole minutes before you got tired or wanted to change activities." The therapist should be sensitive to a child's fatigue level and give him "break time" or change the activity when appropriate.

There has been much discussion on the importance and need for activity modification. Many sources are available in the literature (Mosey, 1986; Pedretti, 1985). Other aspects of activity modification include changing the sequence of the tasks; changing the position of the child; changing the position of the materials; changing the size, shape, weight, or texture of the materials; changing the procedures used in the task; and changing the nature and degree of personal contact (Hinojosa, Sabari, & Rosenfeld, 1983).

### Therapist Verbalization and Cuing

A therapist's voice can be used to elicit attention. A change in volume—either higher or lower—is alerting. Making elaborative sounds associated with the stimuli may make tasks more fun and appealing. Using simple,

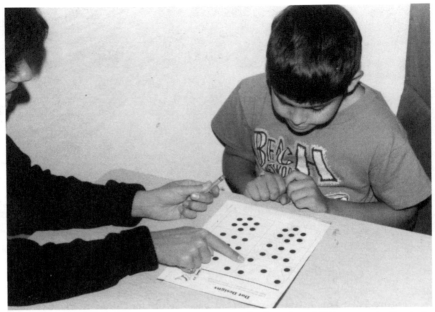

**Figure 7.8**   Visual and verbal cues are given before the child attempts the task.

appropriate labels to reinforce concepts may maintain the child's visual and auditory attentiveness.

A therapist must be careful about the type and amount of verbalization she uses during an activity, because sometimes it may be too distracting (Fig. 7.8). A therapist should focus on positive behaviors. For example, a therapist might say, "Look at the paper" rather than "Don't look over there." To reinforce "on-task" behaviors or task completion positively can assist an inattentive child who may receive a lot of negative comments about his inability to attend. A therapist must monitor continually the child's responses to her verbalizations and perhaps adjust them to achieve desired responses. If a therapist concludes that her verbalizations are overwhelming or distracting, she should keep them brief and simple, drawing attention to one feature at a time. If these responses continue to be overwhelming, a therapist should consider nonverbal cues.

Nonverbal cues can alert a child to the salient features of a task. A therapist may point out the important visual information with her finger or with the child's finger. When a child uses his own finger to trace or point, it can be a strong stimulus to increase his visual attention.

Finally, if a therapist explains to a child why he is doing a certain activity, it may stimulate his interest. This is especially effective with older children who may be motivated to improve. For example, a therapist might say, "We are doing this paper because it will help you pay more attention to details, which you tend not to do. You'll do so much better in school."

## Visual Memory

Several techniques can be used by a therapist to assist a child's registration of information into his memory. Repeated and consistent experiences with specific visual objects and symbols increase the opportunities for a child to recognize and remember them. A therapist should accompany visual stimuli with appropriate and simple labels. When talking about the object, a therapist can associate it with its function or its physical characteristics (such as shape, color, size, texture, or temperature). Finally, associations with previous experiences can help a child remember things.

Visual stimuli that can be recognized and comprehended are potentially memorable. When a child cannot understand what he sees because it is too complex and has few or no familiar parts, he may overlook the object or figure and not register it in memory at all. Identifying familiar items and parts can assist in visual attention and memory. Investigating unfamiliar stimuli and recognizing their functions or parts also helps to encode in memory.

The memory techniques that follow are discussed as they relate to encoding information. These techniques also rely, however, on semantic coding. The combination of visual and semantic coding becomes especially important for academic performance.

Organizing information into smaller "chunks" may help simplify a complex task. **Chunking** can be used when a child is copying an unknown word. A child looks at the word and instead of copying one letter at a time, chunks it into known syllables or two to three letters at a time.

Rehearsal techniques can be helpful for storing information. **Maintenance rehearsal (repetition)** holds information in short-term memory for immediate use, like remembering a telephone number that one is about to call; however, maintenance rehearsal has no effect on long-term storage. **Elaborative rehearsal** consciously relates new information to knowledge already stored in long-term memory. Before the age of seven, a child does not use elaborative rehearsal spontaneously. By the age of eight years, a child can rehearse more than one item at a time and can rehearse information together, as a set, to remember it. In making associations, it is beneficial for a child to relate ideas to more than one other idea or experience for meaningful encoding (Biehler & Snowman, 1990). For example, for a child to learn the concept of oval, the therapist might say, "This shape looks like an egg," or ". . . a squashed circle." A therapist might add that the object feels smooth, with no points or edges.

Grouping information in ways that provide retrieval cues can help a child remember interrelated data. Categorization develops after information is analyzed and placed in subcategories and interrelationships are understood. Children learn to categorize through direct teaching, as well as through experience. Fruits, vegetables, and other foods are examples of categories. Children see and eat different foods and begin to understand that all these items are foods. Then, through continued experience, they begin to understand that groups of food, such as fruits and vegetables are subcategories of the broader group, called food.

Seriation requires that information be organized in a particular sequence. Because there is a tendency to remember items better at the beginning and end of a series, short lists often eliminate the more difficult to remember middle area. Also, remembering series, such as alphabetical and numerical orders, assists in organization and memory. Spelling often relies on visual memory of a series of letters, not necessarily based on phonetic sounds.

Mnemonic devices are memory-directed tactics that help transform or organize information to enhance its retrievability (Biehler & Snowman, 1990). Some of the more common mnemonic-directed tactics include rhymes, songs, and acronyms.

Some children use visual imagery to relate incoming information into meaningful images. For example, a therapist may model this technique by saying, "I'm going to remember that a 'u' can catch rain like a cup, so imagine drinking water from a cup." A child may have to invent his own **memory hooks** to make things more meaningful.

Compensatory techniques for poor memory can include strategies such as lists and color coding. For example, color coding books and folders can be helpful to some children who forget school work and materials related to that work.

Activities such as Concentration™ or other memory games are good for visual memory. Modifying the statement "I'm going on a picnic" with pictures instead of words can be fun. In this case, a therapist asks a child to describe what he would bring to the picnic. Other games can include copying a sequence of objects, colored blocks, or pictures after viewing them for several seconds, or remembering what was removed from an array that was just examined.

Encouraging a child to develop a set of procedures or a sequence for performing functional tasks can help that child to remember how to do an activity. This can be facilitated by having the child perform the task each time in the same consistent sequence. Learning of routines can be assisted through consistent visual and verbal cues. In addition, routines can be especially useful to prepare a child for transitions, like leaving home in the morning, getting ready to leave school, or completing homework.

Environmental structuring is effective in improving a child's visual memory. Once a child has learned to anticipate the structure of a session, then the therapist can build in memory demands. After the joint planning of a treatment session, the therapist can write down the sequence of the tasks. During the treatment session, the child can be asked to remember what comes next. In addition, the child can be asked to check his answer on the written plan.

## Visual Discrimination

A clearly organized environment with appropriate amounts and types of visual stimuli can help a child attend to the relevant cues. Visual stimuli should be available but not overwhelming. The child who needs to be able to function within that environment really is the only one who can determine what is overwhelming. The therapist should be aware of cues from the child that he is feeling overwhelmed. Such cues include increased levels of distraction or inattention, increased gross or fine motor activity, and frequent changing of physical position.

Visual stimuli that are familiar to the child tend to be inhibited more easily; novel stimuli gain attention. New changes, therefore, should be introduced with adequate time for the child to explore them. Later, a child may find it easier to ignore new stimuli when he needs to attend to other things in the environment.

Reducing stimulating sensory input (auditory and visual input) can help focus the child who is unable to screen out such stimuli. One modification may be to have a distraction-free place in which ambient stimuli are minimized. A study carrel makes a good "office" when visual attention needs to be more focused. Lighting should be direct and should not produce glare. This becomes extremely important when computer screens are used for visual perceptual tasks. (Be aware also of sunlight glare from the windows.) Fluorescent lighting may produce glare, especially on certain surfaces such as formica

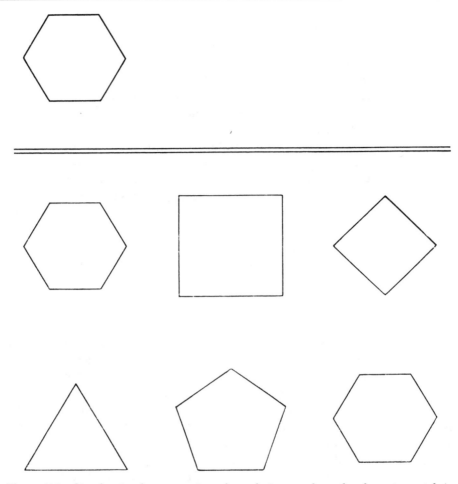

**Figure 7.9** Simple visual presentations: boundaries are clear, the shape to match is presented above the choices for visual comparison. Choices are limited and clearly organized in rows and columns.

desks or shiny paper. (This can be offset with additional incandescent lighting.) Headphones may assist in screening out auditory stimuli as long as the tactile sensation of the headphones is not distracting.

In simple visual presentations, shapes or figures should be defined clearly. This requires clear boundaries with no competing background (Fig. 7.9). In a simple visual presentation, the internal details included in the shape or figure emphasize the distinctive characteristics of the object. Early children's books demonstrate these principles well. Outlining the important visual cues in

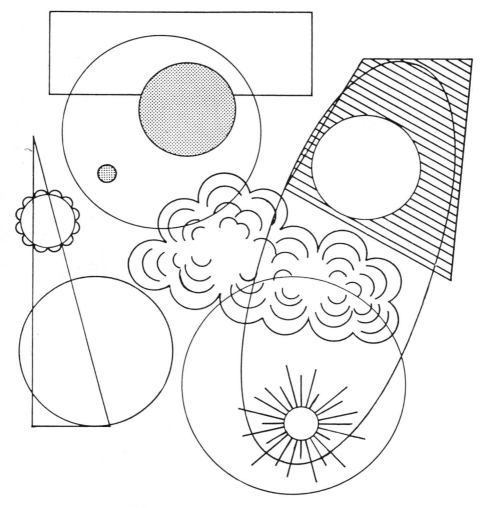

**Figure 7.10**   Complex visual presentation. Familiar shapes (circles) overlap and are embedded.

heavier lines simplifies visual presentation. As the child's ability to discriminate detail improves, complex visual presentations that have overlapping or embedded figures set amid a lot of foreground and background detail should be used (Fig. 7.10.). The amount of internal detail from the stimuli should be increased and presented in such a way that the child is able to inspect things visually, to distinguish differences.

It is important to position the materials so that a child can see them comfortably. This may not always be at midline. A therapist might ask the

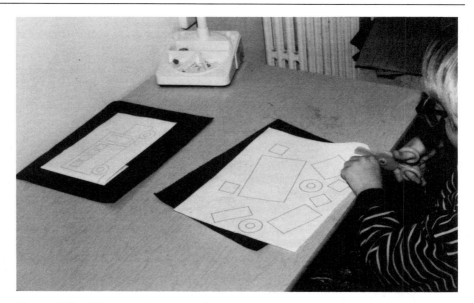

**Figure 7.11**    Mat is used to create high contrast and assist in visual attention. Task requires construction of parts into a whole by attending to positional relationships among the parts.

child where he sees things most easily and assess to see if that is indeed the most functional location. An easel, which positions the work on a vertical plane, is sometimes helpful for improving visual perception. Visual stimuli should always be oriented according to the child's vertical/horizontal axes.

When using activity worksheets or other graphic materials, the guidelines that follow might be helpful:

- Extraneous distractions should be kept to a minimum. Everything should be cleared from the child's work surface, except for the activity.
- The amount of material on a page should be sequenced carefully so that selective attention can be used to the best of the child's ability.
- High contrast and defined boundaries attract the eye and provide clear input.
- Purple reduplication ink or type with a low contrast colored paper should be avoided. Clear copies with distinct figures and no extraneous marks should be used.
- Outlining in heavy lines can attract visual attention to the appropriate details.
- A contrasting colored mat, black or red, behind a white worksheet can sometimes simplify the visual field and attract attention (Fig. 7.11).
- "Masks" that reveal only one line or one figure may help focus some children's visual gaze.
- Covering work that is finished, or not yet finished, may reduce visual distractions.

Some children cannot ignore an incorrect answer that they have made and may even rip the paper in trying to erase it. White-out products can help a child correct errors without overattention to conflicting visual stimuli.

The position of items within a visual array also can assist performance, in that items arranged vertically for comparison/discrimination are simpler to see than items organized horizontally. Organize the array visually by grouping items that go together in an obvious way, such as by placing them next to each other. For example, begin with a simple linear arrangement, with one complete activity to a line and a few activities to a page. Worksheets then can progress to columns and other more complicated arrangements, such as combinations of rows and columns. A training period may be needed to follow increasing amounts of work on a page so that the child can organize himself independently. Drawing lines to separate items and give visual boundaries can assist a child who is disorganized and skips around the page because he cannot group the work easily on his own. Often children who have perceptual problems may be able to do the academic work and are moved to more advanced worksheets only to fail or become "sloppy" because the increased amount of work or the way in which the information is presented visually interferes with progress.

## Specific Visual Discrimination Skills

Many of the techniques already discussed for attention and memory can be used to improve visual discrimination skills. Discrimination tasks should be presented along the same continua as for other skills—general to specific, whole to parts, familiar to unfamiliar, and concrete to abstract.

Young children tend to identify and match stimuli by general characteristics or by global form, not by detail. Begin with object recognition and then proceed to function, and, finally, move on to characteristics. Match identical objects that are meaningful to the child. A therapist may then decide to match similarly shaped objects, one of which may differ in color, size, or internal detail. From there, draw attention to the differences between objects rather than focus only on the similarities. The next step is to match tasks with objects; for instance, color matching (Teddy Bear Bingo); size matching (graduated pegboards); shape matching (formboards and puzzles with outlined shapes); positional matching (pointing out the spatial differences with the same shape or using objects or flannel board pieces that can be placed in

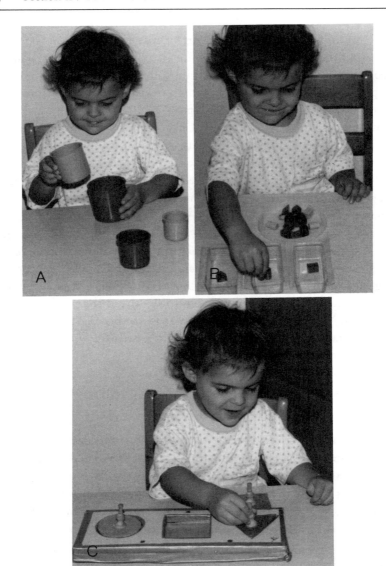

**Figure 7.12**  Examples (**A, B, C**) of size and shape matching tasks at a simple level.

different positions, such as upside down, reversed, or angled) (Fig. 7.12). A child can watch the change in position as pieces or objects are rotated, or he can move the things himself to reorient the piece to match a stimulus. The child does not usually develop the ability to do mental rotations at this point; that skill comes later.

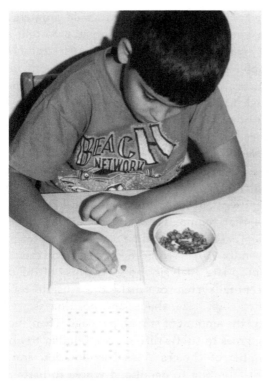

**Figure 7.13**  Constructional tasks require step-by-step organization and analysis of whole-to-parts relationships.

Active exploration of objects that have interrelated parts can focus the child's attention to the details of objects. For example, the child can manipulate take-apart toys such as cars, ring sticks, and puzzles. A therapist can also talk about the toy and how its parts go together as the child "plays" with it. It usually is easy for a child to take things apart and not know how to put them back together. Constructional tasks, such as block, parquetry, peg, bead, and pegboard designs, encourage the child to analyze the whole configuration through its parts and then synthesize parts back into a whole (Fig. 7.13). Constructional tasks require flexibility in that a child must be able to go back and forth to view the stimulus' parts and check that they retain their relationship to the whole design. In addition, he must compare his own reproduction to the sample as he goes along with the task. Activities should begin with simple three-dimensional designs, pegboards, blocks, parquetry, and designs that use one line going in one direction (either vertical or horizontal) and the border as a guide. These things then would progress to more complex designs, such as two lines that must be related to one another, diagonals, the use of empty (null) space, shapes that are inset and not on the border, and, then, overlapping shapes. Colored pieces can provide early, helpful organizing cues. Later, plain wooden cubes and three-dimensional card designs can be copied. Other activities can include copying Lego™, Tinkertoy™ structures, or other constructional toys. At first, the child may have to copy the design piece-by-piece, imitating the therapist; but later, he should be able to copy from a completed model or from pictorial directions. Cutting and pasting shapes to copy a design is also a good constructional task, beginning with a matching space for the cut-out and then moving to reconstruction of the design without given boundaries.

Two-dimensional tasks that require visual matching abound in many worksheet books and perceptual programs. Some perceptual motor programs (see Resource List in Appendix 7.B) have been criticized for their ineffectiveness; however, the appropriate analysis and graded use of the demands placed on the child's perceptual system can make these useful tools. First, analyze for content areas of color, size, shape, and position as well as for configuration of choices and the amount of stimuli per page. Then, move from simple to complex figures, gross to subtle differences, familiar to unfamiliar shapes, and a greater number of choices. Visual exploration and manual manipulation can highlight attention to detail and whole to parts relationships. Use of three dimensional objects for construction usually precedes the copying of graphic, symbolic designs.

When two-dimensional worksheets are used for whole to parts relationships, the amount of internal detail within a figure should be monitored. Begin with gross differences and move to the more subtle. Gross differences include totally different shapes, whereas subtle differences include similar shapes or differences in internal features with the external configurations remaining the same (Fig. 7.14). Internal details may differ in shape, number, or spatial orientation. A therapist needs to be aware of details that are different as a result of inversions, rotations or tilt, because these are the last differences that to develop. It should be noted that a therapist may have to provide additional structuring and cuing when doing these types of tasks (Fig. 7.15). Furthermore, a therapist may elect to teach systematic visual analysis by showing ways to analyze the whole to parts relationship. The following cues may help a child: Choose a starting point to begin, give a reference point, and be consistent. Cue the child to ask himself, "Where do I start?" In most constructional tasks, begin at the bottom; in writing tasks,

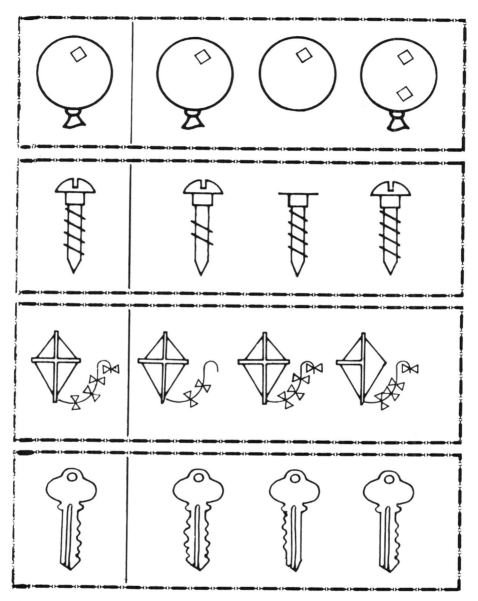

**Figure 7.14**   To notice change in internal features is critical to this matching task. The overall configuration of choices is similar. Presentation is low in number, simply arranged in horizontal rows, and divided by high contrast lines. Figures are familiar objects.

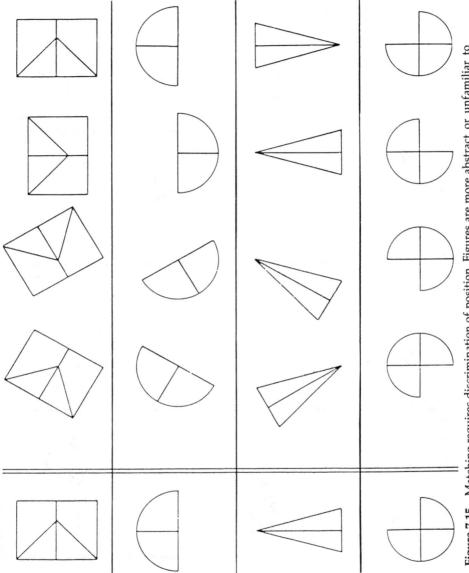

**Figure 7.15** Matching requires discrimination of position. Figures are more abstract or unfamiliar to younger children. Arrangement is clear and simply presented in horizontal rows.

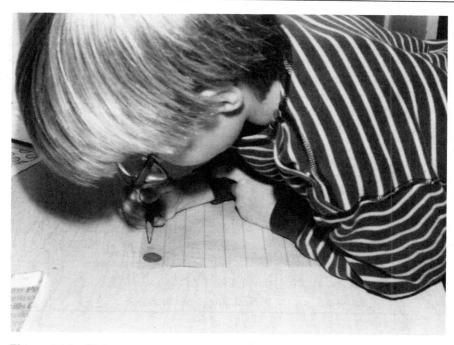

**Figure 7.16**  Giving cues as a consistent reference point may help children orient more easily when they begin a visual motor task.

begin strokes on the top line. Move sequentially in one direction at one time, usually beginning on the left and working right. Adding a visual cue like a sticker or a happy face in the upper left corner may cue a child visually to remember where to begin writing (Fig. 7.16). Many children who have perceptual difficulties choose random starting points, which often confuses the task from the outset. One such example is when children begin to write on the right side of the paper and write backwards from there.

When working with complex visual stimuli, pick out a familiar shape and add onto it. Once the child can find a meaningful whole shape, it becomes easier to look at more details. Carefully grade the amount of additional details. Label, point to, and discuss the different relationships. The child may find that counting internal items helps to analyze the parts-to-whole relationships. Spatial concepts are important to the development of whole-to-parts relationships because the child can use these concepts and verbal labels to follow other directions and to cue himself verbally. The therapist needs to be aware of the development of spatial concepts to know how to give directions appropriate for the child's developmental level. Many children who have visual perceptual difficulties often have language delays as well. The chart that follows gives the concepts and labels that develop first and can be used to give simple spatial directions. This progression indicates the age at which a child is expected to understand how to place one object in relation to another according to the spatial concept/label. For some concepts, the understanding and use of spatial words in relationship to self develops at a younger age.

| Age (yrs) | Spatial Concept/Label |
|---|---|
| 2.0 to 2.6 | in, off |
| 2.6 to 3.0 | on, under, out of, together, away from |
| 3.0 to 3.6 | up, top, apart, toward |
| 3.6 to 4.0 | around, in front of, high, in back of, next to |
| 4.0 to 4.6 | beside, bottom, backward, forward |
| 4.6 to 5.0 | down, low |
| 5.0 to 5.6 | behind, ahead of, first, last |

Once matching progresses and the child can identify similarities and differences among objects and pictures, sorting tasks should be included. These entail activities that require a child to decide which object is different. Begin with objects or pictures that can be moved around and grouped physically for closer inspection. For example, worksheet pages can be cut up and given to the child to sort (Fig. 7.17). When the child is ready, let him look at groups of three to four items to identify the different one. Again, grade from simple to complex.

When a child repeatedly experiences particular visual stimuli, the stimuli will become familiar and recognizable. The items then can be matched more easily, perceived within a background, and recognized in various environments and spatial orientations. Figure-ground worksheets can be used to find a familiar shape, such as circles, within a competing background (see Fig. 7.10). Finding familiar shapes in the environment is based on detecting similar shapes that may differ in color, size, internal detail. Begin with concrete (three-dimensional) objects. Present them in a variety of ways. Change their sizes, general shapes, and spatial orientations. Shape change may be done with objects such as cups. They share a general characteristic but may be slightly different in that some have handles and some do not. Make sure that the cups have been observed from various angles so that all surfaces have been seen. This helps detect the invariant features that make the objects

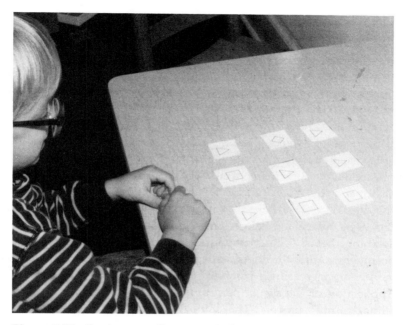

**Figure 7.17**  Sorting two-dimensional shapes cut from worksheets to make them moveable and allow them to be manipulated for closer visual comparison if necessary.

similar. Use all the senses to explore and discuss various attributes such as shape, color, texture, and function. When the child finally can recognize objects in a variety of contexts, the therapist may want to move toward books and pictures. A developmental progression may proceed from clearly defined color photographs to realistic drawings with relevant details and from line drawings to abstract representation to word symbols. This may be a helpful progression when choosing picture icons for a communication board.

## Summary

Visual perception is the child's ability to interpret and use what is seen. It is an interactive result of sensory input received through the visual system, intersensory integration, and cognitive analysis. The information processing model is one way to explain cognitive analysis so that visual information is understood and becomes meaningful.

The theoretical base of this frame of reference includes three major assumptions. First, visual perception is learned through interaction with the human and nonhuman environments. Next, acquisition of visual perception skills is a complex process affected by learning and moves from general to specific, whole to parts, concrete to abstract, and familiar to novel. And, finally, although each visual perception skill develops in its own sequence, the acquisition of each skill affects the acquisition of other skills. Fundamental to this process are visual attention, visual memory, and visual discrimination. Specific visual discrimination skills result in the visual perception skills of recognition, matching and sorting.

This frame of reference contains function/dysfunction continua, which include visual attention, memory, and specific visual discrimination abilities. The function/dysfunction continua describe the behaviors that are observed clinically and that may indicate what difficulty the child is having in processing visual information.

The 19 postulates regarding change in this frame of reference draw heavily on learning theory. These postulates concentrate on the structuring of the environment so that the child can learn to discriminate visual information in ways that are increasingly complex.

Application of the visual perceptual frame of reference is based on the teaching/learning process. The child first works on visual attention, then moves onto visual memory followed by visual discrimination, and, finally, focuses on specific visual discrimination skills. In this frame of reference, the therapist plays a major role in creating an environment and structuring activities so that the child benefits from the therapeutic experience.

## Outline of the Visual Perception Frame of Reference

   I. Theoretical base
      A. Visual system
      B. Visual perception
      C. Information processing model
         1. Input
         2. Processing
         3. Output
         4. Feedback
      D. Processing skills for visual perception
         1. Visual attention
            a. Alertness
            b. Selective attention
            c. Vigilance
         2. Visual memory
            a. Coding of information
            b. Visual short-term memory
            c. Visual long-term memory
            d. Retrieval of information
         3. Visual discrimination

          a. General to specific
          b. Whole to parts
          c. Concrete to abstract
          d. Familiar to novel
    E. Learning visual perceptual skills
    F. Specific visual discrimination abilities
        1. Recognition
        2. Matching
        3. Sorting

II. Function/dysfunction continua
    A. Visual attention
        1. Alertness
        2. Selective attention
        3. Vigilance
    B. Memory
    C. Specific visual discrimination abilities

III. Evaluation
    A. Visual attention skills
    B. Evaluation of visual memory
    C. Evaluation of specific visual discrimination skills
    D. Summary

IV. Postulates regarding change
    A. Those that relate to the use of learning within this frame of reference
    B. Those that relate to visual attention
    C. Those that relate to visual memory
    D. Those that relate to visual discrimination

V. Application to Practice
    A. Teaching/learning
    B. Visual attention
        1. Structuring
        2. Activity selection
        3. Activity modification
        4. Therapist verbalization and cuing
    C. Visual memory
        1. Rehearsal techniques
        2. Grouping information
        3. Mnemonic device
        4. Visual imagery
        5. Compensatory techniques
        6. Activities
        7. Environmental structuring
    D. Visual discrimination
        1. Environmental modification
        2. Reducing stimulating sensory input
        3. Visual presentation
        4. Position of the materials
        5. Using activities that involve worksheets or other graphic materials

E.  Specific visual discrimination skills
1. Continua of general to specific, whole to parts, familiar to unfamiliar, and concrete to abstract
2. Active exploration of objects
3. Two-dimensional tasks

## Acknowledgments

The author wishes to thank Kathleen Tsurumi, M.A., OTR whose clarity of vision, relentless questioning, and experience with children who have perceptual problems contributed greatly to this chapter.

## References

Abreu, B. C., & Toglia, J. P. (1984). *Cognitive rehabilitation manual.* New York: Authors.

Anderson, J. (1986). Sensory intervention with the preterm infant in the neonatal intensive care unit. *American Journal of Occupational Therapy, 40,* 19–26.

Ayres, A. J. (1972). *Sensory integration and learning disorders.* Los Angles, CA: Western Psychological Services.

Ayres, A. J. (1979). *Sensory integration and the child.* Los Angeles, CA: Western Psychological Services.

Banus, B. S. (1971). *The developmental therapist.* Thorofare, NJ: Slack.

Biehler, R. F., & Snowman, J. (1990). *Psychology applied to teaching.* Boston, MA: Houghton Mifflin.

Bouska, M. J., Kauffman, N. A., & Marcus, S. (1985). Disorders of the visual perceptual system. In D. Umphred (Ed.). *Neurological rehabilitation* (pp. 552–585). Philadelphia, PA: F. A. Davis.

Chedru, F., Leblanc, M., & Lhermitte, F. (1973). Visual searching in normal and brain damaged subjects. *Cortex, 9,* 94–111.

Collarusso, R., & Hammill, D. (1972). *The motor free test of visual perception.* Novato, CA: Academic Therapy.

DeGangi, G., & Porges, S. (1991). Attention/alertness/arousal. In C. Royeen (Ed.). *Neuroscience foundations of human performance.* Rockville, MD: American Occupational Therapy Association.

Folio, M. R., & Fewell, R. R. (1983). *Peabody developmental motor scales and activity cards.* Allen, TX: DLM Teaching Resources.

Frostig, M., & Horne, D. (1973). *The Frostig program for the development of visual perception.* Chicago, IL: Follett.

Gardner, M. (1988). *Test of visual perceptual skills.* San Francisco, CA: Health Publishing.

Getman, G. N. (1965). The visuomotor complex in the acquisition of learning skills. In J. Helmuth (Ed.). *Learning disorders.* Washington, D. C.: Special Child Publications.

Gianutsos, R., & Matheson, P. (1987). The rehabilitation of visual perceptual disorders attributable to brain injury. In M. J. Meier, A. L. Benton, & L. Diller (Eds.). (1987). *Neuropsychological rehabilitation* (pp. 202–241). New York: Guilford Press.

Gibson, E. J. (1963). Perceptual development. In H. W. Stevenson (Ed.). *Child psychology.* Chicago, IL: University of Chicago Press.

Gibson, E. J. (1969). Principles of perceptual learning and development. New York: Appleton, Century, Crofts.

Gibson, J. J. (1966). The senses considered as perceptual systems. Boston, MA: Houghton Mifflin.

Hinojosa, J., Sabari, J., & Rosenfeld, M. S. (1983). Purposeful activities, *American Journal of Occupational Therapy, 37,* 805–806.

Kephart, N. C. (1971). *The slow learner in the classroom* (2nd ed.). Columbus, OH: Charles C. Merrill.

Levine, M. (1987). *Developmental variation and learning disorders.* Cambridge, MA: Educators Publishing Service.

Luria, A. R. (1980). *Higher cortical functions in man.* New York: Basic Books.

Meldman, M. J. (1970). *Diseases of attention and perception.* Oxford, England: Pergamon Press.

Miller, L. J. (1982). *Miller assessment for preschoolers.* Littleton, CO: The Foundation for Knowledge in Development.

Miller, P. (1983). *Theories in developmental psychology.* San Francisco, CA: W. H. Freeman.

Mosey, A. C. (1986). *Psychosocial components of occupational therapy.* New York: Raven Press.

Mussen, P. H., Conger, J. J., & Kagan, J. (1969). *Child development and personality* (3rd ed.). New York: Harper Row.

Pedretti, L. W. (1985). *Occupational therapy: Practice skills for physical dysfunction* (2nd ed.). St. Louis, MO: C. V. Mosby.

Piaget, J. (1963). *The origins of intelligence.* New York: Norton.

Posner, M. I., & Rafal, R. (1987). Cognitive theories of attention and the rehabilitation of attentional deficits. In M.J. Meier, A.L. Benton, & L. Diller (Eds.). *Neuropsychological rehabilitation.* New York: Guilford Press.

Richmond, P. G. (1970). *An introduction to Piaget.* New York: Basic Books.

Ruff, H. A. (1980). The development of perception and recognition of objects. *Child Development, 51,* 981–992.

Short-DeGraff, M. A. (1988). *Human development for occupational and physical therapists.* Baltimore, MD: Williams & Wilkins.

Toglia, J. P. (1989). Visual perception of objects: An approach to assessment and intervention. *American Journal of Occupational Therapy, 43,* 587–0595.

Warren, M. (1990). Evaluation and treatment of vision and visual perception in the neurologically impaired adult. Philadelphia, PA workshop notes.

Warren, M. (1990). Identification of visual scanning deficits in adults after cerebrovascular accident. *American Journal of Occupational Therapy, 44,* 391–398.

*Appendix 7.A*   Pediatric Clinical Vision Screening for Occupational Therapists. Scheirman, M., Pennsylvania College of Optometry, 1991, reprinted with permission from Dr. Scheirman.

## Visual Efficiency Screening

A. **Accommodation**
   1. Materials: $+2.00/-2.00$ flip lenses (from Bernell Corporation, 1-800-348-2225), target.
   2. Procedure: target held at 16 inches, place lenses in front of child and ask child to clear print, flip lenses to other side and repeat as many times as possible for 1 minute. Record number of cycles per minute (cpm). One cycle equals two flips.
   3. Expected value: 8–10 cycles per minute.
   4. Observations: double vision, effort, squinting, discomfort.

B. **Binocular Vision**
   1. Materials: penlight.
   2. Procedure: hold penlight about 12 inches from eyes. Ask child to look at light and slowly move it toward nose. Ask child to tell you when he sees double, record the distance. Now move penlight away from child and ask child to report when he sees single again. Record this distance.
   3. Expected value: double vision at 2–4 inches, single vision (recovery) at 4–6 inches.
   4. Observations: effort, squinting, discomfort, eye moving out without report of double vision.

C. **Ocular Motility**
   1. Materials: Developmental Eye Movement Test (DEM). Available from Bernell (1-800-348-2225).
   2. Procedure: ask child to call off numbers on plate one, two, and three as quickly as possible without using fingers. Record time.
   3. Expected values: norms available in manual. Normed by age and grade level.
   4. Observations: head movement, working distance, uses fingers.

*—continued*

## Observations of Visual Function in Children

| Behaviors | Yes | No |
|---|---|---|
| Turns head, tilts head, thrusts head forward | [ ] | [ ] |
| Shuts or covers eye | [ ] | [ ] |
| Rubs eyes | [ ] | [ ] |
| Excessive head movement | [ ] | [ ] |
| Excessive blinking | [ ] | [ ] |
| Excessive distractibility | [ ] | [ ] |
| Watery eyes | [ ] | [ ] |
| Squints or frowns excessively | [ ] | [ ] |
| Irritability after sustained visual work | [ ] | [ ] |
| Fatigue after sustained visual work | [ ] | [ ] |
| Limited attention span for visual tasks | [ ] | [ ] |
| Holds objects close to eyes | [ ] | [ ] |
| Misses the mark when starting to cut a line | [ ] | [ ] |
| Unable to see objects clearly at a distance | [ ] | [ ] |
| Loses place when reading | [ ] | [ ] |
| Skips or repeats words or lines when reading | [ ] | [ ] |
| Skips or repeats letters, words, or lines when copying | [ ] | [ ] |

| Appearance | | |
|---|---|---|
| Eyes cross or diverge | [ ] | [ ] |
| Eyes are inflamed or watery | [ ] | [ ] |
| Eyes are red-rimmed, crusty, or swollen | [ ] | [ ] |

| Complaints | | |
|---|---|---|
| Blurry vision | [ ] | [ ] |
| Double vision | [ ] | [ ] |
| Headache, nausea, dizziness following close work | [ ] | [ ] |
| Itchy, burny, scratchy feeling in eyes | [ ] | [ ] |

*Appendix 7.B*

## RESOURCES FOR VISUAL PERCEPTUAL ACTIVITIES AND WORKBOOKS

Continental Press
520 East Bainbridge Street
Elizabethtown, PA 17022

Frostig Program for the Development of Visual Perception
Modern Curriculum Press
13900 Prospect Road
Cleveland, OH 44136

Coleta Union School District–Sensorimotor Activities for the Remediation of Learning Disabilities
Academic Therapy Publications
Novato, CA

Judy Instructo
4325 Hiawatha Avenue South
Minneapolis, MN 55406

Perceptual Skills Curriculum
Jerome Rosner
Walker Educational Book Corporation
750 5th Avenue
New York, NY 10019

DLM
1 DLM Park
Allen, Texas 75002

Frank Schaeffer
26616 Indian Peak Road
Rancho Palo Verdes, CA 90274

Visual Perceptual Development Remedial Activities
Visual Motor Developmental Remedial Activities
Health Publishing Company
P. O. Box 3805
San Francisco, CA 44136

# 8

# Biomechanical Frame of Reference

CHERYL ANN COLANGELO

The biomechanical frame of reference is applied when a person cannot maintain posture through appropriate automatic muscle activity because of neuromuscular or musculoskeletal dysfunction. Consequently, artificial supports are provided, temporarily or permanently, to substitute for lack of postural control and to provide the most efficient positions of the body for functional activity.

Every time a person moves in relation to another person or object, the person must first move in relation to a greater force, **gravity.** This movement is done in a very subtle way. Each time a person eats a sandwich, embraces a child, or reaches for a book, he must always relate first to the earth's gravitational pull. For controlled movement, the human body must provide a stable center from which the head and limbs can move. Every peripheral movement creates a shift in the center of gravity that requires a compensatory postural reaction (Fig. 8.1) to prevent falling in the direction of the movement.

Gravity affects the human body on physical, mechanical, and physiological levels. Physically, gravity pulls the body toward the earth. It makes a person tend to fall down. It also makes the movement of limbs away from the earth's surface more difficult to execute. Mechanically, each time a person extends a limb away from the center of the body, such as when reaching, a lever arm is created that tends to topple the body by pulling the trunk in the direction of the limb. Fortunately, there are physiological mechanisms that help the body to adapt to the forces of gravity. Receptors, triggered by changes in

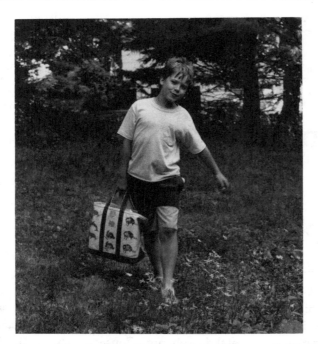

**Figure 8.1.** Because the weight of the bag pulls his body to his right, the child regains his center of gravity by flexing his trunk to the left and abducting his left arm

speed, direction, and joint position, stimulate an equilibrium reaction that allows the body to remain upright or balanced. Through interaction of these receptors with a healthy nervous system and responsive muscles, the human body reacts to the forces of gravity in a predictable and functional way.

The general goals of the biomechanical frame of reference are twofold. The first goal is to enhance the development of postural reactions by reducing the demands of gravity and by aligning the body. The second goal is to improve distal function and skilled activity by reducing the need for, and the demands on, postural reactions by providing external support.

The biomechanical frame of reference frequently is used as the main approach with children who exhibit severe physical disabilities. In addition, this frame of reference is used in combination with other frames of reference. For example, often it is used in conjunction with dynamic therapeutic handling (neurodevelopmental treatment, Brunnstrom and proprioceptive neuromuscular facilitation). When applied in this way, it allows for a carryover of goals throughout the day in the absence of constant physical handling.

# Theoretical Base

The biomechanical frame of reference draws from theories in physics and physiology. It addresses the implications of physical and physiological principles on motor development. Two assumptions are accepted by the biomechanical frame of reference in terms of normal development: (1) motor patterns develop from sensory stimulation, and (2) automatic motor responses, which maintain posture, develop in a predictable way. This frame of reference also contains an additional assumption related to atypical development—that dysfunction of or damage to the musculoskeletal or neuromuscular systems can interfere with effective postural reactions.

## *Motor Patterns Develop from Sensory Stimulation*

In infancy, motor behaviors most often are reflexive. Reflexes are stereotypical reactions that occur in response to specific stimuli that generally are tactile, proprioceptive, or vestibular in nature. These motor patterns, once executed, provide additional sensory input, which contributes to the modification of reflexes and development of motor control. One example of a stereotypical reflexive reaction is the asymmetrical tonic neck reflex (ATNR). The ATNR is elicited by turning the head, producing extension and abduction of the arm on the face side with flexion and adduction of the arm on the skull side. When a baby extends an arm as part of this reflex and touches an object, then the baby receives simultaneous sensations from proprioceptors in the shoulder related to reaching, tactile receptors in the hand, and visual awareness of the hand and object. The baby ultimately associates these sensations with the experience of touching an object, and, by reproducing the "feeling" of shoulder and arm movements, may reach successfully and touch the object again. The implication is that motor patterns develop from sensation.

## *Automatic Motor Responses That Maintain Posture Develop Predictably*

The most sophisticated postural responses, righting and equilibrium reactions, are well developed by the second year of life. Righting reactions are movements which maintain alignment of the head in space and of the trunk in relation to the head. For example, if a seated child leans forward to rest his arms on a desk, neck extension is the righting reaction used to maintain his head in an upright position despite the forward tilt of his trunk. Equilibrium reactions are movements that help to maintain balance when the child's center of gravity is disturbed by an external force. External forces that provoke equilibrium reactions occur (1) when a child is pushed, or (2) when a child is carrying or manipulating a heavy object. Equilibrium reactions are manifested by movements of the trunk and extremities in the direction opposite to the displacing force, to reestablish the center of gravity. If a seated child is pushed backward, his trunk curves forward, accompanied by forward thrusting movements of the limbs. This may involve shoulder flexion with elbow extension or hip flexion with knee extension. If the child is pushed toward the left, the equilibrium reaction is demonstrated when the child's trunk curves against the force to the right. This reaction may also involve abduction and extension of the right arm and leg.

Equilibrium reactions often are accompanied by protective reactions. Protective reactions are limb movements that occur in the same direction as the displacing force. The primary purpose of these reactions is to protect the body from harm by breaking a potential fall. When the seated child is pushed to the left, the equilibrium response causes the right limbs to extend to regain the center of gravity. Concurrently, the left limbs may extend and abduct protectively. Equilibrium reactions also may be seen alone. This occurs more frequently with slow or gentle displacement. These reactions may be replaced entirely by protective reactions when the displacement is more vigorous. In the previous example, if the seated child had been pushed hard to the left, then the left limbs would have extended and adducted to protect against a possible fall.

Righting and equilibrium reactions form the foundation for movements from one position to another. They assist in the maintenance of body position when the center of gravity is changed by moving or by engaging the limbs with objects. Before these reactions can develop, the child must integrate specific lower level reflexive responses, which are primarily for survival, such as flexor withdrawal or rooting (turning the head more in the direction of a stimulus to the mouth or cheek). Further, higher level reflexive responses, such as the ATNR and positive supporting reactions, provide movement and proprioceptive input. Development is overlapping, so that as one level approaches completion, the next has already begun to develop. These levels continue to develop sequentially, both within the body in a cephalocaudal fashion and in space from a horizontal to vertical position. For example, a child in a prone position may respond to lateral tilt with neck, trunk, and limb reactions, whereas in the upright position, the child may demonstrate righting only in the neck as his body is tipped laterally.

Another developmental sequence that is relevant to the biomechanical frame of reference has been described as **motor patterns,** which were investigated by Margaret Rood (Stockmeyer, 1967). Along with cephalocaudal and horizontal-vertical sequences, postural reactions can be viewed within this third category.

Motor patterns include sequences of motor development that go from unorganized to skilled movement, including the maintaining of posture and the ability to reestablish a center of gravity. Skilled motor patterns depend on the ability to bear weight without collapsing, and the ability to shift weight from one part of the body to another.

The process of motor development begins with mobility during infancy. Phasic movement, the lowest level of muscular control, consists of large undirected movements such as spontaneous kicking, waving, and banging. Muscles that primarily perform phasic movements tend to be superficial and distal members of the flexor group and often crossover more than one joint. They are used more for "light" work, movement of distal parts, than for "heavy" work (prolonged contractions needed for posture). Later in development, phasic movements are under more voluntary control and therefore are used in skilled movements.

After the child has acquired mobility, he begins to develop stability. Stability refers to the child's ability to maintain a weightbearing position by the cocontraction of agonist and antagonist muscles around a joint. Muscles that primarily perform tonic contractions tend to lie more deeply and proximally and generally are extensors that crossover only one joint. They are responsible for sustained tonic contractions around a joint. These muscles are under greater reflex control than phasic muscles.

Once a child has developed stability, he is able to bear weight, that is, to maintain a posture. From there, he begins to play with movement in that position. For example, take the prone-on-elbows position. At first the child supports himself on his arms, but if he begins to move, he may collapse. Soon he can rock from side to side without falling over. This grading of movement indicates that the child can create movement in a joint without losing the joint's capacity to support; this is referred to as **mobility superimposed on stability.** Functionally, this appears as weightshifting—the ability to transfer some or all of the weightbearing load to another joint or to maintain support in one joint as the body's center of gravity changes slightly. When the baby rocks laterally in a prone position, the weight is partially shifted back and forth between the two shoulders. A complete shift of weight to one shoulder frees the other side for reaching. Even then, the weightbearing shoulder must

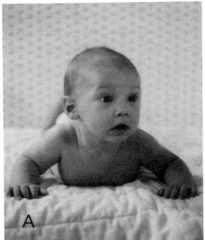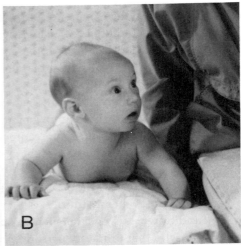

**Figure 8.2A,B.**    The infant weight shifts toward his right side **(A)** to keep from rolling into the depression created when his mother sits on the bed **(B)**.

engage in weightshifting activity because movements of the freed arm cause the body's weight to move slightly over the weightbearing shoulder.

The ability to superimpose mobility on stability can be demonstrated in two ways when a baby in the prone position is observed while propped on a bed: (1) If an adult sits alongside the baby, the adult's weight depresses the mattress and the baby must shift weight away from the mattress depression to avoid rolling over; (2) when this same baby reaches for a toy in the prone position, he must readjust his center of gravity toward one shoulder for weightbearing. These movements free the baby's other arm to reach for the toy (Fig. 8.2A, 8.2B).

This reaching out action demonstrates the baby's transition to another level of motor development: the acquisition of skilled movement. Skill is the highest level of motor function. In the previous example, the distal portion of the baby's arm is free, and this serves as the basis for volitional, coordinated movement. The shoulder's ability to hold the arm out in space and yet direct placement of the hand reflects the development of stability on mobility. Phasic movements have been refined into skill through their interaction with tonic movement, weightbearing, and weightshifting.

## Components of Postural Control and Skill Development in Developmental Positions

The biomechanical frame of reference focuses on function within a relatively static position rather than on transitional movements. It is essential, therefore, to examine the developmental sequence of motor behaviors characteristic of various positions.

### Supine Position

Although flexor tone predominates in the newborn, it is modified by the influence of the tonic labyrinthine reflex (TLR), which causes an increase of extensor tone in the supine position. Gravity also influences strongly the movements of the newborn; the head is held to the side and the scapulae are retracted and accompanied by shoulder elevation and external rotation. Despite increased extensor tone, the hips are flexed; gravity pulls them into abduction and external rotation. Because of the influence of the ATNR, the newborn experiences more extensor tone on the face side and more flexor tone on the skull side of the body. The flexor pattern on the skull side causes shoulder retraction and lateral trunk flexion, which moves the infant's center of gravity over to the extended face side. This provides the initial sensation of weightshifting and weightbearing on the extended side. Each time the infant turns his head, he shifts weight slightly to the other side.

Flexor activity contributes to emerging midline control as the baby manages to center his head. Eventually, the baby is able to flex his neck against gravity enough to achieve a chin tuck, at which point the chin comes in contact with the chest. Later, this controlled flexion, when combined with neck extension, provides head control in an upright posture.

In the supine position, the infant develops the ability to bring his hands to the chest and then reach upward by using a succession of movements, producing internal rotation, then shoulder flexion, and, finally, protraction against gravity (Fig. 8.3A, 8.3B). The ability to reach out in a directed and controlled fashion, which is a skilled movement, begins at the same time that the infant masters weightbearing in the prone-on-elbows position (mastery of mobility superimposed on stability in the shoulders). As the infant reaches upward and outward, a stable base of support is needed to keep from flipping over. Initially, abdominal support is low, and the legs are held off the floor because of the flexed, abducted, and externally rotated hips. The development of the abdominal musculature in conjunction with a decrease in hip flexor tone allows the infant to plant the soles of his feet firmly on the supporting surface, contributing to trunk stability during reaching. It is important to be aware that directed reaching in the supine position can be mastered with limited demands on head and trunk control because the child is supported fully, whereas reaching in the upright position requires additional control of the head and trunk to maintain a vertical position.

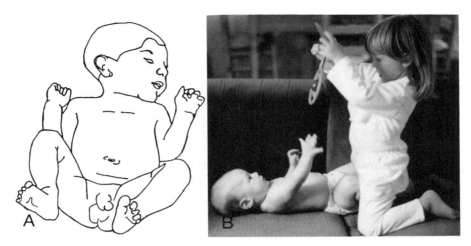

**Figure 8.3A,B.** In the newborn, the head is held to the side, scapulae are retracted, hips are flexed, abducted, and externally rotated **(A)**. As he develops, the infant gains the ability to reach upward by using shoulder flexion **(B).** He will later develop protraction against gravity.

During infancy, eye movements are not separated from head movements. Visual fixation and tracking are influenced by the development of head control. Similarly, oral-motor control is influenced by the force of gravity on the jaw and tongue and the development of postural tone. Initially, in the supine position, the infant's tongue goes toward the back of his mouth, and the lips and jaw are slightly open. As the ability to flex against gravity develops in the neck, a similar development occurs orally: the jaw closes, the lips come together more easily, and the tongue comes forward. A more mature sucking pattern is now possible.

### Prone Position

Following several crowded months of flexion in the womb, the effects of the TLR in the prone position increase flexor tone even more in the newborn. This results in a little ball of a person in the prone position. Hip flexion places the buttocks high in the air, so that body weight is distributed over the chest/face area. The newborn's head is turned to the side for breathing. The infant must hyperextend his neck to raise the head or turn it from side to side, because the spine is descending from the pelvis toward the neck. Maintaining the head in a righted position using hyperextension requires a great deal of energy, therefore mobility of the neck in a hyperextended position is limited. Because of this, head righting does not develop until the hips begin to extend.

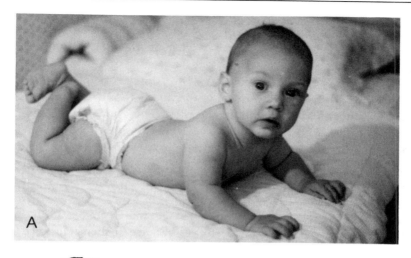

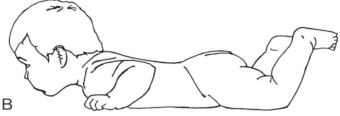

**Figure 8.4A,B.**  Before protraction develops in the prone position **(A)**, elbows are behind shoulders, trunk is horizontal, and neck hyperextension is necessary to right head **(B).**

Gradually in the prone position, the pelvis then comes in contact with the supporting surface, and the spine becomes more horizontal, with weight distributed along the trunk and pelvis. This postural change decreases the amount of neck extension needed to right the head. At first, headrighting is accompanied by unopposed extension of the upper trunk. This prepares the neck and back extensors for additional heavy work in any upright position.

When infants prop on their arms, flexor muscles work in conjunction with extensor muscles. The chest muscles bring the arms forward and down, so that elbows that were previously behind the shoulders now come directly beneath the shoulders in a tonic, weightbearing position. Once the upper trunk can be supported on the forearms and back extension is modulated by interaction with flexors, graded movements of the neck can be accomplished by the interplay of flexion and extension (Fig. 8.4A, 8.4B). This allows the infant to have volitional head movement. From this base, directed head movements and skilled eye and oral movements can develop in upright positions. Independent jaw and tongue movements then depend on the stability of the head and neck.

Once the infant has developed stability in the shoulders, he begins to weightshift. Weightshifting requires the infant to move his chest over the weightbearing arm to maintain equilibrium. This allows the infant to maintain balance on an unstable surface or to reach out with the opposite arm. This action curves the spine, elongating the weightbearing side of the body and shortening the nonweightbearing side. *The pattern of extension on the weightbearing side and flexion on the mobile side can be seen during weightshifting activities in all positions as the child matures.*

Although the focus of this section for the most part has been on movements of the head and upper extremities because of their relevance to functional activity in a static posture, the biomechanical frame of reference also recognizes the critical role of the pelvis in the maintenance of stability. This is different from the frequent concentration on the development of pelvic movements on end-goal ambulation. *Lower trunk and pelvic stability in the supine position allows for controlled head and arm movements,* preventing the child's body from rolling whenever the head is turned or an arm reaches out. In the prone position, balanced interaction of neck flexion and extension for head control, and placement of shoulders and elbows for weightbearing, depends on the position of the pelvis and legs.

### Sidelying Position

The tonic labyrinthine reflex has no influence in the sidelying position; therefore, asymmetrical movements can be executed more easily. Sidelying provides dramatically different sensory input to either side of the baby's body to help develop a sense of laterality, or the awareness of and control of the separate sides of the body (Fig. 8.5).

In the prone and supine positions, the infant masters the coordination of dorsal extensors with ventral flexors for trunk stability. Sidelying requires more sophisticated control, because the flexors and extensors on *one side* of the body must work together *and* in opposition to the coordination of flexors and extensors on the other side. Lateral headrighting is a good example: the neck flexes to the side through the activation of flexors and extensors on that side and against relaxation of the corresponding muscles on the other side. This general pattern of movement is compatible with the principles of extension and elongation on the weightbearing side and of flexion on the nonweightbearing, mobile side of the body.

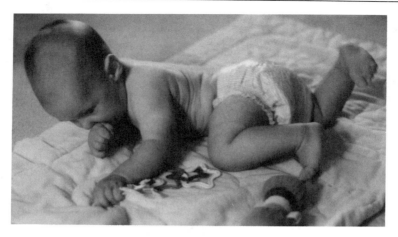

**Figure 8.5.**    In sidelying, the weightbearing side is extended and supporting, and the nonweightbearing side is flexed and mobile.

The lateral neck flexion against gravity that develops in sidelying as the child rights his head contributes to neck stability and head control in the upright posture. For example, in sitting or standing, every shift in weight to one side of the body necessitates lateral neck flexion to maintain the head in a righted position. The repeated movement of the head against gravity in the sidelying position helps this movement become effortless in the upright position. The same principle applies to the lateral trunk flexion that appears later in sidelying, when the child begins to prop on one arm.

The interaction between dorsal trunk extensors and ventral flexors bilaterally is also essential in sidelying. Too much extension pulls the child onto his back; too much flexion causes him to roll forward. This interaction is particularly important as the infant experiments with head and arm movements, because each of these movements shifts the infant's center of gravity. Once stable in sidelying, the infant has an excellent opportunity to try out skilled arm and hand movements of the nonweightbearing arm. This horizontal position demands less trunk control than sitting, reducing the stress of controlling posture and skilled movements simultaneously. No weightbearing demands are made on the shoulder of the up-side arm, as opposed to the prone position, nor does the infant have to work against gravity to use his hand in front of his face, as in the supine position. When the infant reaches out toward an object on the floor, his hand naturally falls toward the midline and into the visual field.

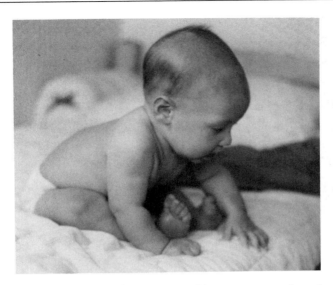

**Figure 8.6.**   The infant must use his arms to prop in early unsupported sitting. His hands are not free for exploration, and the pelvis is forward for stability.

### Sitting Position

Sitting is the infant's first independent upright position. Head and shoulders have become stable in the horizontal positions, and, although the demands of gravity on neck extension decrease when upright, the infant still must master the interaction of muscle groups in the neck to produce controlled head movements in the new position. Until that point, the infant often uses elevated shoulders to nestle the head to help steady it. This shoulder elevation frequently limits arm mobility.

Infants use **ring sitting** (hips abducted and externally rotated, knees flexed), which provides a wide base of support and a low center of gravity. The back is rounded, and lower back extension has yet to develop (Fig. 8.6). The shoulders and arms provide postural stability in one of two ways: (1) shoulders can be retracted to assist upper back extension to compensate for the rounded lower back, or (2) arms can be extended and used as props in front of the infant to keep him from tumbling forward. In the latter sitting posture, known as **tripod sitting,** neck hyperextension is required to right the head and often is accompanied by an open jaw. In either scenario, the hands are not free to engage in play. As head and trunk control develop, the back straightens and elevated and retracted shoulders come down and forward. As the pelvis becomes stable, the wide base in no longer necessary and **long sitting** is possible. In long sitting, the legs come together, putting the hip joints in a more neutral position. This makes weightshifting easier, because one hip can move into extension and external rotation, while the other flexes and rotates internally.

The ability to weightshift over the hips has implications for midline crossing with the arms, allowing for more functional activity with the arms. As the child rotates the trunk and reaches toward the contralateral side, weightshifts over the hips toward the contralateral side to maintain the center of gravity. The mature sitter can reach with a fully extended arm in all planes and still maintain posture and equilibrium.

### Standing Position

In the biomechanical frame of reference, standing is viewed as an alternate postural base for skilled movements of the head and arms rather than as a dynamic prerequisite for walking. The standing position is used with a large percentage of children in the context of this approach, regardless of whether or not ambulation is a probable goal. In fact, supported standing is particularly important for those children who are least likely to stand or walk independently.

The standing position is unique because of the amount of extensor activity required to maintain the posture. As in sitting, when the child begins to stand, he uses scapular retraction to assist with upper back extension. Scapular retraction also compensates for the lordosis created as the lower back is pulled forward by the weight of the abdominal cavity. As abdominal control develops, the pelvis tilts posteriorly into a neutral position, the spine becomes straighter, and the arms are liberated for skilled use.

When the standing posture is fully developed, a child can maintain a resting position of erect spine, neutral or slightly posterior pelvic tilt, and hips extended with neutral rotation. This neutral rotation of the hips involves placement of the knees and feet directly below the hip joint, without extreme abduction or adduction of the lower extremities. The knees are extended but not hyperextended. "Locking" of the knees may be used in the absence of muscular stability to provide mechanical stability. Ankles are at 90° of flexion and in neutral alignment laterally. If irregularities occur in the distal parts of the lower extremities during standing, proximal stability is influenced.

It should be noted that mobility in and out of positions has not been discussed. Although an understanding of these concepts is critical to the knowledge base of the occupational therapist, these concepts are not used in the biomechanical frame of reference. In this frame of reference, posture is looked at in a relatively static way, emphasizing those components that contribute to a stable, relatively immobile trunk as a basis for distal movements.

## Interference with Postural Reactions That Result from Damage or Dysfunction

Dysfunction of the musculoskeletal system has serious implications for postural control. As discussed in the previous section, mobility of all major joints is essential to weightshifting and equilibrium reactions. Fixed bony deformities and muscle contractures clearly would interfere with this freedom of movement. Lack of proper bone formation similarly can affect the balanced interaction of the movements needed for a child to keep himself righted in space. For example, incomplete development of the spinous processes on one side can result in a fixed lateral flexion of the spine. The fixed lateral flexion of the spine interferes with weightshifting onto the affected side in sitting. Without lateral movements to the opposite side, the child is unable to reestablish his center of gravity and is likely to fall to the affected side.

A compensatory movement or posture is the body's attempt to correct an error. In the previous example with fixed lateral flexion of the spine, compensatory positions are necessary in both the neck and in the hips. Two possible compensations are: (1) the child flexes the neck or nonaffected part of the spine in the opposite direction, creating an S-curve while keeping himself upright; or, (2) the child uses one arm as a prop to support the tipping trunk. In the first situation, neck mobility is limited, with possible negative effects on visual and oral-motor function. In the second situation, bimanual activity is impossible. Compensations often decrease mobility in joints that are not affected directly by the initial deforming process, because the compensatory positions must be maintained to provide a stable posture. They may occur not only in the presence of bony deformities but also in any situation in which normal movement patterns are compromised.

Motor problems that result from the neuromuscular dysfunction caused by central nervous system (CNS) deficits, such as cerebral palsy or static encephalopathy, may be more diverse and complex. Motor problems may be more diverse because such neuromuscular dysfunction is more global and is rarely isolated to one specific site in the body. Similarly, motor dysfunctions may be more complex because the manifestations of these deficits can fluctuate in relation to many factors, including changes in the child's position in space, effort in activities, affect, and stimulation in the environment.

Neuromuscular dysfunction often affects muscle tone. Muscle tone refers to the muscle's responsiveness to stretch, or its "contractability." This is not a matter of strength, rather, it is more the ability to contract on command and maintain or cease activation appropriately. A common error is to confuse high tone with strength and low tone with weakness. Normal tone gives muscles the ability to contract on command and to maintain or cease activation as necessary. Normal tone depends on the integrity of motor neurons and muscle fibers. More specifically, normal muscle tone depends on CNS ability to receive and respond to proprioceptive cues with the simultaneous excitation of certain muscles and inhibition of others. Normal muscle tone allows the muscle to react immediately with enough tension for weightshifting and support yet still have enough "give" to allow for quick changes in movement (Scherzer & Tscharnuter, 1982; 1990).

Muscles with low tone, or hypotonia, produce delayed responses. Children who have hypotonic musculature are "floppy" and tend to succumb to gravity. Their shoulders and backs often are rounded and their hips generally are abducted and externally rotated. Their joints are very mobile, and they may develop compensations for inadequate antigravity responses in the upright position, such as shoulder retraction and lumbar hyperextension. Despite low muscle tone, the compensatory muscle groups might be shortened or contracted because they often are used to maintain posture. Prolonged shortening or contraction of the muscle groups because of such compensation may result in decreased range of motion and deformity.

Muscles that exhibit high tone, or hypertonus, often are described as spastic. They exhibit a hyperactive stretch reflex. Clinically, this means that the muscle shows increased resistance to passive stretch. Functionally, these muscles generally respond to activation with full, rapid contractions, whereas antagonist muscles are relatively inactive. This results in ungraded movements that are maintained with the muscle in a shortened state. Hypertonicity appears primarily in antigravity muscle groups; however, all muscles in the group may not be hypertonic, even though it may appear otherwise. When the muscles work together as a group, the hypertonic muscles influence those muscles that have normal tone to produce atypical postural patterns. Two atypical postural patterns are (1) a flexion pattern of flexion, abduction, and external rotation in the upper extremities; and, (2) an extension pattern of extension, internal rotation, and adduction in the lower extremities. Children who show hypertonicity resist gravity and do not succumb to its force. They also have limited ranges of motion because of the overactivity of certain muscle groups. In addition, it is important to note that muscles that may not be hypertonic can become shortened because they are part of a pattern of movement initiated and maintained by hypertonic muscles.

It is also possible to have fluctuating muscle tone. This condition is commonly referred to as **athetosis**. In this case, antagonistic muscle groups contract and reflex almost in turn rather than interactively. This causes exaggerated movements with little control in the midranges.

In addition to muscle tone, it is important to consider the effects of the action of the muscles on the joints. One example of this is the multiarthrodial muscles—those muscles that cross over more than one joint. When children have high tone or shortened muscles (secondary to hypertonia), the control of such joints may be particularly affected, and this has implications for postural control. For example, the hamstrings, which run across both hips and knees, often are shortened in children who have hypertonus. It is difficult for these children to elongate those muscles over both joints simultaneously, making it difficult for them to combine hip flexion with knee extension. It is hard for these children to sit for long periods, because hip flexion often is compromised and the pelvis is pulled into a posterior tilt. To stay upright, these children develop a compensatory forward curve of the trunk.

When children have intact central nervous systems, their movements and and postures are effected by touch, proprioception, sight, sound, smell, health, and attitude. The influences of these factors are exaggerated in children who have tone problems. Postural stability in children who have CNS dysfunction may be influenced by movement, position in space, position of the head, tactile stimulation, stress or effort, temperature, surface support, intensity of environmental stimulation, and affect.

**Movement** includes active and passive movement, as well as movement of individual joints or of the body through space. Rapid passive movement of a joint in a hypertonic child may increase tone, as might efforts to initiate active movement. Rapid changes in speed can increase tone, particularly when unexpected. Slow, gentle rocking often decreases tone.

**Position in space** refers to changes in position of the body (e.g., upright, supine, tipped back, and so forth.) These positions are registered through vestibular, proprioceptive, and tactile receptors, that stimulate reflexive responses. Mature, functional responses include righting and equilibrium reactions. In children who have CNS dysfunction, reflex activity—involuntary, stereotypical movements in response to specific stimuli—often is primitive or pathological. A primitive reflex is one that normally occurs before the development of righting and equilibrium reactions and, therefore, should not recur after the first year of life. Such reflexes sometimes continue to happen in children who have CNS dysfunction and who have not developed normal postural reactions. A reflex is pathological when it occurs with greater persistence and when the child cannot willfully move out of the stereotypical pattern. An example of a primitive reflex influenced by the body's position in space is the TLR, which is triggered by increased flexor tone in the prone position and extensor tone in the supine position. A pathological manifestation of this reflex might be a total extension pattern in the supine position, with the child unable to tuck his chin, close his jaw, or bring his hands together or up to his mouth.

**Position of the head** in relation to the body may affect reflex activity. Examples include (ATNR) and the symmetrical tonic neck reflex (STNR), each of which creates different movement patterns, depending on whether the neck is rotated, flexed, or extended. The ATNR interferes with midline activity, whereas the STNR interferes with freedom of arm movements and pelvic stability for sitting. In addition, changes in head position can produce stereotypical, whole-body reactions in the presence of neuromuscular dysfunction. For example, head extension in a hypertonic child can create a strong, total extension pattern with shoulder retraction, arched back, and extended hips. Conversely, when that child's neck is flexed passively, then the entire body relaxes.

**Tactile stimulation** includes both light touch and deep pressure. Light touch often elicits phasic movements, which are undesirable in maintaining posture. Reflexes such as rooting and the Gallant are elicited by light touch and affect head or body position. The rooting reflex response takes the head out of the midline and may also elicit an ATNR, causing the entire body to be asymmetrical. The Gallant reflex causes trunk incurvation toward a source of touch on the lateral trunk, creating a temporary asymmetry of the spine.

The amount of **stress or effort** that an activity requires influences a child's movement and posture. An isolated movement that is difficult to execute may be accompanied by a total body reaction. For example, a child who easily is able to right his head when tipped forward 5° may have more difficulty when his head is tipped forward 20°. When the head is tipped forward 20°, the child may respond with total body extension because of the effort needed to meet the increased demands on neck extension. Furthermore, strenuous activity or emotional stress also may exacerbate associated reactions. An associated reaction, such as tongue protrusion when a child concentrates on a fine motor task, may be more pronounced in a child who has neuromuscular difficulties. For example, when a child with neurological impairment engages in a writing task with the dominant arm, exaggerated mirror movements may occur in the other arm. In the extreme case, the associated reaction may result in the nondominant upper extremity retracting and flexing, accompanied by fisting of the hand. This asymmetrical posture would interfere with bilateral use of hands, such as holding down the paper as the child writes.

The **temperature** of the environment also may influence movement and posture. Cool temperatures can increase muscle tone. Neutral warmth—temperature that approximates body temperature (provided by warm clothing or ambient temperature)—tends to reduce muscle tone.

**Surface support** refers to the surface on which a child is placed. Hard surfaces tend to be alerting and, therefore, may increase muscle tone. Hypertonic children may relax on well-cushioned but firm surfaces, whereas children who have lower tone may sink into the embrace of heavily upholstered surfaces and respond with more active postural control to a harder surface.

Frequent changes and high **intensity of environmental stimulation** increase tone, whereas monotony and low levels of intensity have lulling effects and generally are associated with a reduction of muscle tone.

**Affect** also may influence posture and movement. Affect refers to the child's state of mind and his emotional responses to events that occur in the environment. Strong affectual responses increase tone, regardless of their positive or negative associations. The strong positive emotions associated with motivation and particularly well-being obviously should not be discouraged for the sake of modifying hypertonus.

The last major assumption related to the effects of neuromuscular dysfunction on postural reactions and function applies to Rood's concept of phasic and tonic muscles and their appropriate purposes (Stockmeyer, 1967). Tonic muscle groups are best suited to postural maintenance and are located more proximally. Physiologically, these muscle groups are better suited for sustained contractions. When these muscles are unable to perform their tasks adequately, the phasic muscles act as substitutes. Because the primary functions of phasic muscle groups are mobility and skill, they are ineffective in postural maintenance. For example, children who have CNS dysfunction may use their shoulders and arms to "hold themselves up" because of inefficient tonic muscle groups that cause poor postural tone. The result is not only fatigue but also a lack of development in volitional skills for the extremities. Fatigue occurs because the phasic muscles are not well equipped for sustained contraction. Volitional skills do not develop because the extremities are used to maintain posture and are not free to engage in skilled activities.

The fundamental goal of the biomechanical frame of reference is to provide an artificial posture base from which the child can attend freely to his environment. An additional goal is to liberate the distal extremities so that the child can use them to interact with the environment. For one child, this might mean providing enough head control to make and maintain eye contact with a care provider or enough tone reduction to breathe deeply and easily. For another, it may mean the physical capacity to manipulate toys. This approach assumes that all children need consistent, effective postural responses for optimal manipulation of and interaction with their environments. When children are unable to do this effectively, therapists who use the biomechanical frame of reference can help the child develop those postural responses or can provide external substitutions for them.

## *Review of Assumptions*

As previously discussed, the biomechanical frame of reference maintains the following five major assumptions:

1.  The biomechanical frame of reference contributes to independence by providing external supports to substitute for inadequate or abnormal postural reactions and therefore
    A.  Facilitates the development of some postural control by reducing the effects of gravity, or,
    B.  Provides a permanent support when potential to improve seems negligible.
2.  Children learn to move effectively through sensory feedback, especially through the proprioceptive, vestibular, tactile, and visual systems. They repeat successful movements based on the sensory cues that the movements provide.
3.  Normal motor development is predictable and sequential. The development of motor abilities depends on a stable base of support and on the righting and equilibrium reactions that allow a person to respond unconsciously to the forces of gravity.
    A.  Posture depends on the body's response to gravity.
    B.  Postural reactions develop sequentially. Each new skill is based on a previously developed skill.
4.  Dysfunction or abnormalities of muscle, bone, or the CNS may impair the development of normal postural reactions.
    A.  Tone affects posture; tone is influenced by many internal and external factors, all of which can be modified.
    B.  If normal postural reactions have not developed, the body compensates by using substitute movements, more effort, and more conscious attention. All of these things may interfere with function.
5.  Occupational therapists must determine the level of postural dysfunction as well as the external factors that may affect performance. Treatment needs to provide substitutes for absent skills yet still make demands on the child's existing capacity to function.

# Function/Dysfunction Continua

Many things cause delays or dysfunction in a child's ability to interact with his environment. Only those things related to compromised postural reactions that interfere with skill development are appropriate targets for the biomechanical frame of reference. For example, the inability to use both hands at midline may be related to delayed sitting skills, which may cause retracted shoulders or the need to always prop on one arm for support. Conversely, that same inability may be the result of perceptual processes such as poor bilateral integration or tactile defensiveness and may exist regardless of postural competence. On the one hand, lack of fine motor control in ocular, oral, or hand skills may be related to head and shoulder instability. On the other hand, the problem may be specific to isolated distal muscles, or it may be come from a lack of organizational skills unrelated to posture. The first area to assess then is the child's general ability to make rapid, unconscious, and effective postural changes in relation to the forces of gravity.

The therapist should consider several questions. First, does the child respond to changes in position of head or trunk with readjustments throughout his body to keep his head righted and body balanced? Or, are these reactions present but delayed or weak so as to be ineffective? Or, are these reactions exaggerated and ungraded, so that the reaction causes movement in the opposite direction, throwing the body off balance? Or, are these reactions carried out primarily by more distal, phasic muscles that normally mobilize the shoulders and hips rather than by the central, tonic musculature in the trunk meant to maintain posture?

If postural reactions are delayed, weak, exaggerated, or performed by improper muscle groups, then the biomechanical frame of reference should be considered.

## *Range of Motion*

| Full Passive Range of Motion | Contractures, Deformities |
|---|---|
| FUNCTION: Full active range of motion | DYSFUNCTION: Limitations in range of motion or contractures |
| BEHAVIORS INDICATIVE OF FUNCTION: | BEHAVIORS INDICATIVE OF DYSFUNCTION: |
| Full, active range of motion | Functional limits of range of motion |
| | Fixed contractures |

# Head Control

In this continuum, function is represented by the child who can maintain his head in a righted position, regardless of movement and position in the rest of the body, and who can direct head movements as desired. This provides stability for ocular tasks such as eye control and visual fixation and for oral-motor control, as well as mobility for turning the head toward a source of stimulation. Dysfunction is represented by limited mobility or stability. This may occur primarily through inadequate muscular control or secondary to compensatory movements, such as stabilizing the head through use of shoulder elevation, which limits active range in both the neck and shoulders.

| Good Head Control | Poor Head Control |
|---|---|
| FUNCTION: Normal head control and mobility | DYSFUNCTION: Poor head control and mobility |
| BEHAVIORS INDICATIVE OF FUNCTION: | BEHAVIORS INDICATIVE OF DYSFUNCTION: |
| Head is righted and mobile in all planes | Able to maintain head in an upright position but loses head control when initiating a movement |
| | Unable to right head or control any head movements |

# Trunk Control

The functional end of this continuum is represented by the child who demonstrates equilibrium reactions in the trunk in an upright position and who has full thoracic range for inspirations and expirations. Here, respiration is only considered related to tone and position of the trunk. With less trunk control, dysfunction appears as (1) an inability to remain upright once distal limb movements are initiated, or (2) an inability to maintain any upright position at all. Abnormal muscle tone in the trunk can compromise respiratory capacity. Trunk deformities may occur from the force of gravity curving the trunk or from constant use of compensatory movements. Lateral or forward curvature of the spine reduces the thoracic space and may impair respiration, with detriment to health, energy, and phonation.

| Good Trunk Control | Poor Trunk Control |
| --- | --- |
| FUNCTION: Good trunk control | DYSFUNCTION: Poor trunk control |
| BEHAVIORS INDICATIVE OF FUNCTION: | BEHAVIORS INDICATIVE OF DYSFUNCTION: |
| Child's trunk is righted and stable in an upright position and is symmetrical when the child is seated or standing on a horizontal surface | Trunk is righted but unstable when limb movements are initiated |
|  | Trunk is not righted; is unable to remain upright or remains upright with asymmetry |
| Able to take advantage of a normal respiratory capacity | Respiratory capacity is compromised by decreased size of thoracic cavity because of trunk/shoulder position |
|  | Respiratory capacity is decreased because of abnormal muscle tone on respiratory muscles, such as the intercostals |

## Control of Arm Movements

The child who can reach in all planes, regardless of position, and who can maintain his hands where he would like them is at the functional end of the continuum. Dysfunction is represented by an inability to direct the hands because shoulders are involved in supporting the trunk, because tone in the arms is abnormal, or because arm movements against gravity are difficult to execute. Providing trunk support or changing the child's position in space can enhance function.

| Good Control of Arm Movements | Poor Control of Arm Movements |
| --- | --- |
| FUNCTION: Ability to reach in all planes | DYSFUNCTION: Inability to reach in all planes |
| BEHAVIORS INDICATIVE OF FUNCTION: | BEHAVIORS INDICATIVE OF DYSFUNCTION: |
| Able to place, maintain, and control his hands where he pleases when in an upright position | Child's arms are not liberated in an upright position: either they are needed for propping, or shoulders are retracted to aid in upper trunk stability, bringing the hands back with them |

Child cannot move his arms in gravity—resisted planes of movement—and therefore cannot place or maintain his hands where he wants them

## Mobility

The ability to move through space to attain a goal, explore an environment, or experience movement in many planes is at the functional end of the continuum. Mobility that is stressful or slow is dysfunctional, because the child often may feel that the effort is not worth the goal, or he may be too fatigued to interact with the person or object once he attains his goal. Lack of mobility is also dysfunctional in that the child is deprived of essential sensory experiences, particularly vestibular and proprioceptive, which are provided by movement through space.

| Mobility | Immobility |
|---|---|
| FUNCTION: Mobility through space | DYSFUNCTION: Slow, effortful mobility, or immobility |
| BEHAVIORS INDICATIVE OF FUNCTION: | BEHAVIORS INDICATIVE OF DYSFUNCTION: |
| Child is mobile through space in all planes (walking; climbing in, out of, and over obstacles) | Child can only locomote by rolling |
| Able to locomote in a horizontal position (crawling or creeping) on a flat surface | Child cannot move his body through space |

## Functional Performance Behaviors

The functional goal of the biomechanical frame of reference is to provide an artificial postural base from which the child can engage in functional activities. Other function/dysfunction continua are directed toward providing a secure postural base. The following function/dysfunction continua—eating and toileting—are two important examples of functional performance behaviors.

### Eating

The functional end of this continuum includes adequate oral-motor control to ingest food safely in an average amount of time without choking. Although feeding difficulties may exist despite the development of postural control, the absence of good head and trunk control exacerbates oral-motor dysfunction. Dysfunctional eating patterns (lack of jaw stability, poor tongue, cheek, and lip control, and disorganized swallowing) are affected by an unstable neck, compensatory movements in the shoulder girdle, impaired respiration, and abnormal tone associated with certain postures.

| Safe Eating | Unsafe Eating |
| --- | --- |
| FUNCTION: Safe, efficient eating | DYSFUNCTION: Difficulty with chewing and swallowing |
| BEHAVIORS INDICATIVE OF FUNCTION: | BEHAVIORS INDICATIVE OF DYSFUNCTION: |
| Child can chew and swallow food successfully without aspirating | Child is unable to grade jaw movements or control lips and tongue when eating |
| | Child frequently aspirates food |

## Toileting

Function in toileting includes the ability to void when seated on a toilet and the ability to sit independently on a toilet or commode. Dysfunction, with its concomitant lack of comfort and dignity, is represented by a lack of awareness or control of the voiding process or the inability to relax enough to void when sitting unsupported on a toilet. Awareness and control may be affected by abnormal tone, and postural control has a direct effect on the ability to relax when sitting independently.

| Continence | Incontinence |
| --- | --- |
| FUNCTION: Independence on toilet | DYSFUNCTION: Inability to void in toilet |
| BEHAVIORS INDICATIVE OF FUNCTION: | BEHAVIORS INDICATIVE OF DYSFUNCTION: |
| Child can empty bowel and bladder when seated on a toilet | Child can only void when lying down |
| | Child can maintain balance on a toilet but cannot direct the flow of urine into the bowl |
| | Child has no conscious bowel and bladder control |

Each of these functions depends on the interaction of numerous factors. Cognition, perception, and behavior, as well as organization and fine motor abilities, contribute to these skills. Evaluation of the postural components necessary for function will determine whether, and, specifically, which biomechanical assists are appropriate.

# Evaluation

The purpose of the evaluation is to assess the postural components of a given dysfunction to plan intervention. This can be done by using the function/dysfunction continua.

Within the biomechanical frame of reference, the child's potential for change in the area of postural reactions is a major concern. This requires the use of professional judgment and may require ongoing assessment over a period of months. The child's potential for change is an important factor, because it helps determine what type of postural aids should be used and how they will be most effective.

At times, the assessment of a child's needs within this frame of reference may be done by a therapist who has particular expertise in this area or through a clinic. The therapist who treats the child should be actively involved in equipment decisions because of her long-term interaction with the child and her understanding of the child's potential for change.

The assessment of the child begins by considering age, therapeutic history, physical status, prognosis, and environment, because they all contribute to the child's potential for change. Age is an important consideration because of the plasticity of the CNS. Therapeutic history is important because it indicates the types and focus of the child's previous contact with therapy and the child's responsiveness to intervention. Physical status indicates the child's general health, medication regime, and surgical history. Prognosis indicates the sequelae of the child's diagnosis. The environment influences the child's potential for growth and motivation.

When a child is evaluated for positioning options, the therapist needs to observe carefully any sequence of specific elements of postural control. The outline in this section is intended to assist with this process. It is important during this scrutiny to remember, however, that all elements of movement are interrelated, and that the therapist must step back and view the child's body as a whole. To take this further, it is imperative to apply the evaluation and intervention process to the child's life—the end goal is not that the child look good posturally in the therapist's eye but that he can **do** something that is important to **him.**

The assessment of the child should be done with the child involved in activities. This provides the therapist with an opportunity to analyze movement as it relates to posture and gravity. It is important to look at the child's ability to make rapid, unconscious, postural changes within the context of an activity. References and charts are available to assist in this evaluation of the sequential development of motor skills (Bly, 1983; Fiorentino, 1981; Pratt, Allen, Carrasco, Clark, & Schanzenbacher, 1989). In addition, wheelchair assessment forms are available from wheelchair manufacturers and are found in textbooks (Barnes, 1991; Bergen & Colangelo, 1985). Concentration is on those central postural skills needed to support movement of the head and limbs to manipulate the environment.

The following questions provide some guidelines for evaluating motor development in terms of functional posture, as derived from the function/dysfunction continua. In all cases, it is important to determine if dysfunctional movement is **delayed, slow to develop,** or **pathological,** influenced by abnormal tone or reflexes. Each question in italics is directed toward the functional end of the continuum.

*Can child move all body parts through full range against gravity?*

This involves the assessment of the child's passive range of motion and the presence of fixed or dynamic contractures. Just as important as passive range of motion are the effects of movement and changes in position on functional range of motion. Is muscle tone high, low, or fluctuating? What kinds of stimuli increase pathological tone and, possibly, interfere with active range of motion? Does the effect of gravity prevent certain ranges of movement mechanically or physiologically and can movement be enhanced by changing position to decrease the effects of gravity or by using gravity to assist movement? What movements or positions elicit reflexes that compromise full range?

If functional range is influenced by position, then the therapist needs to know how much of each day the child spends in different positions. A **positioning log** can be completed with the help of parents, care providers, and educators. How is the child fed, transported, toileted, and positioned for rest, recreation, and school? Which positions have been selected with function in mind, which can be modified to enhance movement, and which are selected to reduce stress on the family or care providers? In addition to the time spent in school chairs, high chairs, and wheelchairs, the child's time in backpacks, baby swings, car seats, beanbag chairs, floor, and bed

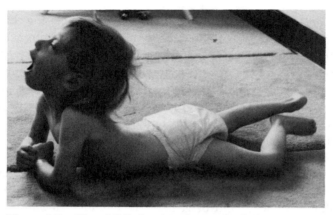

**Figure 8.7.** The child's head is thrown back for stability. Note the position of the mouth because of hyperextension.

should also be assessed. From the positioning log, the therapist can make modifications or suggestions to promote independent movement for the child and to ease caretaking for his family and school staff.

*Can child right his head and is it mobile in all planes?*

In the **supine** position, can the child maintain his head in midline, turn it to either side, and tuck his chin to observe people, body parts, and what might be in his hands? Is development delayed yet following a normal sequence, or is pathology present (Fig. 8.7)? Is difficulty with movement caused by low-tone struggle against gravity, or is immobility caused by high tone? Is there increased extension in this position because of the influence of the tonic labyrinthine reflex? This might include neck hyperextension, an open jaw, retracted lips, or upward gaze. Does the rooting reflex cause the child to press one side of his face against the floor? Does the inability to maintain head in midline elicit an asymmetrical tonic neck reflex? When attempting to lift his head from the supine position, does the child use peripheral, phasic musculature, such as the sternocleidomastoids, to substitute for deep tonic work?

In the **prone** position, can the head be lifted to 90°, or can it be turned freely to either side and be isolated from body movements so that the child does not flip over when he turns his head? Can he raise and lower his head with graded movements? Functionally, can he turn his head to examine his world visually, and can he control his mouth for age-appropriate speaking and swallowing in this position? If delay or pathology is present, is neck hyperextension necessary to keep the head upright? If so, is it accompanied by extension throughout the body? Can the child close his mouth when his head is righted, or is the jaw pulled into extension? Does the child simply collapse to lower his head?

In **sidelying,** where the effects of gravity on the head are minimized, can the child look up and to the side without flipping into a prone or supine position? Can he use lateral neck flexion against gravity to right his head or initiate movements of his body?

In the **upright** position—either sitting or supported standing—is the child's head aligned in space? Is it aligned with his body? It should be noted that the head may be righted, but the neck may be flexed laterally or hyperextended to compensate for poor trunk position, such as in scoliosis or kyphosis. If head control is poor, is shoulder elevation used to "nestle" the head for stability, thereby limiting neck mobility? Or, is the head generally thrown back or flopping forward? What is the controlled range of head movements? Can the child flex his neck forward 5° and right it again but loses control if he flexes 10° or more? If head control is inadequate, does tipping the trunk slightly forward or backward activate righting reactions or change muscle tone so that head stability is enhanced? If head control is minimal, how far back must the therapist tip the child's seat or stander until his head rests on a supporting backpiece without flopping forward? If the therapist supports the head by tipping the seat back in space, is this a functional position for viewing the world and a safe position for swallowing?

*Can child right his trunk and maintain stability?*

For therapeutic purposes, the trunk is seen not in terms of mobility but as a stable base of support for the head and arms, the primary parts of the body for seeking stimuli and manipulating the world. *This is not meant to minimize the importance of the whole body in learning but to establish priorities for someone who is very limited in functional movement.* The therapist, therefore, looks at the trunk's capacity to stay upright in response to displacement and its ability to support the head and arms as they change position in relation to the trunk (Fig. 8.8). The roles of the pelvis, legs, and feet are observed in conjunction with the trunk as part of the support basis for the body rather than in their roles of providing mobility through space.

A functional trunk also provides the base for good respiration: the rib cage is mobile and no fixed or functional contractures exist to reduce the thoracic space in which the lungs expand. For example, a fixed scoliosis may reduce the capacity of the lung on the flexed side.

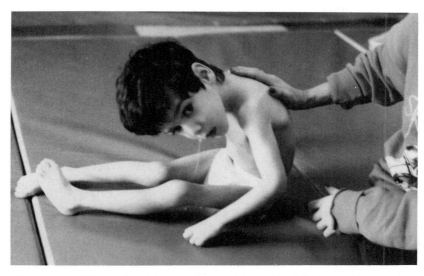

**Figure 8.8.**   When placed in a sitting position, this child is unable to right his head or trunk. Protective extension is absent.

Although the ultimate goal is a trunk that works well in an upright position, that capacity is based on postural skills that have developed first in a horizontal position. Attention to this area is particularly important in a dynamic approach when goals include improving motor skills in a developmental continuum.

In the **supine** position, is the trunk free from the influences of abnormal tone or pathological reflexes? Is the back hyperextended or asymmetrical? Are the legs stuck in a frog-like position or extended and adducted? Can the trunk maintain the body's position when the head turns and the arms reach away from midline, or does the child inadvertently roll over during head/arm movement? Is the pelvis mobile enough to allow the child to play with his feet? Or is it tilted anteriorly as part of an extension pattern so that there is a space between the lumbar spine and the floor? If the child needs extra stability, can he plant his feet on the floor?

In the **prone** position, is the child trapped by increased flexor tone or by the inability to extend against gravity? Is the pelvis flat on the floor, or does hip flexion push the center of gravity toward the chest so that it is difficult to raise the chest off the floor? Likewise, do exaggerated hip abduction and external rotation tip the pelvis in the anterior direction? Do the arms help support the chest, or does the child need to use back hyperextension to raise the chest and to reach out? When lifting the head

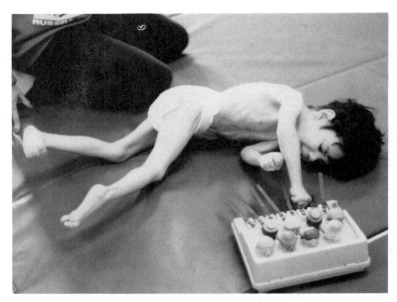

**Figure 8.9.** In an effort to maintain sidelying, tone is increased. The lower extremities are not available for stabilization and the hands are fisted.

and chest, is there associated hyperextension in the neck, lower back, and legs? When reaching upward, is there adequate abdominal activity to keep the child from rolling onto his back?

In the **sidelying** position, can the child maintain the position without bracing himself with arms or legs forward to keep from rolling? Can he look and reach in all planes and still maintain the position? Does an increase in extensor tone create arching and flipping back? Are there any trunk asymmetries that are exaggerated when lying on one side (Fig. 8.9)?

In an **upright** position (seated or standing), is the trunk righted, stable, and symmetrical at rest? Are adequate space and mobility evident in the chest for effective respiration? Can the child sit in various positions, or is he limited to one because of the stability it provides, such as ring sitting or "W" sitting? Are equilibrium reactions fully effective, or only within a limited range of displacement? Are arms liberated; can the child reach in any plane without losing balance, or is activity in the shoulder girdle or arms necessary to maintain an upright trunk? For example, retracted shoulders may assist upper back extension, or there may be a need to prop on one or both arms. Can the trunk support the head and itself but not the weight of the arms? This can be determined if the child can sit erect only when resting, **not when leaning,** with his arms placed lightly on a tabletop.

How do the positions of the pelvis and legs affect the trunk? Is weight distributed equally to both sides of the pelvis? Is the pelvis relatively neutral or tilted in the anterior or posterior direction? Is the pelvis too far forward, requiring compensatory lumber hyperextension or shoulder retraction to remain upright? Does a pelvis tilted toward the posterior create a rounded back, possibly with protracted shoulders and a hyperextended neck?

In the **sitting** position, does hip extension cause the child's back to press against the back of the chair, sliding him toward, or off the front edge of the chair? Are the hips adducted in such a way that the child has no lateral stability, or abducted in such a way that he has little anterior stability? Can hips, knees, and ankles be maintained in a position that allows feet to be planted firmly on the floor? Does the child seem to be more functional in a standing or sitting position?

*Can child place, maintain, and control position of his hands?*

In this area, the therapist's concern is not fine motor skill per se but the ability to **get** the hands where they need to be, **keep** them there as long as necessary, and **change their position** through controlled movements of the shoulders and arms from a stable base. Improving function in this area may have secondary effects on fine motor skills in two ways. First, modification of muscle tone in the trunk and shoulders often improves tone in the extremities. Second, control of hand placement provides more opportunity for manipulation and the sensory experiences that contribute to fine motor control.

As with previous areas, the clinician must look at the quality of muscle tone. How can gravity impede or improve movement mechanically and physiologically? Mechanically, the concern is how gravity weighs limbs down in various positions. Physiologically, the concern is how it elicits righting or reflex activity in various positions. Also, what compensatory movements or associated reactions interfere with function?

In the **supine** position, can the child reach in all planes against gravity and maintain his hands away from his body without the need to stabilize by grasping an external object? For example, can he reach up and touch a mobile or does he need to hold onto it to keep his hand in that position in space? Can he bring his hands to the midline, or does gravity or the

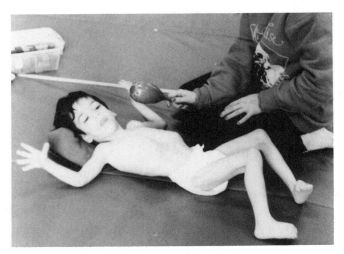

**Figure 8.10.** Because of the influence of the tonic labyrinthine reflex, this child is rendered dysfunctional by extensor tone.

activity of an ATNR or TLR prevent this (Fig. 8.10)? Can he get his scapulae off the floor by protracting for an upward reach? Can he look at and reach his tummy, knees, or toes, or must he look up and initiate a STNR to reach down?

In the **prone** position, can the child lift his chest off the floor by using interaction of his flexors and protractors to bring arms forward as supports, or with his extensors to bring his head and back up so that his elbows are beneath the shoulders (Fig. 8.11)? In the absence of flexor activity, is the chest raised by back extensors with little or no weightbearing on the forearms? Can the child shift weight onto one arm to reach out with the other? Does he collapse onto his chest when attempting to reach out, or compensate with neck and back hyperextension to keep from collapsing? Is shoulder stability adequate for sustained play in this position?

In the **sidelying** position, is the upper arm fully mobile in the sagittal plane? Can the child reach up from the floor against gravity? Are shoulder movements isolated, or does he need to initiate them with changes in the position of his head? Is his shoulder trapped in an internally rotated position by the effects of gravity in this position?

In an **upright** position, are the shoulders and arms free to move in all planes? Are there compensatory movements such as elevation, retraction, and external rotation, or protraction and internal rotation to assist an ineffective head or trunk? Is the shoulder girdle mobile enough for full

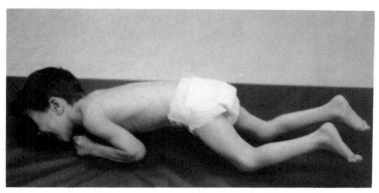

**Figure 8.11**  Hip flexion causes the center of gravity to shift toward the child's chest. He is unable to bring his arms forward to prop.

range but stable enough to maintain a position against gravity? Can the child use his arms only when supported by a tabletop? How does the position of the shoulder girdle affect mobility of the humeri and forearms? For example, protraction often is accompanied by internal rotation, adduction, extension, and pronation in children who have tone problems. How do the positions of the trunk and pelvis affect the position of the shoulders?

*Is child mobile through space in all planes?*

In this area, the concern of the therapist who uses the biomechanical frame of reference is not ambulation but mobility through space for two purposes. First, can the child move to attain a goal such as a toy, person, or food? Second, can the child move to provide proprioceptive and vestibular input to enhance the development of body schema and spatial awareness? The clinician looks at how the child moves independently through space and if mechanical assistance would be beneficial.

Can the child get to a desired goal by walking, creeping, crawling, or rolling? If so, does this process require pathological movements? Is the amount of time needed for the movement too extreme, or is the effort too exhausting? What alternatives for goal-oriented movement are realistic? Does the child have the potential to propel a wheelchair (either mechanical or powered), tricycle, or scooterboard, based on what the therapist knows about his functional range, postural reactions, and ability to maintain and control his hands? If he has independent but not optimal locomotion, is the potential improvement gained through a piece of equipment worth the extra training and hardware on child, family, and care providers? If the child has no independent movement through space, which one of several methods is most appropriate for his physical and emotional growth and his life style? In addition to goal-directed movement through space, what kinds of passive movement through space can be provided? How can the child's position be modified so that he feels comfortable and secure?

*Can child chew and swallow food successfully without aspirating?*

Feeding skills are assessed by the impact of posture on oral-motor function. The assessment of hand placement and control, as previously discussed, should yield similar information in relation to self-feeding skills. Although assessment of posture is critical to effective feeding intervention, it is only one part of a sophisticated evaluation of sensory, fine motor, cognitive, and behavioral skills that goes beyond the scope of this chapter.

Without describing an in-depth feeding evaluation, the following explanation gives examples of how posture and tone are incorporated into oral-motor assessment. Are the trunk and neck stable to provide a base for movements and stability of the jaw? Can the head be maintained in a neutral or slightly flexed position? Is the neck extended so that the airway is open and aspiration of food is more likely, or is it flexed in such a way that swallowing is difficult? Is the trunk in an optimal position for respiration, so that the coordination of swallowing and breathing is enhanced?

Does the presence of hypertonicity contribute to such oral reflexes as rooting or the bite reflex? Does it prevent isolated movements, such as separation of the tongue from the jaw? Are the tongue and lips retracted in association with extensor tone, so that the tongue cannot come forward and the lips cannot come together?

Is gradation of oral movements affected? Does the jaw just open and snap shut when food is presented? Can support of the head and trunk or changes in body position in space modify high tone so that oral control is enhanced?

How does gravity affect oral-motor control in the presence of hypotonicity? Does the child bite on the spoon because of ungraded jaw movements or because he is trying to keep his head from wobbling? Do the tongue and lips fall backward in a passively retracted position when the head is tipped back, and forward when the neck is flexed? Can the child create enough lip pressure to keep food from falling out of his mouth? Is there enough activity in the cheeks to keep food from spilling over the teeth and pocketing in the cheeks? Does the child manage better in supported standing or reclined sitting positions? Does a change in position increase postural tone or is extra support needed to accommodate for lack of tone?

*Can child void when seated on a toilet or potty?*

As with feeding, the biochemical frame of reference is only part of a complex evaluation of independent toileting. Information about the child's levels of cognition and sensory awareness is essential. Furthermore, it would be helpful for the therapist to know about the child's diet and behavior patterns.

The postural component addresses comfort, trunk stability, and the ability to relax hip extensors and adductors that otherwise might interfere mechanically with controlled elimination. The assessment is the same, then, as an evaluation of the child's capacity to sit in a stable, comfortable position with hips flexed and slightly abducted. In addition, the child should be assessed for the ability to direct the flow of urine into the toilet rather than onto the floor. This can be an issue with boys and girls alike and often is related to pelvic position.

An additional, extremely important component of the assessment is consideration of the family's or care provider's acceptance of any toiletting aid or device in terms of size, management, and cosmesis.

# Postulates Regarding Change

The biomechanical frame of reference uses external devices to promote the child's functioning. Based on the evaluation data, the occupational therapist establishes functional goals for the child that may be developmental or task specific. For example, a functional developmental goal might be to provide the child with a device to facilitate weightbearing on the forearms in preparation for controlled mobility. Another task-specific goal might be to provide the child with a switch plate to activate his communication device.

Postulates regarding change define relationships between concepts that structure the environment for change. These postulates help the therapist determine how and when to use adaptive equipment. In the biomechanical frame of reference, specific guidelines for the design, fabrication, and fitting of special devices are found in the application to practice section.

1. If practice time for a skill is increased, then the skill is developed more rapidly.

During therapy sessions, the therapist often handles a child so that he is better able to perform a task. A great increase in therapeutic handling time generally is as impractical for the staff as it is intrusive for the child. Adapted equipment can help the child practice certain skills because equipment "reproduces" the therapist's hands, albeit in a static fashion, to enhance function.

Regarding this postulate—that an increase in practice results in an increase in skill—the therapist must remember that *there is a point of diminishing return.* Judgment must be exercised in determining how often the child uses equipment and at what point its use causes stress. *Without moderation, a good tool can become abusive.*

2. If the therapist combines knowledge of the developmental progress of postural skills along with an awareness of the effects of gravity and sensory stimulation on normal and dysfunctional movement, then the therapist can determine appropriate positions to enhance a child's function.

The therapist needs to determine at what point in the development of the child's postural skills that dysfunction occurs and then how this dysfunction affects goal achievement. For example, the goal may be to bring the hand to the mouth in midline. The child cannot bring his hands together against gravity in the supine position and demonstrates compensatory shoulder retraction and external rotation in supported sitting. The therapist may choose sidelying, a position in which reflex activity is reduced and the effects of gravity are minimized. Or the therapist may find that correcting the child's seating position liberates the arms. If neither of these changes works, then the therapist may facilitate midline activity in sitting by guiding the shoulders and arms forward by using humeral "wings" attached to a laptray or table. These solutions are task-specific. The therapist may also choose to evaluate the child's capacity to maintain a prone-on-forearms position, understanding that this is believed to enhance shoulder mobility-on-stability, which is essential to directed hand movements.

Another important consideration for the therapist is to explore which positioning options are most effective for a specific child. In the previously mentioned situation, sidelying, corrected sitting with arm support, and the prone-on-forearms position were theoretically appropriate. The therapist may discover, however, that the child is unable to maintain a righted head in a horizontal position. The prone position, then, is not a good alternative for equipment, although the therapist may work toward that goal through active handling. Modified weightbearing on forearms could be considered in a more vertical position, such as supported standing at a 60° to 75° angle with forearms on a tabletop.

3. If the therapist handles the child in a variety of ways, she can determine how best to enhance normal postural responses in any one position.

Once the therapist determines an appropriate position, she often finds that the child cannot maintain the position independently without using compensatory movements. Because compensations defeat the purpose of using a position to enhance function, the therapist must identify the best way to help the child maintain a position correctly and still engage in as much normal postural activity as possible. This should be done by providing as much support as the child needs, but no more.

For example, to be able to use his arms, one child may need a seat belt and hip supports to stabilize his pelvis, lateral trunk supports, and a high back. A second child may self-correct when seated on a chair with a nonskid surface to maintain pelvic position, provided with back support only to the lumbar area. Adding other supports for this child is counterindicated, because it would increase dependence on a support surface. Active handling of these two children would determine their different needs.

The process of determining an effective way to correct a child's position includes a combination of handling, an understanding of theoretical information, and trial and error. The understanding of theoretical information helps the therapist gain insight into what might be happening as a child moves or is moved; she should not depend exclusively on that insight, however, to predict what will happen. Objective observation is essential, so that the therapist *sees and responds to what is happening, not what is expected to happen.* This is the point at which trial and error become important: the therapist makes an adjustment in the child's position based on theoretical principles and then evaluates the child's response. If the response is not a desired one, the therapist continues to experiment and evaluate until the desired response is attained. Although the many principles for correct positioning are discussed in the application section, *no* rules should be accepted without question.

What follows are postulates that may be helpful when handling a child to determine how to facilitate an effective position:

4. If the therapist first provides control centrally, then the distal parts of the body may be freed from the task of assisting the trunk or from the influence of associated reactions.

For example, if a child cannot prop in the prone position, it may be because his body weight is shifted onto his chest. Before supporting him under the chest, the therapist should extend the child's hips fully by pressing down on his buttocks. With weightshifting back over the hips, the child may now be able to bear weight on the forearms.

5. If the therapist uses the effects of gravity to the child's benefit, then the therapist may reduce the need for more intrusive pieces of equipment.

For example, a child in a prone stander may have poor head control. A prone stander provides full support to the child's ventral body surface, with a slightly forward tipping. When the child attempts to right his head, a full extension pattern appears, so that his neck becomes hyperextended, his arms retract actively, and his back arches. With a supine stander, the child can use slight neck flexion to right his head and lean back against the head support when fatigued, thus eliminating the need for the additional head and back controls in the prone stander. A supine stander provides support to the child's dorsal surface, with the body tipped back slightly.

6. If the therapist modifies the child's sensory environment, she may enhance the positive effects of adapted equipment.

If the therapist observes how the child responds to factors such as ambient noise and light, temperature, and the texture or firmness of a supporting surface, she should make changes in the environment to complement the postural device. For example, a child who responds to being placed on a cold plastic chair with a startle reaction and accompanying increase in extensor tone may be more posturally competent with a lightly padded surface. A child who becomes lethargic in the presence of soft, slow music may maintain an upright position more easily with an increase in the volume and tempo of the music.

7. If the therapist can identify an effective position through handling, she can reproduce that position by using an adapted device.

The therapist can "translate" a position from handling to a durable piece of equipment by recording what supports she provides with her hands or body and at exactly which points the supports contact the child's body. This record provides a blueprint for constructing or ordering equipment. Although specifications for measuring are included in the following section, some general principles that apply to all positioning devices include the following:

- The surface of support units should be solid and stable so that it does not "give" or change with the child's movements. Flexible surfaces such as beanbags or sling seats on wheelchairs accommodate to the child's weightshifting and can exacerbate asymmetries or dysfunctional postures.

- Ancillary supports, such as lateral trunk supports, leg adductors, or humeral "wings," should be large enough to distribute pressure over the surface of the body part. In this way the controlling support does not dig in and cause discomfort or, in some cases, active resistance. Whenever possible, blocks rather than straps should be used to control. For example, a therapist may feel the need to strap a child's arm to the laptray because a dysfunctional movement pattern of shoulder extension and internal rotation causes the child's fingers to become entangled in the wheelchair wheels. A more comfortable solution, and one that allows movement in functional patterns, would be to block the humerus forward, preventing horizontal abduction and shoulder extension and thereby keeping the fingers safe.

- The positioning devices should be fitted to the child; the child should *not* be fitted to the device. It may be tempting to place a child in a piece of equipment, to see how it "fits." Once in the equipment, ill-fitting parts may be difficult to observe. For example, a child initially may look well-supported in a wheelchair, when, in fact, the seat is too deep, causing a posterior pelvic tilt that is difficult to see. The better approach is to *measure the child first, then compare the ideal measurements to those provided by the equipment.*

8. If the therapist considers the needs of the child's care providers, she may provide equipment that is more likely to be used effectively.

Factors that influence care providers' attitudes include cosmesis, how much space the equipment fills, how difficult it may be to place the child in and out of the equipment, and how the device enhances or interferes with social interaction. For example, does the adapted commode fit in the bathroom at home? Or, does the chrome and plastic standing device look too industrial? If the equipment is offensive to those persons expected to use it, it is less likely to be used.

9. If the occupational therapist engages in team decisionmaking, then the child's equipment program will be more effective.

Working with family members, physical therapists, speech pathologists, teachers, physicians, and equipment vendors as a team provides more information about the child and makes the problem easier to solve. Each member of the team has a unique area of expertise and concern for the child. Accordingly, each team member provides distinctive input. All team members, including the family, should participate whenever appropriate in goalsetting and problemsolving.

# Application to Practice

Application to practice is divided into two sections. The first section discusses common positions in which central stability is provided artificially. The second section deals with postural components or pieces of equipment as they relate to functional skills.

## *Central Stability*

Any one position may be appropriate for a variety of goals, depending on where supports are provided and how the equipment, and, therefore, the child's body are oriented in space. Is the equipment perpendicular or parallel to the floor or tilted, and how does this affect the child? The following section provides an outline of what general goals may be approached in various positions, and how to fit equipment to the child. The box that starts each section contains a brief review of expected skill development in each position, along with the therapeutic advantages of the position.

### Supine Position

---

— Flexor activity develops

— Head control: midline control and chin tuck

— Shoulder protraction and flexion against gravity

— Hands to midline

— Reduced demands on trunk; more effort can be given to head, oral, ocular, and shoulder control

---

Although not normally very functional past infancy, for children who have physical impairments, practicing some movements in a restful supine position may be beneficial. Keeping in mind how gravity affects the child who has low tone and how reflex activity may increase hypertonicity in the supine position, the therapist may alleviate these effects by providing passive flexion. A pillow may be placed beneath the head and shoulders of a child so that it not only enhances neck flexion but also supports the head laterally and protracts the shoulders passively. A roll beneath the thighs can place the hips in a flexed position and yet allow the soles of the feet to be in contact with the floor.

### Prone Position

---

— Headrighting in a horizontal plane

— Interaction of dorsal extensors and ventral flexors for propping on forearms

— Shoulder stability during weightbearing (propping) and mobility-on-stability during weightshift

— Increased range of shoulder flexion when reaching from horizontal position

— Decreased effects of gravity on lateral asymmetries

— Hands more likely to be in visual field by nature of shoulder position when propping

---

A wedge provides the basic support unit to enhance prone positioning for a child who cannot prop independently. The wedge should be wide enough so that it does not tip if the child starts to roll over. The length of the wedge is determined by the point of support at the chest and hips. The lower the contact of the wedge on the chest, the greater the demands on the shoulder girdle for weightbearing. If the front edge is too far back, the child may flex his trunk and curl over it. The front edge of the wedge, where it contacts the child's chest, may also affect respiration (Fig. 8.12).

If a child tends to be kyphotic in the upright position but has a mobile spine, then the lumber spine can be extended passively by having the back edge of the wedge end at the child's waist. Conversely, a lordotic child who lies in the prone position with an anteriorly tipped pelvis should be provided with a wedge that extends well beyond the hips so that the lumbar curve is not exaggerated. The pelvis can be flattened further by **strapping** an "X" across the buttocks, each strap beginning at the iliac crest and crossing down to the opposite hip. This pelvic position, assisted by the straps, keeps the center of gravity at the hips. The straps also can prevent the child from pulling himself forward over the front edge of the wedge. It should be noted that the use of a single strap often results in the strap sliding up to the lumbar area, causing an increase in lumbar extension and pelvic tilt (Fig. 8.13A, 8.13B).

The distance of the front edge of the wedge from the floor determines the demands placed on the shoulder girdle. A very low wedge provides support

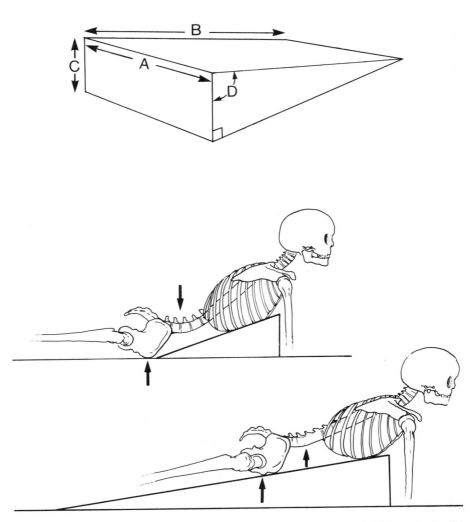

**Figure 8.12**    Measurements to consider for a prone wedge. **(A)**, Width: unit should be wide enough so that it will not tip over if the child rolls over when strapped to it. **(B)**, Length: Contact of the front edge with the chest will determine how much shoulder stability is needed; the lower on the chest, the more the child is taxed. Where the back edge ends in relation to the child's trunk or legs will determine lumbar curve and pelvic tilt. **(C)**, Height of wedge will determine if weight is borne on forearms or extended arms. **(D)**, Depending on which side of the wedge is chosen as the top surface, shoulders will be placed in either 90° flexion or a lesser degree of flexion.

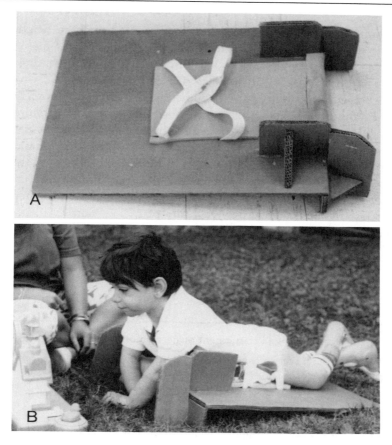

**Figure 8.13.**   The prone lyer **(A)** provides hip control, lateral controls, and wings to prevent shoulder abduction and extension, keeping the arms forward of the shoulders **(B)**.

to the chest as the child fatigues but places high demands for weightbearing on the arms and allows more upper trunk mobility for weightshifting. A higher wedge that fully supports the chest but is low enough so that the forearms contact the floor reduces stress on the shoulders, provides proprioceptive feedback, and allows the less stable child to reach out without collapsing. A very high wedge may be used to eliminate demands on upper extremity weightbearing. In this position, a child's arms may dangle downwards, in the same direction as the force of gravity. As the influence of gravity is minimized on the arms by the position, when the child makes a slight shoulder movement it results in a larger movement of his hands in his visual field. It is important to remember that the activity provided and the height of the activity relative to the child determine how the child uses his arms. For example, the child may play with small figures when weightbearing on both elbows but must weightshift to place rings on a stackpole.

When used in conjunction with hip straps, lateral supports to the trunk can help align the spine in the prone position. With some children, head raising in a prone position is accompanied by associated extensor patterns in the lower extremities, including hip adduction and ankle plantar flexion. This pattern can be modified by placing an abductor between the knees, distributing pressure along the inner legs. Too much abduction creates an anterior pelvic tilt. A small roll beneath the ankle supports the instep so that the ankles are not stretched passively into plantar flexion.

Maintaining the head upright when in a horizontal position can be stressful. *The therapist must monitor carefully the amount of time a child is required to be in this position.*

### Sidelying Position

---

— Lateral headrighting (a component of neck stability in the upright position)

— Differentiation of two sides of the body (bottom side weightbearing, top side mobile)

— Hands easily placed in visual field

— Hypertonicity reduced; tonic labyrinthine reflexes inhibited

— Effects of gravity on shoulder flexion/extension reduced

---

The child who cannot maintain the sidelying position independently requires front or back supports to prevent inadvertent rolling (Fig. 8.14). The back support can be a wall or a board perpendicular to the floor. The front support can be a block that contacts the trunk but allows movement of the shoulders and hips. This block is preferred to straps because it distributes pressure more evenly.

The child's head should be supported by a pillow or padded block that keeps the head and neck aligned laterally with the spine, to prevent asymmetry and to facilitate lateral headrighting. This also helps relieve pressure on the downside shoulder. It is important to make the pillow deep enough so that the child's head does not fall when he flexes his neck. If he tends to extend his neck, slight padding can be attached to the back support behind his head to encourage a neutral anterior/posterior neck position.

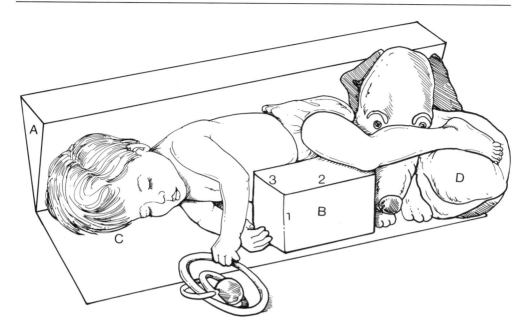

**Figure 8.14.** Possible components of a sidelyer: **(A),** Wedged back tips child forward and assist in passive protraction. **(B),** Chest block/ leg support. (1.) Height determines the position of the upper hip (adduction/ abduction; internal/external rotation). (2.) Length determines if chest alone is supported or if hip, leg, and foot of upper leg are supported while lower leg is held in extension. (3.) Depth is an issue only if the block also is used to maintain the position of the lower arm in shoulder flexion and elbow extension. **(C),** Surface is padded beneath this child's head, but no pillow is used because his head is proportionately large in relation to his body. A pillow would flex his neck laterally. **(D),** Stuffed animal acts as a leg block to extend the lower leg while supporting the upper leg in flexion. A longer chest block/leg support could have been used.

If the child tends to retract his shoulders, the therapist can use gravity to facilitate protraction by rolling him slightly forward. This can be done by angling the back support slightly forward. As the child's upper arm falls toward the floor, the shoulder tends to adduct horizontally and rotate internally. If this is not a desirable position, the top of the trunk support block can be used as an armrest. This does, however, eliminate functional hand use in this position.

The downside leg generally is extended and the upside leg is flexed. If necessary, the weightbearing leg can be extended by blocking the knee, distributing pressure along the thigh and skin. The child who has lower tone generally does not need this blocking at the knee, because the upside leg can be flexed easily, adducted, and rotated internally. This is important because the child who has low tone tends to position his hips in abduction and external rotation. When placing the child who shows extensor hypertonicity in sidelying, his hips generally are positioned more appropriately in neutral abduction/adduction and neutral rotation. This is accomplished by supporting the knee, tibia, ankle, and foot with a long block to position the hip properly and, simultaneously, to prevent the tibial torsion and ankle inversion/plantar flexion caused by lack of support to the foot.

It is important that the child be positioned in sidelying on both sides equally, in most cases. A sidelyer can be provided with detachable parts so that head and leg supports switch, allowing the child to be placed on either side. One exception is the child who has a functional scoliosis; generally the scoliosis is reduced when the "C" curve faces down and is exaggerated when the "C" faces up. Another consideration for determining on which side to place a child is hand use: the upside arm is more liberated and most likely to be used.

### Sitting Position

---

— Anterior/posterior and lateral stability of neck and trunk

— Weightshift on hips; hips in a slight anterior tilt

— Arms liberated; shoulder position independent of trunk

— Shoulders provide stable base for arm movements

---

The child who is unable to sit independently basically needs stability in the pelvis and lower body to use the upper trunk, arms, and the head actively (Fig. 8.15). Compensatory movements often occur in response to an inadequate central base of support. The therapist must first correct or support any inadequacies in the base, especially at the pelvis, hips, or legs. This may decrease compensatory movements or associated reactions elicited by stress, giving the therapist a better idea of what corrections need to be made in the more mobile, upper parts of the body.

Another way to modify tone to enhance the child's function is to consider the padding on the support unit. Sitting on a hard support tends to increase arousal level. Adding a medium density foam to create a softer support, which conforms to and supports the curves of the child's body, tends to reduce postural stress and hypertonicity.

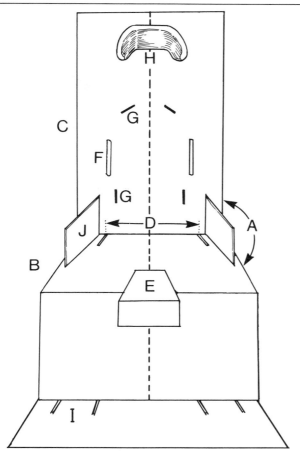

**Figure 8.15.** Possible components of an adapted chair: **(A),** Hip angle is commonly 90°, open more if hamstrings are very tight; close angle slightly if it helps to reduce extensor hypertonus. **(B),** Seat depth should support thighs fully without digging into calf behind knee. **(C),** Seat height is determined by need for trunk/head support. **(D),** Hip straps generally come from seat bottom to hold bottom of pelvis back. Slots or attachments should be placed directly alongside the body to prevent lateral shifting of pelvis. **(E),** Abductor serves to keep legs centered; amount of abduction is determined once pelvis is secured in seating unit. Abductor starts at midthigh, distributing pressure out to the front of the knees, beyond the front edge of the seat. **(F),** Lateral trunk supports are placed only as high as necessary to assist with trunk control. They should not interfere with humeral mobility because of height or thickness. **(G),** Slots or attachments for harness come in contact with shoulders without digging into the child's neck, and lower placement should be below the rib cage to allow for thoracic expansion during respiration. **(H),** Placement and angle of head support should be determined after hip and trunk controls are provided, in conjunction with decisions regarding tilt in space. **(I),** Footstraps may be needed if knee extension keeps feet from providing a base of support. **(J),** Hip guides may be necessary to keep pelvis centered and may help keep pelvic weightbearing symmetrical.

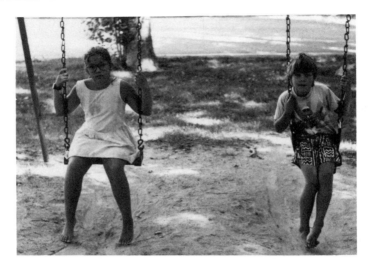

**Figure 8.16.**   A solid seat (left) allows the hips to assume a relatively neutral position. The sling seat (right) forces the hips into adduction and internal rotation.

The child's pelvis should be supported on a solid surface—padded if necessary—that extends to just behind the knees to support the thighs. Careful measurements must be taken when designing and ordering seating equipment. A seat that is too deep causes the edge to dig in behind the child's knees, pushing the legs and the bottom of the pelvis forward. A seat that is too shallow does not support the child's thighs, and the weight of his legs pulls his thighs downward and the bottom of his pelvis forward (Fig. 8.16).

The back support should be no higher than necessary to discourage postural dependency. Some children do better with a back support that stops at the level of the pelvic crests, or with no back support at all. If a full back that also supports the head is necessary, attention should be given to the shape of the child's head. Young children, and those with hydrocephalus, often have large occipital regions. The high back support may push a large head forward, causing compensatory curve in the neck. In such cases, recessing the head support allows for correct cervical alignment.

The position of the child's pelvis also is controlled by the angle of seat-to-back (the angle of hip flexion) and the angle of the seating unit in space (amount that it tilts backward). These two factors should be explored simultaneously. The hip angle generally is most effective at 90°. Increasing hip flexion or decreasing the angle of seat-to-back may reduce **severe extension hypertonicity.** Once that high tone is reduced, however, only minimal postural tone may remain in the trunk. In another situation, when a child has

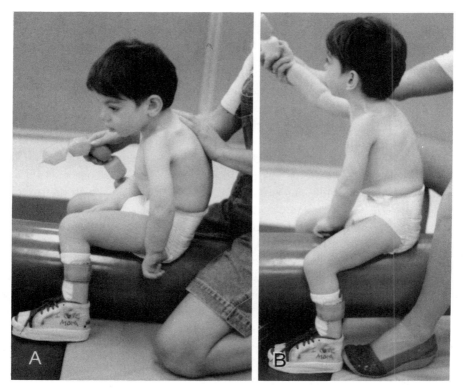

**Figure 8.17A,B.** **(A),** Tight hamstrings pull the pelvis into a posterior pelvic tilt. **(B),** By decreasing the angle of hip flexion on an elevated roll, the pelvis assumes a neutral position, enhancing a sitting posture.

very tight hamstrings, extending the hips slightly (5°–10°) may reduce the posterior pelvic tilt caused by the pull of his hamstrings. Opening the seat angle also can be effective with a low-tone child if the back is perpendicular to the floor and the seat slopes down from the back. The increased proprioceptive input to the feet may facilitate postural alertness (Fig. 8.17A, 8.17B).

To secure the child's pelvis, a seat belt is used. Coming up from the point at which the seat meets the chairback, the belt is at a 45° angle to the hips and holds the pelvis in place. Rather than coming from the outside edge of the seat, it should be attached alongside the hips to keep the child's pelvis centered. If the belt comes from the back support parallel to the floor, it holds back the top of the child's pelvis. This is helpful when an exaggerated anterior pelvic tilt exists, but, in most cases, it is contraindicated. A strap that comes from the seat perpendicular to the floor holds the pelvis back well but may cause more hip adduction than desired. The belt itself should be wide enough so that it does not dig into the child's flesh, but narrow enough so that it places control only where desired. A too-wide strap placed at a 45° angle causes a posterior pelvic tilt by pulling the top of the child's pelvis backward.

If the child's pelvis tends to move laterally on the seat despite the seat belt, pelvic blocks can be used for centering. These blocks angle slightly out from the seat back to nestle the child's pelvis in place.

Depending on the degree to which it is done, tilting the seat unit slightly backward may increase or decrease postural demands. The stress and extensor tone that accompany an upright position can be decreased with a backward tilt. This provides the child with a back support on which he can lean intermittently. The same position may encourage activity in the neck or trunk flexors when the child comes forward into an upright position from a partial recline (Fig. 8.18). When a reclining position is used to reduce the effects of gravity on the trunk and the child is incapable of flexing his neck or trunk forward into a righted position, it is important to support his head so that it is upright. This allows him to look forward rather than at the ceiling.

The child's thighs contribute to his base of support. Too much abduction reduces anterior/posterior stability. Too much adduction reduces lateral stability, as well as contributes to a pattern of extensor hypertonicity. Supports that run laterally along the child's thighs reduce abduction (Fig. 8.19A, 8.19B, 8.19C). In general, the child's hips should be in neutral abduction/ adduction. For some children, moderate hip abduction may be used to provide a wider base of support or to help reduce extensor tone in the hips. A rhombus-shaped wedge can be used to abduct the child's hips. When used, it should start at the middle of the child's thighs and extend to his knees, beyond the edge of the seat, to distribute pressure. A rhombus-shaped wedge also may be needed to keep the child's thighs symmetrical if one hip tends to abduct or to rotate externally while the other adducts or rotates internally (Fig. 8.20A, 8.20B, 8.20C).

Care must be taken that the seat is not too high from the floor so that the child's feet can be placed firmly on the floor or on the foot support. Having knees and ankles at 90° is a good guideline. Foot orthotics should be considered to correct ankles that are unstable or pathologically positioned so that the child's feet can contribute to stability.

Once the child has been positioned so that his pelvis is aligned properly, the therapist is better able to determine the positioning needs of the trunk, shoulders, and head. Trunk supports provide lateral stability as well as some shoulder correction. Lateral supports should contact the child's trunk only

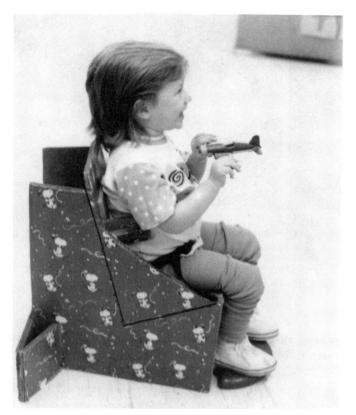

**Figure 8.18.**  This child feels secure and is able to use her hands for play in a slightly reclined seat. Note that lines on the chair indicate seat angles.

when necessary. *If lateral supports are placed slightly away from the body to encourage the child to do more postural "work," it is critical to determine if this demand compromises functional use of his arms.* A child may not be able to control his trunk and arms simultaneously. The higher the lateral supports, the more control they provide. The two supports should be opposite each other, unless tone in the trunk is asymmetrical; in that case, the supports should be low on the convex side and high on the concave side to correct the scoliosis. Care should be taken that the supports are not so high that they press into the axilla, nor so far apart that they hold the humeri in an abducted position. *Improperly placed lateral supports interfere with shoulder mobility and hand use.*

Laptrays or table surfaces can be designed to contribute to the child's correct shoulder and trunk positioning. *It is important that they be provided only*

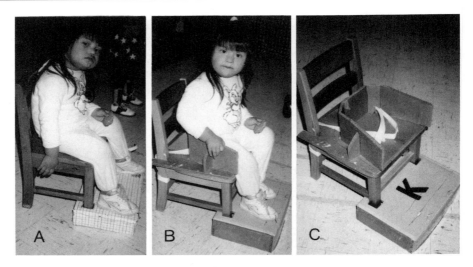

**Figure 8.19.**   By providing support to the lower back **(A)** and adducting the thighs **(B)**, this positioning device enhances an upright posture **(C)**.

*after optimal positioning has been attained through design of the seating or standing unit.* With an improperly fitted basic unit, a child may use a laptray to "hang" by his arms or to rest his head and upper trunk, rather than enhance arm position and function.

A laptray should provide enough surface area to support the full length of the child's arms during all movements. Hands or fingers do not hang off the edge of the tray. If the tray "wraps around" the child's trunk, the cutout should be large enough so that it does not dig into the child's chest or interfere with his breathing or slight weightshifts. It should be snug enough so that his arms do not slip between the trunk and the tray and become wedged. In general, it is preferable to provide a transparent tray for two reasons: First, a child can see the rest of his body, and second, in a wheelchair, a child or care provider can see the floor through the tray to maneuver more easily through space.

A harness made of a chest plate with four straps can prevent the child from falling forward. Often, when a harness is used, the child's sitting unit is tipped slightly backward so that the child rests against the back and does not hang into the harness. The top two straps attach to the back support directly over the shoulders. Slots may be cut into the back for proper strap placement. This ensures a snug fit and, simultaneously, discourages shoulder elevation. It also discourages lateral upper trunk flexion by keeping the shoulders at the same level. The lower straps should attach to the back or through

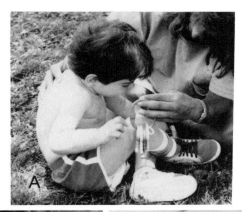

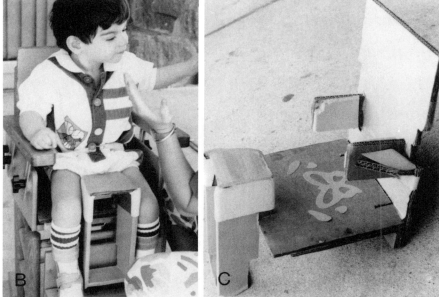

**Figure 8.20.** Correction of this child's sitting posture requires appropriate seat depth, high back support, seat belt at 45°, an abductor running from thighs to ankles, and lateral trunk support. In the sitting device, the child's arms are free for play **(A-C).**

slots on either side of the trunk, below the level of the rib cage so that they are less likely to interfere with thoracic expansion during respiration. The chest plate should be at midchest so that there is no danger of it digging into a child's neck (Fig. 8.21).

If the harness causes the shoulders to become retracted, small wedges attached to the back support at the level of the scapulae can be used to nudge

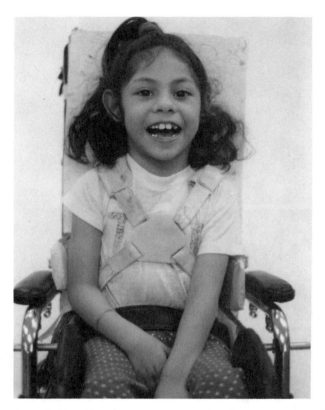

**Figure 8.21.**   This harness prevents shoulder elevation and provides trunk support.

the shoulders forward. Care should be taken that the sizes or positions of the wedges do not create rounding of the upper trunk. If retraction is mild and the scapulae are mobile, then the protraction wedge may be used without a harness.

The child's use of a laptray can enhance arm and hand function by diminishing pathology in his shoulders. Although it cannot directly affect humeral rotation by flexing the shoulders, the pattern of internal rotation, extension, and protraction is modified. In addition, the humeri can be adducted horizontally, bringing the arms toward the midline, by using humeral wings. These also help to correct the position of humeri that are extended as part of a retraction/external rotation pattern. The "wings" are surfaces attached perpendicular to the laptray. They push the humeri forward, preventing humeral extension or horizontal abduction. They should provide contact along the length of the humeri and be high enough so that the child cannot lift his arms over them and get trapped behind them. By holding the child's arms in the desired position and running a pencil mark along the humeri on the tray, proper placement of the "wings" can be marked.

The child's use of a laptray can contribute to trunk control by supporting his arms, thereby relieving the trunk of the weight of the arms. In this situation, the tray supports the arms, **not the trunk.** In addition, passive shoulder flexion that places the humeri in an almost horizontal position helps to elongate the thoracic spine as long as the child is not hanging by his arms on the tray. Position of a laptray or table surface can range from midtrunk to just below the axillae, depending on the child. It may be difficult for children who demonstrate inadequate shoulder flexion or tightness in shoulder extension to keep their elbows and forearms on the tray surface, because the arms are inclined to slide back from the tray edge. Two possible solutions include the use of a "wrap-around" tray or the use of humeral wings. Using a harness in conjunction with "wings" helps to stabilize the chest and position the arms effectively.

Two issues prompt concern when using a laptray on a seating or standing unit that tips back. First, if the laptray is perpendicular to the back of the unit, it will be angled toward the child in an easel-like fashion when the unit is tilted back. The tilt of the laptray can be controlled with adjustable hardware to keep it horizontal when the unit is tipped back. Second, by tipping the child slightly backward, gravity tends to push the humeri backward. It may be necessary to consider humeral wings that might not be otherwise needed when the child sits in a full, upright position.

The therapist may choose to tilt the laptray like an easel if it helps correct trunk or head position. By resting his forearms on an easel surface, the child may use greater degrees of shoulder flexion. This may elongate the upper trunk, enhancing the upright position. Also, tilting the laptray places visual stimuli closer to eye level. This may encourage the child to keep his head in a more upright position, rather than to look downward and initiate a flexion pattern in neck and trunk when reading or drawing (Fig. 8.22A, 8.22B).

Because of the complexity of the head, shoulder, and arm interaction, the therapist must be flexible and try several approaches to meet the child's needs. Correction in the child's shoulders may provide more freedom of head movement or, conversely, may create a need for external head support. For example, by correcting a pattern of shoulder retraction and external rotation and straightening of the upper back, the child may no longer need compensatory neck extension to align his head with his body. Another child, with the same corrections, however, may require a head support.

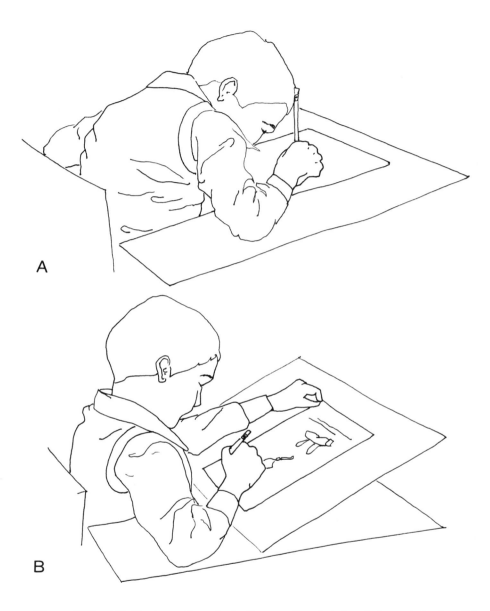

**Figure 8.22.**  **(A),** Flexion pattern, including overflow into hands is created when this child looks down at his work. **(B),** Angling the work surface changes the position of the head and modifies associated tone.

The first approach to improve inadequate head control or dysfunctional positioning of the head caused by tone problems is to correct total body position. Given enough external body support and reduction of physical stress, the child may be able to exercise control over his head on his own. Alignment of the child's body, as well as modification of tone, can reduce associated reactions and the need for compensatory movements in the neck. It should be remembered, however, that many pathological reflexes are elicited by head movement. In such cases, correction of head position can enhance body position. For example, slight flexion of a hyperextended neck may reduce extensor tone throughout the body, and maintaining the head in midline may eliminate body asymmetry caused by the influence of an ATNR.

Head position also is related to the source of visual or auditory stimulation. Most children hyperextend their necks when seated in a chair to look at and speak with an adult who stands before them. The position of the child in the environment, or the stimulus in relation to the child, must be considered when attempting to correct head position.

The simplest support for the head may be a high seat back. This provides a "resting" place but no lateral or anterior controls. In conjunction with a slight tip-back of the unit, gravity assists in preventing passive, floppy forward flexion yet still encourages active neck flexion against slight resistance. The latter example may enhance active control of the head in some children. Another child may use an undesirable pattern of total flexion to right his head when tipped back. Three drawbacks to the high back for head support are (1) the hard flat back may not provide enough surface support for the rounded back of the head; (2) the point of contact of the seat back with the head may provide a tactile cue that stimulates neck extension against the surface; and (3) if the child's occipital area is big, the head will be forced forward and out of alignment with the back, causing neck flexion with a downward position or compensatory extension at the base of the cranium.

Another simple control consists of lateral head supports in conjunction with a high back. Care should be taken that these supports not interfere with the visual field or not cover the ears. In addition, if the lateral supports touch the cheeks, a rooting reflex may result.

Neck rings and neck collars contribute to head control with no interference to sensory receptors on the head and face. A neck ring attaches to the seat back and cradles the base of the cranium. It should be placed at a height that provides slight traction on the neck, elongating the neck and providing constant contact with the base of the skull. The neck ring reproduces the shape of the therapist's hand were she to place her thumb and forefinger around the back of the child's neck with the occiput resting on the web space and the base of the temporal bones on thumb and fingertips. A neck collar made of medium density foam, cut in width to fit between the shoulders and the base of the skull snugly, supports and elongates the neck and can be used independent of the seating unit. To allow for slight neck flexion or jaw movements, the front of the neck collar should be connected in a yoke-like fashion.

Some supportive headrests are sculpted so that they conform to the head and neck. If a child requires the support of a sculpted headrest, or, in some cases, the less supportive head ring, it is likely that he will be unable to prevent his head from falling forward when in an upright position. A slight backward tilt of the seating unit assists in keeping the head in contact with the support. When a child is tipped back more than 5° or 10° for the sake of trunk control, however, it is necessary to right the head as much as possible by angling the head support or pushing it forward to flex the neck and align the head in space. The therapist must experiment with the child to find the optimal relationship among head, trunk, and angle in space.

In extreme cases, a child may have a complete lack of head control. Three options can be explored, all of which have possible drawbacks. The first is a full neck collar. This immobilizes the head and may interfere with jaw movements or swallowing. The second is a severe recline of the seating unit (up to 40° tipped back) in conjunction with a head support. This limits the child's visual field or possibly compromises swallowing. The third choice involves stabilizing the head in a slightly reclined position by strapping the forehead to the seat back or by wearing a helmet-like device with a chin strap attached to the back of the seat. A forehead strap alone may result in passive compensatory neck extension because the head slides down out of the strap. The helmet may be hazardous to the integrity of the cervical spine if the child's body slides down when the head is immobilized, or pressure from the chin strap may create problems with swallowing.

In general, demands on active head control in the severely involved child should be minimized when the child is seated so that efforts can be directed toward intake of information, interaction with the environment, and fine motor or oral-motor skills. The therapist should keep in mind that developing active components for head control may be addressed by using various positions and equipment such as standers, scooterboards, and prone wedges.

## Supported Standing Position

— Erect spine, liberated arms
— Neutral or slightly posterior pelvic tilt
— Hips extended with neutral rotation

— Knees stable but not locked in hyperextension

— Ankles in 90° flexion, neutral eversion/inversion

— Improved circulation and bone growth from upright weightbearing

— Increased alertness from upright position and extensor activity

— Decreased effects of flexor hypertonicity in neck and trunk when weightbearing on extended hips and knees

The supported standing position should not be used for potential ambulators exclusively (Fig. 8.23). In fact, this position provides increased opportunities of function for those children who are least likely to walk by enhancing circulation, growth, and alertness; it also provides opportunities for head and arm control for children who have moderate to severe disabilities.

The therapist first must decide which surface of the child's body is to be supported in standing. Providing support to the ventral surface by using a "prone" stander at an 80° to 85° angle to the floor provides a close-to-normal standing position and requires slightly more extensor activity. If upright at 90°, the prone stander tends to throw the child's body backward in space, and he may flex over the top edge of the stander to compensate. A supine stander provides dorsal support for children who show very high or very low tone. For example, when slightly reclined in a supine stander, the very floppy child who has minimal head control is provided with total support. The child who has too much extensor tone and who throws his head, shoulders, and upper trunk back in a prone stander is encouraged to use flexion to right himself intermittently in a slightly reclined supine stander.

Through a series of trials and observations, the therapist can determine the optimal angle of standing board to floor. Postural demands and postural responses change as the stander is tipped farther forward or backward. In a prone stander, demands on headrighting are less in an upright position than in a horizontal position. The child who cannot maintain a righted head in a prone lying position may be successful in a prone stander at 75°. In this case, with head control and tolerance in the prone position as the primary goal, the prone stander actually may be lowered as the child masters head control in increasingly higher horizontal positions.

The height of the stander determines how much support is provided to the trunk (and head in a supine position) and how much postural work must be done by the child. The therapist's goal is to make some postural demands without causing fatigue or undesirable associated reactions that result from physical stress.

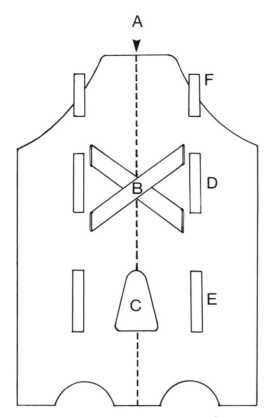

**Figure 8.23.** Possible components of a prone stander. **(A)**, Height is determined by child's need for ventral support, anywhere between the waist and sternoclavicular joint. When the support is cut high (as in this example), sides must be cut out to allow for shoulder mobility. **(B)**, Hip straps come through slots right alongside the hips. They cross from the posterior crest of one side to the hip joint of the other side, placing pressure over the sacrum. **(C)**, Abductor wedge keeps the legs aligned symmetrically and determines the amount of hip abduction. It runs above and below the knees but does not come in contact with the perineum. **(D)**, Hip guides may be added for additional lateral stability, especially in the presence of a functional scoliosis. **(E)**, Lateral leg guides prevent the external rotation/knee flexion pattern that often causes children with low tone to collapse in standing. **(F)**, Lateral trunk supports may be necessary and should be placed as low as possible.

As with sitting, the hips and legs should be positioned first. In the prone stander, crossed straps should stabilize the pelvis in the same way as in the prone position. If lateral shifting of the pelvis occurs, which would create a compensatory curve in the trunk, lateral pelvic blocks similar to lateral trunk supports should be placed on either side of the pelvis. With hips in neutral, the knees are directly below the hips. Occasionally, some hip abduction is desired. In either case, depending on the degree of abduction desired, a rectangular- or trapezoid-shaped block should be placed between the knees. This spacer, or abductor, should extend above and below the knees to distribute pressure. Its primary purpose is to keep the legs aligned and symmetrical. If the child abducts and rotates his hips externally, knee flexion no longer is blocked by the surface of the stander, because the knees will be facing laterally. Lateral supports at the level of the knees bring the hips into a more neutral abduction/adduction position and prevent collapse at the knees.

Padding in front of the knees on the prone stander relieves pressure and prevents knee flexion. Too much padding causes the knees to hyperextend. If the knees hyperextend regardless of padding, the joint can be flexed by realigning the feet so that the ankle is slightly back of the knee. If the child wears foot orthoses, then the upper straps must be loosened, because this position requires some ankle dorsiflexion.

Holes must be cut in the bottom of the standing board to accommodate the toes. Care must be taken to align these cut-outs with the hips and legs. Blocks placed laterally or medially to the child's feet can maintain the foot position if necessary. A nonskid surface could be just as effective (Fig. 8.24A, 8.24B).

The integrity of the ankle and foot must be evaluated in standing. Although this skill is beyond this chapter, ankle/foot orthoses must be provided for standing if pathology exists in that area.

The need for and placement of lateral trunk supports can be determined once the lower body position is corrected and stable. The chest support, or upper edge of the prone stander, may end anywhere between the bottom of the sternum to just below the clavicle, depending on need. If the chest support is cut high, it should be curved down away from the midline—something like the end of an ironing board—to free the shoulder girdle for movement.

As in the sitting position, height and angle of the laptray contribute to correcting posture. A low laptray may encourage weightbearing on extended arms. A child who has inadequate extension, however, may flex over the top of the chest support in an attempt to rest on the laptray. In such cases, a laptray at nipple level helps elongate the upper trunk and provide support for the arms as the child masters head control. The need for humeral wings should be assessed if the child retracts and extends his shoulders.

In the supine stander, a hip strap is unnecessary because the child is extended against the back support when chest and knee straps are applied. Care should be taken that the chest strap not dig into the axillary area.

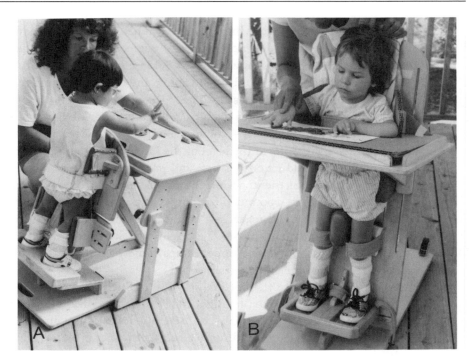

**Figure 8.24.**   Two examples of standers. **(A)**, Prone stander. **(B)**, Supine stander.

Hip blocks may be desirable to prevent lateral movement and any resultant asymmetries. As with the prone stander, abductor/spacer blocks or lateral adductors should be considered to align hips and legs. Padding should be placed behind the knees if there is any indication of hyperextension at that joint. Ankle straps that comes from behind the heel over the instep at a 45° angle or medial or lateral foot blocks may be needed to maintain foot placement.

A laptray that has a supine stander not only supports the arms and provides a working surface but also encourages the child to use some active neck and upper trunk flexion to right his head and come forward to the working surface. Because the supine stander is tilted backward to some extent, humeral wings may be necessary to assist the child in keeping his shoulders and arms forward against gravity. If head supports are needed, this is determined in the same way as for the partially reclined sitting position.

## Functional Skills

The previous section discussed common positions in which central stability is provided artificially to decrease pathological movement, encourage components of postural responses, and liberate the head and arms. The first few function/dysfunction continua that relate to range of motion, head control, and trunk control are addressed directly as the therapist determines the appropriate position and equipment. The last few function/dysfunction continua that relate to hand control, mobility, feeding, and toileting involve more than postural responses. These functions also require cognition, perception, attention, motor planning, and fine motor skills. Postural control is a foundation for the development of these functions. The absence of postural control impedes the development of skills in these areas. The sections that follow describe postural components or equipment related to these functions.

### Ability to Place, Maintain, and Control Hand Position

Although it is desirable to have shoulder and arm mobility in all planes, this is not always a realistic goal. If expectations must be limited, then the most functional ranges of shoulder and arm movement are those that contribute to midline activity, so that the child can bring objects toward his eyes, ears, and mouth for learning and survival. In this case, desirable ranges of volitional movement include neutral toward slight protraction; neutral toward internal rotation; 0° to 90° shoulder flexion, abduction, and horizontal adduction; and midranges of elbow flexion/extension and forearm rotation. The development of control in these ranges can be addressed in two ways: first, by establishing skill in shoulder and elbow mobility and stability in developmental positions (enhancing the development of components of movement); and, second, by providing as much support as necessary to the body and arms so that the child can perform a few isolated movements. (This improves distal function by reducing the need for postural reactions through external support.)

With a child who has moderate to severe disabilities, the therapist may choose to devise a specific pattern of movement related to one function. Examples of specific patterns of movement may be a hand-to-mouth pattern for feeding or a simple elbow movement to activate a switchplate. The first step is to provide an optimum base of support to modify tone and reduce demands on the rest of the body and yet enhance attention to task. Sidelying, sitting, prone standing, and supine standing should be considered. The second step is to determine how many arm movements the child can control, and which ones need to be supported artificially by a laptray or other equipment components. For example, humeral wings eliminate the child's need to protract actively or to adduct horizontally when bringing his hand to his mouth. If the therapist raises the laptray to axilla level, the child's movements are then limited to the horizontal plane, and demands for movements against gravity are eliminated.

In extreme cases, if a child has no control over arm movements (i.e., such as a child who has severe athetoid movements), one arm can be positioned so that movement is channelled in one direction. For example, blocks may be placed laterally and medially along the child's arm, creating a channel on the laptray. With such an arrangement, the hand can move only in the vertical plane, regardless of extraneous shoulder, elbow, or forearm movements. In this way, the child may successfully depress a switchplate. Following a training period, supports should be withdrawn.

### Ability to Move Through Space

Devices can be provided that facilitate mobility for the child who has severe disabilities and who cannot move through space. Those children who have less severe involvements and who cannot move fast enough or efficiently enough to attain an end goal or who cannot keep up with peers also may benefit from such devices.

If pathological tone is increased through passive movement because of the intensity of the stimulation but affectual responses are positive, it is up to the therapist's creativity to provide a position in which unwanted overflow of tone can be controlled. For example, a child who hyperextends when swinging may be nestled in a flexed position within an inflatable tube placed on a platform swing.

Scooterboards may be effective in enhancing self-initiated movement in a child who has moderate to severe disabilities. They can also provide weightbearing, weightshifting, and rapid movement through space for the child who has milder disabilities. The scooterboard consists of an appropriately fitted prone wedge placed on highly responsive ball-bearing casters (Fig. 8.25A, 8.25B). Several modifications to the prone wedge can enhance its effectiveness. These include a chest wedge to provide the correct shoulder-to-floor distance and a front wedge cut away to support only the chest and liberate the shoulder girdle (which is "ironing-board"-shaped). The back edge of the wedge should end before the ankles so that the child's feet can hang freely over the end of the board. The child who has severe disabilities may need an extension of the front edge of the wedge for intermittent head support. Directed, forward movement is not the goal in this case. Rather, the child begins to initiate movement through space whenever his hand contacts begin to bear weight through his arms. For the child who cannot roll or crawl,

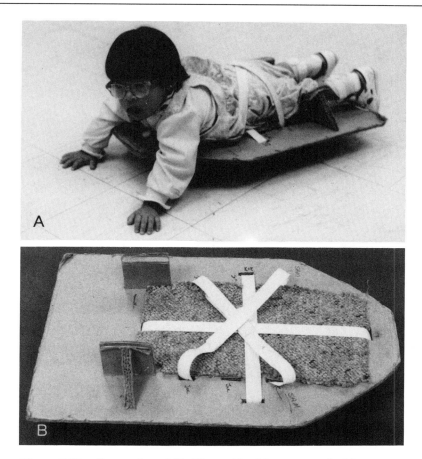

**Figure 8.25.** Scooter board **(A, B)** provides hip straps and adductors to prevent this low tone child from externally rotating her hips and dragging her legs on the floor.

this may be his only opportunity to experience active movement through space.

Children who are nonambulatory or who walk slowly with crutches may be less taxed when using a tricycle. A tricycle also allows them to engage with peers in gross motor activity. Tricycles can be purchased with back supports, hip straps, abductors along the handlebar uprights, and footplates with straps (Fig. 8.26). The therapist needs to determine that the tricycle measurements and supports provided coincide with the child's sitting skills. Arm and hand positions also should be assessed. The handlebars can be raised to encourage an upright trunk. Adapted vertical handgrips that place the

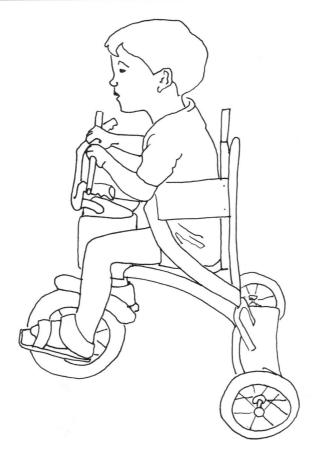

**Figure 8.26.** Adaptive tricycle provides back support, lateral trunk support, hip straps, abductors, foot straps, and horizontal bar to hold onto. Grasp on the original handle bar had encouraged shoulder elevation, internal rotation, elbow flexion, and ulnar deviation.

forearm in a neutral rotation also encourage an erect trunk, provided there is forearm mobility.

A powered wheelchair provides rapid mobility for the nonambulator who finds a manual wheelchair painstakingly slow to propel and requires excessive effort to move. Because switches offer great sophistication, powered chairs can be propelled by severely involved persons provided that they have an awareness of space and good judgment with regard to their safety and the safety of others. Just as an 18-month-old child can direct his body through space with reasonable safety, so can a child of the same maturational age learn to direct a powered chair. By providing for positioning needs in a wheelchair, the therapist combines the optimal sitting position with the most functional position of laptray and arm guides.

### Ability to Feed

Positioning in a feeding program is designed to reduce the influence of low or high muscle tone on oral-motor activity, to prevent situations that might trigger primitive reflexes and to provide central stability to enhance controlled distal mobility. This promotes skills such as sucking, biting, chewing, and swallowing.

Tone can be modified through the choice of position and supports. A child who has very high or very low tone may need total support, such as that provided by reclined sitting or supine standing with a harness to provide shoulder control and thoracic support. A child who has slightly low tone may respond well to increased postural demands, such as a seat with low back support or a prone stander. In other cases, the best positioning device may be the therapist's body. The child who is positioned properly in an adult's lap benefits from physical warmth and touch and social interaction, all of which may be the most effective therapy during his feeding.

Head support may be needed to provide a stable base for jaw movements. A neutral or slightly flexed position of the neck contributes to controlled swallowing, reduces extensor hypertonicity, and prevents a child who has disabilities from throwing his head back and "bird-feeding," which is uncontrolled swallowing that uses gravity rather than musculature to get the food down. If the child has poor lip closure or lip pressure, however, keeping food in his mouth may be facilitated by a slight tipping back of his head. *It is important that the neck not be extended.* The appropriate position of the head can be accomplished by reclining the trunk partially and bringing the head forward to an almost-righted position.

The head support should not contact the face, to avoid a rooting reflex. Activation of the rooting reflex turns the child's head away from the source of food and also may initiate asymmetries because the turning of the head can produce ATNR activity.

Special attention should be paid to shoulder position during feeding. High tone in elevation, retraction, protraction, or humeral rotation can compromise swallowing and the coordination of swallowing with respiration.

### Ability to Void When Seated on a Toilet or Potty

The primary goal of equipment in this area is to provide support and modify tone so that the child can relax. Postural challenges should not be the issue here, and comfort is essential. Special attention should be paid to provide adequate hip flexion and abduction in supported sitting.

Potty training for young children who have severe disabilities frequently requires a lot of time. Diversional activities are sometimes helpful to motivate and engage the child. If a younger child's potty training program includes diversional activities, then a laptray can serve the dual purpose of arm support and a play surface.

## Summary

The last part of this chapter has addressed the more technical aspects of the biomechanical frame of reference: that is, the practical problems of translating a therapeutic intention into a piece of equipment. This process requires some mechanical skills and an ability to manipulate three dimensional space mentally. Although it is only one component of treatment implementation, the actual prescription or design of equipment often makes the greater demands on the novice therapist. A frequent hazard involved in this process is that concentration becomes too focused on the product (adaptive device) and the multitude of other factors that enhance posture and function can be overlooked.

The diagram illustrates an approach to postural control that is more complete than a simple device to support the child. It should be viewed as a series of "ex-centric," rather than concentric, circles, with the supportive device in the center. The circles widen to demonstrate a more holistic approach to biomechanical intervention. As the circles grow from the center, the factors produce effects on posture and function that are less direct and specific, but that are greater in scope.

The first, smallest circle represents the most direct approach: the positioning device that physically supports the child—the "hardware" that taxes the therapist's mechanical and spatial skills. The next circle includes the physiological reactions that modulate posture, for example, reactions to tactile cues provided by the equipment or reactions to changes in head or body position in space. The next circle represents effort—the amount of work the child must do to stay upright and interact with his environment. Too much effort may cause fatigue or frustration; too little effort may limit the potential for growth and change.

The circle that represents environmental factors includes those things that influence levels of arousal, attention, and tone, and indirectly enhance or disrupt postural reactions. Temperature can be changed to enhance posture

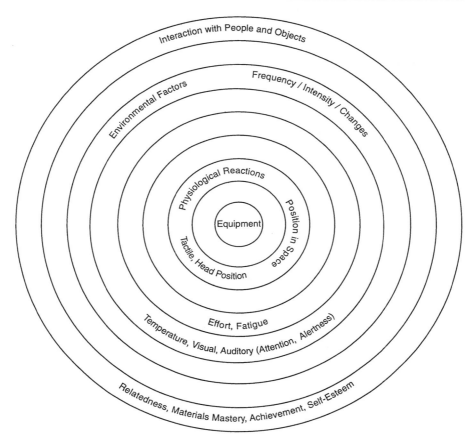

**Diagram 8.1** An approach to postural control that is more complete than a device that merely supports the child.

by altering the heat in the room, by adding or removing layers of clothing, or by providing close physical contact between the child and another person. The position of visual cues may affect how the child holds his head, with resultant changes in tone and posture. The element of motion with visual stimulation can enhance attention or increase fatigue, depending on the child's head control and ocular-motor skills. For example, practical implications include where the teacher stands or sits in relation to the child and whether she moves about as she speaks. Another aspect of this circle is auditory stimulation. Background noise and changes in volume or tempo of voice or music enhance alertness, elicit dysfunctional startle responses, or cause a child to "shut-down," depending on the person. These factors and many others in the physical environment have subtle yet cumulative impact on posture and function and should be incorporated into the therapist's treatment plan.

The outermost circle encompasses opportunities for interaction with people and objects. Although this appears to be the least direct channel to modify posture and function, changes often include observable phenomena. For example, significant improvement in posture may be noted when a child is drawn into a song made up about himself and his friends, or when he is given the opportunity to apply finger paint to his therapist's face. Interaction with people, animals, and materials and the associated senses of mastery and self-esteem represent not only goals but also therapeutic tools.

The occupational therapist can act as consultant to the team to help modify the child's internal and external environment throughout the day. As part of the biomechanical frame of reference, the therapist must learn to identify and use the many forces that are greater than the force of gravity.

## OUTLINE OF BIOMECHANICAL FRAME OF REFERENCE

I. Theoretical base
   A. Motor patterns develop from sensory stimulation
   B. Automatic motor responses develop in a predictable way
      1. Equilibrium reactions accompanied by protective reactions
      2. Righting and equilibrium reactions are the foundation for movements
      3. Developmental sequence
         a. Motor patterns
         b. Cephalocaudal
         c. Horizontal-vertical
      4. Process of motor development
         a. Phasic movement
         b. Stability
         c. Weightbearing
         d. Skill
   C. Components of postural control and skill development in developmental positions
      1. Supine
      2. Prone
      3. Sidelying
      4. Sitting
      5. Standing
   D. Interference with postural reactions resulting from damage or dysfunction
      1. Compensatory movement or posture
      2. Global neuromuscular dysfunction
      3. Neuromuscular dysfunction often affects muscle tone
      4. Movements and postures affected by touch, proprioception, sight, sound, smell, health and attitude
         a. Movement

        b. Position in space

        c. Position of the head in relation to the body

        d. Tactile stimulation

        e. Temperature of the environment

        f. Surface support

        g. Affect

  E. Assumptions

    1. External supports to substitute for inadequate or abnormal postural reactions

        a. Facilitating development of postural control

        b. Providing permanent support

    2. Learning to move effectively through sensory feedback

    3. Motor development is predictable and sequential

        a. Posture depends on the body's response to gravity

        b. Postural reactions develop sequentially

    4. Dysfunction or abnormalities of muscle, bone, or the central nervous system may impair development of normal postural reactions

        a. Tone affects posture

        b. If normal postural reactions have not developed, the body compensates by using substitute movements, more effort, and more conscious attention

    5. Treatment needs to provide substitutes for absent skills while making demands on the child's existing capacity to function

II. Function/dysfunction continua

  A. Range of motion

  B. Head control

  C. Trunk control

  D. Control of arm movements

  E. Mobility

  F. Functional performance behaviors

    1. Eating

    2. Toileting

III. Evaluation

  A. Potential for change in the area of postural reactions

  B. Age, therapeutic history, physical status, prognosis, and environment

  C. Guideline questions for evaluating motor development in terms of functional posture

    1. Can the child move all body parts through full range against gravity?

    2. Can the child right his head and is it mobile in all planes?

    3. Can the child right his trunk and maintain stability?

    4. Can the child place, maintain, and control the position of his hands?

    5. Is the child mobile through space in all planes?

    6. Can the child chew and swallow food successfully, without aspirating?

    7. Can the child void when seated on a toilet or potty?

IV. Postulates regarding change

  A. Those that help the therapist to determine how and when to use adaptive equipment

    B.  Those that may be helpful when handling to determine how to facilitate an effective position

    C.  Those that relate to the efficacy of the child's equipment program

V.  Application to practice
- A.  Central stability
  1. Supine position
  2. Prone position
  3. Sidelying position
  4. Sitting position
     a. Surface
     b. Supports
     c. Laptrays or table surfaces
     d. Harness
  5. Supported standing
     a. Prone stander
     b. Supine stander
- B.  Functional skills
  1. Ability to place, maintain, and control hand position
  2. Ability to move through space
  3. Ability to feed
  4. Ability to void when seated on a toilet or potty

### Acknowledgments

The author wishes to thank the students, parents, and staff of the United Cerebral Palsy School in Purchase, New York for their cooperation and assistance in providing photographs for this chapter.

### References

Barnes, K. J. (1991). Modification of the physical environment. In C. Christiansen & C. Baum (Eds.). *Occupational therapy: Overcoming human performance deficits.* (pp. 701–745). Thorofare, NJ: Slack.

Bergen, A. & Colangelo, C. (1985). *Positioning the client with central nervous system deficits.* Valhalla, NY: Valhalla Rehabilitation Publications.

Bly, L. (1983). The components of normal movement during the first year of life and abnormal motor development. Birmingham, Al: Neuro-Developmental Treatment Association.

Butler, C., Okamoto, G., & McKay, T. (1984). Motorized wheelchair driving by disabled children. *Archives of Physical Medicine and Rehabilitation, 65,* (2), 95–97.

Fiorentino, M. (1981). *A basis for sensorimotor development—normal and abnormal.* Springfield, IL: Charles. C. Thomas.

Paulsson, K. & Christoffersen, M. (1984). Psychosocial aspects on technical aids—how does independent mobility affect the psychosocial and intellectual development of children who have physical disabilities? Proceedings of the Second International Conference on Rehabilitation Engineering, Ottawa, Canada.

Pratt, P. N., Allen, A. S., Carrasco, R. C., Clark, F., & Schanzenbacher, K. E. (1989). Instruments to evaluate component functions of behavior. In P. N. Pratt & A. S. Allen *Occupational therapy for children.* (2nd ed). (pp. 168–197). St. Louis, MO: C.V. Mosby.

Scherzer, A. & Tscharnuter, I. (1982). *Early diagnosis and therapy in cerebral palsy.* NY: Marcel Dekker.

Scherzer, A. & Tscharnuter, I. (1990). *Early diagnosis and therapy in cerebral palsy.* (2nd Ed.). New York, NY: Marcel Dekker.

Schiaffino, S. & Laux, J. (1986). Prerequisite skills for the psychosocial impact of powered wheelchair mobility on young children with severe handicaps. *Developmental disability special interest section newsletter,* American Occupational Therapy Association, *9,* (2).

Stockmeyer, S. (1967). An interpretation of the approach of Rood to the treatment of neuromuscular dysfunction. *American Journal of Physical Medicine, 46,*(1) 900–956.

# 9

# Human Occupation Frame of Reference

SHIRLEY PEGANOFF O'BRIEN

## Historical Perspective

From an historical perspective, the model of human occupation has its roots in the works of Mary Reilly, Ed.D, OTR, FAOTA, who developed the theory of occupational behavior. Drawing from occupational behavior theory (Reilly, 1962) and systems theory (von Bertalanffy, 1968; Boulding, 1968), Kielhofner, Burke, and Igi (1980) proposed the model of human occupation in a series of four articles in the *American Journal of Occupational Therapy* (Kielhofner, 1980a, 1980b; Kielhofner & Burke, 1977, 1980; Kielhofner, Burke, & Igi, 1980). Together, these articles presented a new, comprehensive model for occupational therapy.

After exploring Kuhn's model of scientific revolutions and the use of paradigms, Gary Kielhofner, Dr. PH., OTR, FAOTA and his colleagues expanded the theory and its application to occupational therapy (Kielhofner, 1980a, 1980b; Kielhofner & Burke, 1977, 1980; Kielhofner, Burke, & Igi, 1980) as it is presented in this chapter. According to Kielhofner (1985), the model describes a global foundation for the provision of occupational therapy services to all age groups, across diagnostic and specialty lines.

Even though a model presents a framework for a profession, as such, it cannot be applied to practice. The perspective taken in this book is that the practical application of the model of human occupation with children is a frame of reference. Whenever a model is applied to any particular population, its application then can be discussed as a frame of reference, and, in this chapter, the frame of reference is intended for pediatric practice. It is important to note that some of the ideas and concepts of the model of human occupation, as proposed by Kielhofner, may not fit neatly into the frame of reference "structure" as defined in this book.

Occupational behavior and systems theory provide foundational concepts for the theoretical base of the model of human occupation. An overview of occupational behavior and systems theory, therefore, precedes the theoretical base of the model of human occupation as it relates to children.

## *Occupational Behavior*

Occupational behavior includes that aspect of growth and development represented by the developmental continuum between play and work as it provides the basis for competence, achievement, and occupational role (Reilly, 1966; Woodside, 1976).

Occupational behavior includes those behaviors associated with the roles of child, student, worker, and adult. Historically, Reilly's writing was influenced heavily by the time-binding model of Adolf Meyer, M.D. and the habit training model of Eleanor Clarke Slagle (Reed, 1984). Meyer's time-binding model focused on the value and use of time and the understanding of the balance needed in the internal rhythms of work, play, rest, and sleep (Meyer, 1922). Accordingly, it was through actual doing and practice that this balance is developed in life.

At approximately the same time that Meyer created his model, Eleanor Clarke Slagle devised a model for occupational therapy that concentrated on human habit patterns. For the hospital patients, habits were defined as reeducation in decent habits of living (Slagle & Robeson, 1941). Slagle believed that habit reactions organized life. When dysfunction was present, she hypothesized that degeneration of the habit pattern was seen, which led to idleness and a preoccupation with morbid thoughts. She also concluded that some of the problems exhibited by psychiatric patients were related to their loss of playfulness, which then led to poor morale and degeneration in their habit patterns. Slagle believed that occupational therapy provided patients with the mechanism to modify some habits, construct new habit patterns, and overcome other habits. Ideally, the reeducation of habits would influence the restoration and maintenance of health positively (Slagle, 1922).

Reilly combined concepts from Meyer and Slagle to develop her own model for occupational therapy/occupational behavior. In occupational behavior, Reilly redefined major concepts, presenting occupation as a meaningful need in life. She focused on the effect that work serves in providing stability to daily life patterns and routines. Her interventions were based on the use of occupation to learn, relearn, or modify life skills. In Reilly's view, occupational behavior incorporated and built on the ideas of her predecessors (Reed, 1984).

The existence of a developmental continuum between work and play was another important concept proposed by Reilly (1962; 1966). Play was seen as the foundation for the practice and development of occupational roles and occurred before the development of work behaviors (Reilly, 1962). Reilly (1969) and, later, Shannon (1972) placed emphasis on the development of play and its effect on occupation in later life. Reilly believed that play skills were critical behaviors that had to be acquired to function in society. She also believed that deficiency in play skills would lead to deficiencies in work skills unless corrective actions were taken.

Occupational roles provide the structure for persons to assimilate into groups that meet the needs of productivity, belonging, and life-structuring activities. Socialization provides a person with a way to learn various role behaviors (Reilly, 1969).

The concept of a hierarchical organization of routines, beginning with exploration and competency and ending in achievement, was proposed by Reilly (1974), based on the works of von Bertalanffy and Boulding (1968), McClelland (1953), and White (1964). According to Reilly, exploration served the purpose of generating skills; competency assisted in the organization of habits; and achievement assisted in learning successful role behavior. As proposed by Reilly, these concepts of occupational behavior provided the necessary foundation to link occupation with developmental stages and elementary decision-making behavior for occupational choices, which then served as the foundation for the model of human occupation (Kielhofner & Burke, 1980).

## General Systems Theory

Reilly's occupational behavior model (Reilly, 1966; Woodside, 1976) recognized that each person needs to master, alter, and improve his environment. Based on the works of von Bertalanffy (1968) and Boulding (1968), Kielhofner took systems theory even farther—as a organizing structure within the model of human occupation. According to general systems theory, each person is an open system. Change is an identifiable process with ongoing adaptations that occur within any open system. Systems theory holds that no system can be understood in isolation of its environment.

As stated by Boulding (1968), general systems theory was used to describe the similarities between different disciplines and sciences, such as physics, mathematics, biology, psychology and sociology, which typically were seen in isolation of each other (reductionistic view). Similarities in the theoretical constructions of different disciplines combine to form a "system of systems" (Boulding, 1968, p. 3) that then provides the basis for a gestalt of theoretical development. Laws of hierarchy exist on which the system is built, with subsystems that function for the whole (gestalt) of the system. This hierarchical nature of systems provides the process by which change takes place within the system, going from simple to complex.

Von Bertalanffy (1968) outlined the concepts of open systems even more as they related to general systems theory. These concepts included homeostasis, laws of organization, and the interdisciplinary nature of pure sciences, as well as the biological, psychological, and sociological disciplines. Open systems are organized with hierarchical processes that are dynamic in nature. These systems maintain a steady state internally through the use of **servomechanisms** for the internal control of homeostasis. Servomechanisms works as follows: A stimulus message to an open system affects a receptor that, in turn, sends the message forward to a control apparatus, that sends the message on to an effector area that then triggers a response of some sort to the original stimulus. This response sends feedback to the original receptor (von Bertalanffy, 1968). This suggests a sensory-motor-sensory feedback loop within an open system. The environment is viewed through its interaction with the open system. It is seen as a possible source of stimulation to the initial receptor in this example—that is, as the focus of the response or the system's output (Fig. 9.1).

## Theoretical Base

Initially, Kielhofner and Burke (1980) (and later with Igi) (Kielhofner, Burke, & Igi, 1980) elaborated and redefined Reilly's conceptualization of occupational behavior within the context of systems theory to formulate the overall structure for the model of human occupation. Building on the concept of occupation, general systems theory provides a mechanism for understanding how information from the environment acts on each person to bring about change. It is proposed that a hierarchy of subsystems exists to organize and regulate the output of the system. The subsystems that allow the child to gain mastery over his environment are those of **volition, habituation,** and **performance.** Motivation is an intrinsic drive that acts on competence,

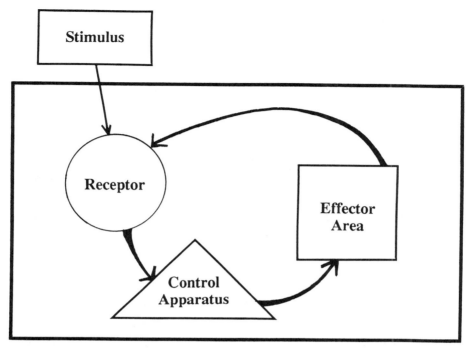

**Figure 9.1.**   Diagram of servomechanism.

achievement, and occupational roles. It energizes the system and powers exploration. In this frame of reference, **the environment is critically important** because it is the setting for the system, providing the input, whereas occupation as the output is viewed in relation to the environment. The theoretical base of the model of human occupation is described as an integration of the biological, psychological, and social aspects of daily life plus self-directed role requirements (Kielhofner, 1980a, 1980b, 1985a; Kielhofner & Burke, 1980; Kielhofner, Burke, & Igi, 1980). General systems theory provides the organizing framework for this model and a way to understand the change process. It is essential, therefore, to understand systems theory as it has been adapted.

From the perspective of general systems theory, the environment includes the physical and social settings in which the system (i.e., the child) operates. The physical and social settings of the environment include the child's culture, people, social groups and organizations, external objects, and actions (as related to task performance). The human system and the environment are

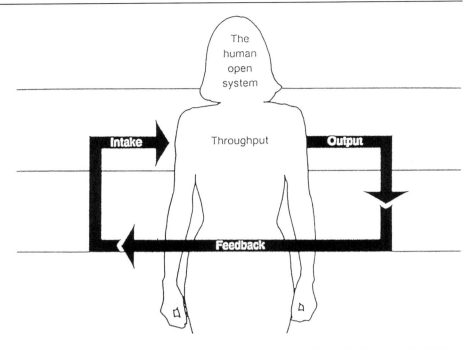

**Figure 9.2.** Concept of the human as an open system. From Kielhofner, G. (Ed.). A model of human occupation. Baltimore, MD: Williams & Wilkins, 1985.

viewed as a dynamic network of interrelated partnerships (Barris, 1982; Barris, Kielhofner, Levine, & Neville, 1985; Kielhofner & Burke, 1980).

As applied in the model of human occupation, general systems theory addresses open systems as follows: An open system consists of four distinct processes that function for maintenance and change in the system. These four processes are **intake, throughput, output,** and **feedback** (Kielhofner, 1985a; Kielhofner & Burke, 1980; Kielhofner, Burke, & Igi, 1980). Intake refers to the importation of energy or information into the system. Throughput refers to the transformation of the energy or information for assimilation by the system and the self-transformation of the system to accommodate the incoming energy or information. Output refers to the external action or behavior of the system—that is, what the system does within the environment and to the environment. Finally, feedback refers to the result of this process and the consequences of the previous actions on the system. Figure 9.2 summarizes the concept of the human as an open system.

An example of an open system is illustrated by the act of eating. A child takes a bite of an apple (**intake**). The apple is chewed and mixed with saliva (**throughput**). The child then swallows the chewed apple mixture, and the food mixture moves through the body toward the stomach, where enzymes are produced to break down the food mixture even more ( **throughput continues**). The child receives satisfaction from the taste of the apple (**output**), and when the mouth is empty (**feedback**), desires more apple (**continued feedback**) and takes another bite of the apple, to continue the process (**starting the action over**). Any intake to the system can bring about change by introducing something new or some feedback into the system. The change process is assumed to take place at the throughput stage, where energy or information is assimilated, leading to self-transformation. Self-transformation is defined as the system's ability to generate new information for change (Kielhofner, 1980b). It refers to the dynamic interaction within the cycle of an open system and its ability to take existing information, produce an output, and thus create new information that may modify the existing system (Kielhofner & Burke, 1980; Kielhofner, 1980b). Through self-transformation, a child can learn from experiences and adapt to situations independently.

Compatible with general systems theory, the model of human occupation accepts the following assumptions:

1. The child is an open system in constant interaction with his environment (Kielhofner & Burke, 1980).
2. A child's occupation is the output of the system's processes (Kielhofner & Burke, 1980).
3. No system can be evaluated or understood in isolation from its unique environment (Kielhofner, 1980b).

These assumptions shape the way in which the model of human occupation is delineated further. The individual child and his family each constitute open systems and need to be thought of with the previously stated assumptions in mind.

## Occupation and Occupational Behavior

Occupation involves the child's purposeful use of time to meet his own needs so that he can explore and master his environment. Occupation includes meeting personal needs as well as the standards of the social group. This concept of occupation, particularly for the child, includes all activities on the continuum of play to work (Kielhofner, 1980a). Occupation, therefore, is a broad concept, essential to the development of the child.

This definition of occupation provides the foundation for the concept of occupational behavior. As stated by Kielhofner and Burke (1985), occupational behavior is "an activity in which persons engage during most of their waking time: it includes activities that are playful, restful, serious, and productive (p. 12)." A child carries out activities of work, play, and daily living in his own way, based on his environment, beliefs and preferences, previous experiences, and patterns of behavior acquired over time (Kielhofner & Burke, 1985).

Occupational behaviors are activities that provide the child with means to master his environment (Keilhofner & Barris, 1985). Three important occupational behaviors are **competency, achievement,** and **occupational role.** These behaviors are organized hierarchically, and motivation contributes to their attainment. The occupational role of the child is to use play as a way to learn about the environment. For example, an infant may explore a toy with his mouth, finger, and eyes. Mouthing the toy brings the infant the most satisfaction, therefore he is motivated to continue. With practice and repetition, the infant becomes competent in bringing the toy to the mouth on presentation, and he achieves the end product of (efficiently bringing the toy to his mouth on presentation). This allows him to meet his occupational role of engaging in sensorimotor play. The desire to explore and interact with the toy is one motivating factor; another motivator is satisfaction.

### Play and Work

Occupational behavior uses play and work to promote growth and development (Kielhofner & Barris, 1985). It is important to clarify the way in which this frame of reference views these two components. **Play** is fundamental to the child. It assists him in organizing his behavior, as well as in initiating change within his system and the environment (Kielhofner, 1980a). Through play, the child practices skills, routines, and other roles. *Play assumes interaction.* Play behaviors incorporate interaction with other humans as well as with nonhuman objects such as toys (Florey, 1971) (Fig. 9.3).

At work, a person is productive for himself (Neff, 1968). For the child, work is participation in self-care activities that serve the purpose of self-maintainence. A child's work includes his interactions at home and in school. Play relates to work because it is the activity through which change takes place in the child's roles and habits.

Motivation is an innate incentive that depends on a reward that exists within the activity itself (Bruner, 1964). *Intrinsic motivation provides a child with the drive to achieve satisfaction for executing an action.* For example, an infant may see

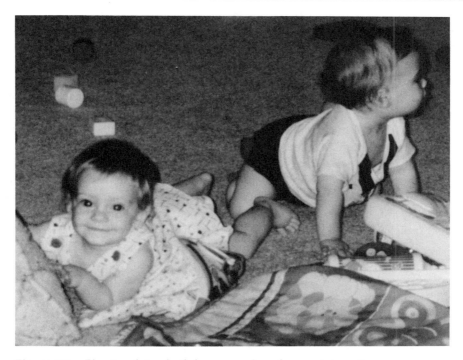

**Figure 9.3.**   Play involving both human and nonhuman interaction.

and try to get a toy that is slightly out of reach. Through weightshifting, he is able to reach and obtain the toy. When the infant obtains the toy, he may feel satisfaction. The action was achieved by the intrinsic motivation to achieve a goal. Satisfaction stimulates the drive even more.

A child's play experiences influence his motivations to participate in activities. A child is intrinsically driven to explore and master his environment. In additional, he makes conscious decisions and independent choices based on his individual needs for exploration and engagement and on his personal beliefs about his abilities. The child's personal belief about his abilities provides his sense of competence, which can lead to a sense of mastery. This interconnection often is achieved through continued practice. A sense of mastery of the environment results in a personal sense of achievement.

Competence is sufficient or adequate performance to meet the demands of a situation or task. The inference is that a child is an active being, able to explore his environment. Competence is assumed to be linked with some degree of confidence in skill development and self-esteem (White, 1971). Self-esteem develops out of positive experiences that result from competent behavior. When a child has a sense of competence, he is motivated to engage in behaviors that are selective, directed, and persistent. This child is able to satisfy his needs to deal and interact with his environment (White, 1959). For example, an infant who is motivated to interact with his environment sometimes engages in exploratory play, which often results in effective grasping strategies. This satisfies the infant's need to interact with his environment. As the infant establishes effective interactions with his environment, he acquires a greater degree of confidence in his ability to interact.

Occupational role refers to tasks and the socially acceptable behavior patterns typically assumed in the performance of most daily routines (Ginsberg, 1972; Reilly, 1969). These tasks may organize most of the child's actions by defining the expectations within a situation. For instance, the occupational role of the school-aged child determines his daily routines—attending school, eating lunch, playing with peers, and doing homework. This organizes the child's time.

### Environment

The model of human occupation addresses the interaction of performance of the system (the child in this example) in the environment (Barris, 1982; Barris, Kielhofner, Levine, & Neville, 1985). The environment includes the physical, social, and cultural settings in which the system (the child) operates. Objects, tasks, social groups, and culture all are components in the environment. Objects are used by persons when they perform tasks, such as when a child uses a rattle to get another toy that is out of reach. Social, physical, and cultural surroundings have strong effects on a person's development and the resultant valued occupation (Klavins, 1972; Shannon, 1970, 1972). The key to understanding human occupation is to see the effects of the biopsychosocial development on the person's sense of occupational behavior and continued adaptation, which occurs from the involvement between the dynamics of human relations and the environment (Burke, 1983). From this perspective, human occupation is the interaction of the system (child) with the environment in its most complete form.

### Hierarchy

In accordance with the laws of general systems theory, one of the major assumptions of the model of human occupation is that hierarchies exist within the system (Kielhofner & Burke, 1980, 1985). The hierarchy within this model consists of three subsystems in the following order: **volition, habituation,** and **performance.** The **volition subsystem** is made up of three components: a sense of personal causation, interests, and values. The **habituation subsystem** views behavior in terms of habits, patterns and roles. This subsystem organizes outputs of the child in terms of patterns of action and roles. And finally, the **performance subsystem** is concerned with skills that provide the foundation for action.

The **volition subsystem** is the highest level of human occupation, and it governs the lower subsystems of habituation and performance. It is based on motivation toward exploration and mastery and consists of innate and acquired urges to act on the environment. Motivation is energizing and determines conscious choices for behaviors. It is based on personal causation, values, and interests (Kielhofner & Burke, 1985).

**Personal causation** is a collection of beliefs and expectations that a child holds about his effectiveness in his environment (Kielhofner & Burke, 1980). Four aspects of a child's sense of personal causation are internal/external control, belief in skill, belief in efficacy of skills, and expectancy of success/ failure (Burke, 1983). Sensorimotor development facilitates the child's growth in these areas. A child acquires a sense of personal causation through early neuromotor behaviors. As an infant begins to roll and realizes that he can do it again, he tests and develops his internal awareness through sensorimotor feedback. From this, he realizes that not only can he do the action, but he also can control it. Another important aspect of the development of personal causation is a nascent sense of autonomy (DeCharms, 1968). The child attempts to influence and gain control over his environment, first through action, then through verbalizations, or a combination of both. Once the child develops values, interests, and a sense of personal causation, these factors serve to control and influence motivation. Motivation then has a strong influence on habits, roles, and performance.

Values are the child's feelings about what is good, right, and important—things that guide human behavior. Four components of values are considered as they relate to occupational behavior: temporal orientation, meaningfulness of activity, occupational goals, and personal standards (Kielhofner & Burke, 1985). Cultural values often shape a child's and his family's internal view of valuable activities.

**Temporal orientation** is defined as the way in which the child views his placement in time, including an understanding of past, present, and future. It is thought that the child also has beliefs about how time should be spent (Kielhofner & Burke, 1985). For example, a child may have a memory of painful events associated with getting a shot at the doctor's office. The child may have a cold, for instance, and the parent calls the doctor for an appointment. Hearing the telephone call, the child may try to mask symptoms to avoid the visit. The child may anticipate the visit and events surrounding the visit with fear because of the previous painful experience.

**Meaningfulness of activity** is defined as the child's internalization of the importance, worthiness, and security of a particular occupation or activity (Kielhofner & Burke, 1985). A child may choose to participate in Little League baseball because of the good sense of self that he receives when he hits a homerun. This activity gives the child a sense of security, and it may become a memory that he evokes as he grows older to reinforce self-worth.

**Occupational goals** are defined as objectives for future accomplishments (Kielhofner & Burke, 1985). For the child, this adds the element of time and future planning into his life. In the previously given example, the child who plays on the baseball team wants to play all season long for the chance to participate in the playoffs. This represents the end goal for a season of hard work.

**Personal standards** are commitments to perform activities in socially accepted ways. This includes morals and time-oriented standards. Perfectionistic behaviors, such as neatness in coloring or in stacking blocks, may be considered in this area.

Cultural values often define a child's and his family's internal views of activities that are good, as well as personal standards (Kielhofner & Burke, 1985). Through reinforcement of acceptable patterns of play, a child learns what is acceptable in a play situation and what is acceptable in the family situation. Interests are the things that children enjoy doing (Burke, 1983); they occur sequentially through the developmental stages of play. If an infant receives pleasure from mouthing a textured toy, then he is likely to continue this exploration of the toy.

During infancy, the volition subsystem is undifferentiated (Kielhofner, 1980a). Through play behaviors, the child's volition subsystem begins to differentiate and becomes organized. Various experiences, particularly sensorimotor ones, facilitate differentiation and organization.

The **habituation subsystem** is the middle level of human occupation and includes components that organize behavior into habits, routines, and patterns of action. The habituation subsystem integrates the person with the environment by linking internal spontaneous urges with external environmental demands (Kielhofner, 1980a). An example is when the infant develops sleep/wake cycles. The infant awakens when he feels some internal cue, such as hunger, or when the parent awakens him to adhere to a schedule. As the child matures, the habituation subsystem guides occupational behavior through the child's habits, routines, and patterns so that he soon responds to self-guided schedules.

Roles are images that the child holds of himself as he attains a certain status or position in a social group. Roles also include the obligations or expectations that accompany these positions. **Perceived incumbency, internalized expectations,** and **role balance** are three components of internalized roles (Kielhofner & Burke, 1985). Some examples of roles are child, sibling, student, and friend. The development of roles during childhood becomes important for later functional interaction with the environment. Roles also provide the child with a way to relate to others in their environments.

Habits guide the child's routines and determine the typical ways in which he performs activities or behaves in particular situations (Kielhofner & Burke, 1985). Habits structure the use of time to achieve more efficacy in daily occupational performance. Early self-care behaviors (self-feeding and toileting) are examples of habits that help the child begin to develop independence.

Through play activities, a child assimilates information. Engaging in play activities, a child acquires a sense of roles and habits (Kielhofner, 1980a). A preschool child may imitate the family roles that he sees at home (Fig. 9.4) When playing house with friends, he pretends to be "the daddy" going to work, thus learning about the adult role of father. A child may have gender expectations about the occupational roles he plays based on information assimilated through his environment as well as from his family's values. Through activities such as daily household chores (for example, setting the table for dinner), the child learns about organizing time for productivity within the family structure. He later can generalize this to social groups. When a child attends school, he accrues other experiences in which he must organize productive behavior, gain a sense of competency, and build habits to maintain the more formal role of student. Competency is optimal for organizing habits. The motive of achievement is optimal for acquiring competent role behavior.

The **performance subsystem,** which consists of the basic capabilities for action in the production of skilled behavior, is the lowest level of human occupation. The performance subsystem consists of skills that provide the basic abilities for action. This subsystem serves as the foundation for the volition and habituation subsystems, which then enable the child to influence his environment. It also provides a child with patterns of skilled action and is responsible for the production of occupational behaviors. This subsystem is considered primary in normal child development.

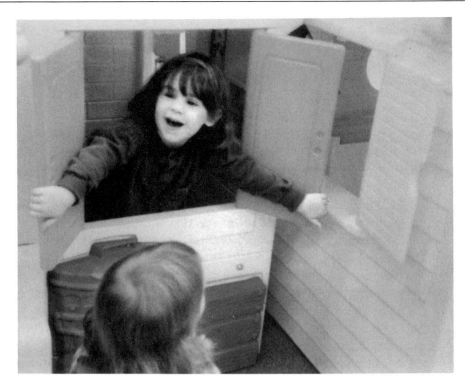

**Figure 9.4.**  Children imitating family roles when playing house.

The performance subsystem in childhood is based on the development of skill constituents that represent the symbolic, neurological, and musculoskeletal bases for the higher level skills. These components depend on the plasticity and learning potential of the central nervous system (CNS). As the child matures, he receives various sensory and motor inputs that become integrated to form complex neuronal models. These models support the formation of perceptual motor, process, and communication skills (Neville, Kielhofner, & Royeen, 1985).

Skills are specific aspects of the performance subsystem that enable the child to engage in purposeful behavior (Kielhofner & Burke, 1985). Skills consist of the following three separate areas: **communication, process,** and **perceptual motor.**

**Communication skills** are used for the child to interact with objects, tasks, social groups, and culture—all environmental components. The way in which the child interacts with others is indicative of the effectiveness of his play and social behaviors. The social smile is an example of a social interaction

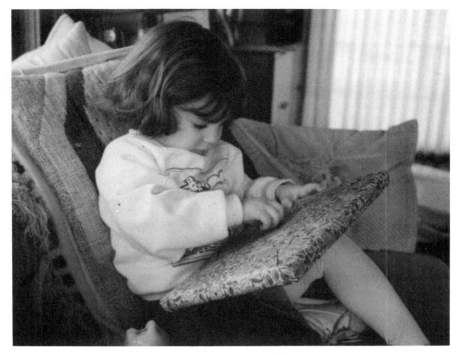

**Figure 9.5.**   Child figuring out how to open a gift.

behavior. A five-year-old child who is an effective communicator about his needs probably does well in a kindergarten setting and plays successfully with other children.

**Process skills** allow a child to plan mentally and to problem solve courses of action (Fig. 9.5). With an infant, this may be exemplified in his ability to develop object permanence and goal-directed behaviors. An example of process skills at an older age is child who works on a puzzle. He knows how to turn the pieces to fit them correctly.

**Perceptual motor skills** require that the child integrate and process sensory information to manipulate objects in the environment. Perceptual motor skills include symbolic images or rules as well as neurological and musculoskeletal components. These skills allow a child to perceive, process, and respond within the skill capacity needed for efficient motor output to accomplish a desired task.

Each subsystem allows for development, differentiation, and integration over time. During childhood, play is the central activity. Skill-building and rule-generating activities that occur during play serve to help the child develop appropriate roles. As the child interacts effectively with his environment, he develops a competent sense of self and a growing repertoire of performance skills. The skills developed in each subsystem depend on previously developed skills from other subsystems. In play, the child explores and develops interests. The family and other institutions socialize the child according to what behaviors are valued, and they provide models for organizing these behaviors. Figure 9.6 depicts the child as an open system and portrays the hierarchical arrangement of the subsystems.

## Change Process

Change is viewed as an identifiable process within the ongoing adaptations that occur in an open system (von Bertalanffy, 1968; Boulding, 1968). By the laws of systems theory, no system can be understood in isolation of its environment. Consideration is, therefore, given in the model of human occu-

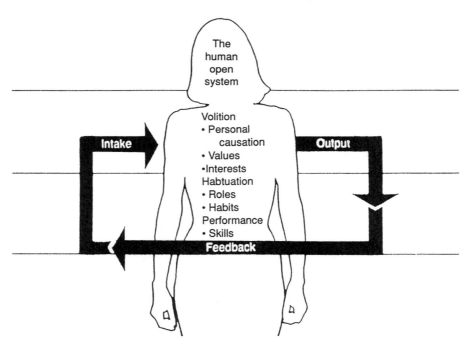

**Figure 9.6.** Summary of the child as an open system and the hierarchical arrangement of subsystems. From Kielhofner, G. (Ed.). A model of human occupation. Baltimore, MD: Williams & Wilkins, 1985.

pation to this established relationship when viewing change within and to the child.

The change process acts within the child (through the subsystems) and through the interaction of the child and his environment, which contributes toward a balance of experiences. The hierarchical nature of systems provides the process by which change takes place in the child, going from simple to complex. It is thus important to remember that the change process is ongoing throughout life and that occupational behavior also participates in this process (Kielhofner & Burke, 1980). Once again, figure 9.6 demonstrates this relationship.

The human occupation frame of reference puts forth the following assumptions (Fig. 9.7):

1. Occupation is fundamental to human experiences and is the essence of existence (Kielhofner & Burke, 1980, 1985).
2. Human occupation emanates from an intrinsic desire to explore and develop mastery in the environment (Kielhofner & Burke, 1980, 1985).
3. A hierarchy of subsystems ranges from volition and habituation to performance (Kielhofner & Burke, 1980, 1985). These subsystems exist within each human.
4. Self-transformation of an open system is hierarchical. This results in change and growth in the open system through the hierarchy of subsystems (Kielhofner, 1985a).
5. Temporality is a universal attribute of work and play and is seen through participation in occupations throughout life (Kielhofner, 1980a, 1980b, 1985a).
6. Modifications within an open system are hierarchical. Adaptive change takes place in the direction of increased complexity and differentiation within the system (Kielhofner, 1980b, 1985a). One must, therefore, recognize the hierarchy of subsystems and levels of differentiation within each subsystem.
7. Work and play are symmetrical. This is characterized by the division of time between work and play on a regular basis (Kielhofner, 1980a; Kielhofner & Burke, 1985).
8. Play supports the work routine by restoring energy within each person, which, in turn, strengthens the worker role (Kielhofner, 1980a; Kielhofner & Barris, 1985). Play, therefore, continues to hold value throughout life in relation to occupational behavior.

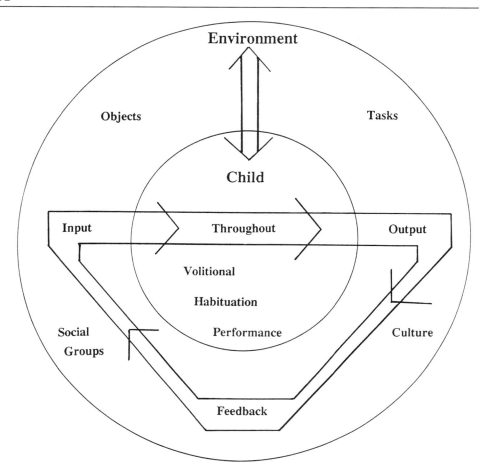

**Figure 9.7.** Change process and the subsystems.

## Summary

The theoretical base of the model of human occupation is influenced greatly by general systems theory and occupational behavior theory. Kielhofner and Burke (1980) began the organization of this model, and Kielhofner continues to refine the model for practice. Important concepts include open systems, occupation, occupational behavior, play, work, motivation, competence, occupational role, environment, and the hierarchy of subsystems and their component parts. The subsystems serve to organize the sections that follow.

# Function/Dysfunction Continua

Function/dysfunction continua provide therapists with descriptions of observable behaviors that are clinically relevant and identify function and dysfunction in children. These things are presented here as they relate to each of the subsystems within the hierarchy mentioned in the preceding section. As growth and maturity occur, each subsystem acquires more meaning for the functional child. When a child functions well, he is an active explorer of his environment, developing skills and competency and a personal sense of achievement. When a child is dysfunctional, he may demonstrate helplessness, incompetence, and inefficacious behaviors (Kielhofner, 1985b).

Among the function/dysfunction continua that follow, distinctions are made for the continua of each subsystem. In reality, all the subsystems are interrelated and interdependent. The human occupation frame of reference presents a specific hierarchy of subsystems; thus, function and dysfunction in any subsystem affects the other subsystems.

## *Volition Subsystem*

The **volition** subsystem represents the highest level in the hierarchy, serving as "overseer" to the two lower subsystems. It addresses the child's motivation toward exploration and mastery of skills. The degree of integration of the lower subsystems (**habituation** and **performance**) also impacts on this subsystem. In a child, the volition subsystem continues to develop and refine with maturation. A child's functional performance is exemplified by his ability to explore his environment, organizing skills into habits and roles and achieving self-awareness and performance. When operational, the volition subsystem guides the child in the initiation of and participation in occupational behaviors. Dysfunction occurs when the child experiences difficulty in exploring the environment. For instance, the child may be unable to achieve self-awareness (Neville, Kielhofner, & Royeen, 1985). The volition subsystem consists of three components: a sense of personal causation, interests, and values. Each area is important and is examined here in terms of function and dysfunction.

As previously mentioned, personal causation relates to the child's expectations and beliefs about his effectiveness in the environment (Kielhofner & Burke, 1980). When functional, the child demonstrates a good sense of self-worth and takes responsibility for his actions. He demonstrates pride in skill mastery, noting competence. A sense of reality also is inferred as the child demonstrates competence and achievement. The child explores his environment actively, which, in turn, can serve to generate more interest, excitement, and motivation. From a developmental perspective, personal causation evolves over time, with maturation. A true internal awareness may not occur until late in childhood, as psychological processes continue to refine and mature. When dysfunctional, the child may have a poor self-image, blaming others for his actions, thus denoting external control of self. He feels bad about himself, which limits him in terms of role and habit formation. He may elect not to explore his environment, detracting from perceptual-motor and communication skill development.

*Self-Image*

| Effectiveness in the Environment | Ineffectiveness in the Environment |
|---|---|
| FUNCTION: Ability to take responsibility for actions and to see himself as having self-worth | DYSFUNCTION: Unable to take responsibility for actions and to see himself as having self-worth |
| BEHAVIORS INDICATIVE OF FUNCTION: | BEHAVIORS INDICATIVE OF DYSFUNCTION: |
| Explores his environment | Does not explore his environment |
| Takes pride in skill mastery, noting competence | Unable to recognize skills and feels incompetent |
| Good self-image | Poor self-image |
| Takes responsibility for actions | Does not take responsibility for actions |
| Demonstrates internal control of behavior | Needs external controls for behavior |

Values determine the child's sense of right and wrong and what is important to him. A child's ability to internalize goals and standards contributes to his development of a value system. As noted in the previous section, values may be shaped by the environment, which includes cultural and social groups. The family provides a structure in which values are fostered. When a child is functional, he demonstrates a sense of right and wrong in his behavior, which fosters the development of exploration, competence, and achievement. When a child is dysfunctional, he is unaware of right and wrong, which interferes with his development of competence and achievement.

*Personal Values*

| Values Congruent with the Environment | Values Incongruent with the Environment |
| --- | --- |
| FUNCTION: Ability to internalize morals toward the development of personal values | DYSFUNCTION: Inability to internalize morals toward the development of personal values |
| BEHAVIORS INDICATIVE OF FUNCTION: | BEHAVIORS INDICATIVE OF DYSFUNCTION: |
| Aware of the rules in the environment | Does not demonstrate awareness of the rules in the environment |
| Adheres to the rules in the environment | Does not follow rules in his environment |
| Alters patterns of behavior consistent with feedback from the environment | Does not alter patterns of behavior in response to feedback from the environment |
| Demonstrates internalization of values through behavior | Does not demonstrate internalization of values through behavior |
| Accepts responsibility for actions consistent with the standards of the environment | Does not accept responsibility for actions consistent with the standards of the environment |
| Demonstrates self-discipline | Does not demonstrate self-discipline |

Interests—things that the child enjoys—continue to develop throughout life. Interests begin in infancy as the child actively explores his environment and satisfies the inner drive of curiosity. At this level, exploration is relatively nonthreatening, because it does not require skills. Through all ages, however, exploration fosters the development of skilled behaviors, competency, and achievement. Exploration can also serve to facilitate the discovery of meaning in actions (Neville, Kielhofner, & Royeen, 1985). The child tends to do and enjoy things in which he is interested. Interests are relative to the child's developmental stages and change over time. A functional child has interests that are developmentally appropriate and consistent with his peers. These interests, however, change over time. A dysfunctional child may have limited interests—interests that are immature for his age or that are not consistent with his peers.

*Age-Appropriate Interests*

| Age-Appropriate Interests | Lack of Age-Appropriate Interests |
|---|---|
| FUNCTION: Selects and engages in various age-appropriate interests | DYSFUNCTION: Limited selection of interests that may not be age-appropriate |
| BEHAVIORS INDICATIVE OF FUNCTION: | BEHAVIORS INDICATIVE OF DYSFUNCTION: |
| Pursues various interests | Pursues a limited amount of interests |
| Engages in various activities reflective of interests | Does not engage in activities reflective of interests |
| Interests chosen and pursued are age-appropriate | Interests chosen and pursued are not age appropriate |
| Interests chosen are accepted by and consistent with the environment | Interests chosen are not consistent with the environment |

## Habituation Subsystem

The **habituation subsystem** integrates the child with the environment by linking internal, spontaneous urges with external, environmental demands (Kielhofner, 1980a). Through feedback from the environment, the child develops socially and culturally acceptable roles. The habituation subsystem consists of two components: **roles** and **habits.** Each component must be addressed when assessing function and dysfunction in children. Roles and habits contribute to the child's interaction with the environment.

Roles—the images that the child holds of himself in relation to social groups—develop through the child's continuous interaction with his environment. The ability to identify and internalize roles becomes important to the development of self, through which control and mastery are achieved in the volition subsystem. Occupational roles, therefore, become important links in assessing the child's performance. When a child is functional, he actively explores his environment, both socially and culturally, to develop role expectations. When dysfunctional, a child may not develop roles that facilitate appropriate interaction with his environment. The child may shy away from association with the human and nonhuman environments alike (Neville, Kielhofner, & Royeen, 1985).

Habits assist in structuring the child's use of time in daily occupational performance. They develop as the child participates in self-care skills, which contributes to his independence. A functional child is able to organize himself enough to perform a skill and, thereby, demonstrate an awareness of temporal orientation. For example, a child knows that on waking (temporal orientation) he walks to the bathroom, uses the toilet, washes his hands and face, and then goes to the kitchen for breakfast. A child who is dysfunctional cannot organize himself enough to establish such daily routines. The dysfunctional child cannot accrue habits or build on the skills needed to develop habits. At that point, the habituation subsystem breaks down into two function/ dysfunction continua, one that relates to roles and another that relates to habits.

*Age-Appropriate Roles*

| Age-Appropriate Roles | Lack of Age-Appropriate Roles |
|---|---|
| FUNCTION: Meets age-appropriate role expectations | DYSFUNCTION: Does not meet age-appropriate role expectations |
| BEHAVIORS INDICATIVE OF FUNCTION: | BEHAVIORS INDICATIVE OF DYSFUNCTION: |
| Responds appropriately to family roles | Indifferent to family roles; may not recognize parents as authority figures |
| Develops an appropriate role within the family (son/ daughter,brother/sister) | Does not recognize or develop an appropriate role within the family |
| Develops appropriate social roles (student, Cub Scout) | Indifferent to social roles; may have difficulty in recognizing socially and culturally acceptable behaviors |
| Plays at an age-appropriate level with others in a social situation | Does not play at an age-appropriate level with others in a social situation |
| Meets role expectations within the environment | Not aware of or does not try to meet role expectations |

*Age-Appropriate Habits*

| Age-Appropriate Habits | Lack of Age-Appropriate Habits |
| --- | --- |
| FUNCTION: Ability to perform daily habits within an appropriate time frame | DYSFUNCTION: Unable to perform daily habits within an appropriate time frame |
| BEHAVIORS INDICATIVE OF FUNCTION: | BEHAVIORS INDICATIVE OF DYSFUNCTION: |
| Develops habits at an age-appropriate level | Habits are maladaptive or not age-appropriate |
| Behaviors indicate an awareness of temporal adaptation as it relates to the performance of habits | Behaviors indicate a lack of awareness of temporal adaptation as it relates to the performance of habits |
| Demonstrates age-appropriate self-care habits | Demonstrates a lack of age-appropriate self-care habits |
| Demonstrates the ability to follow school routines | Demonstrates difficulty in following school routines |

## Performance Subsystem

The **performance subsystem** facilitates the child's ability to act on his environment and helps the child to develop patterns of skilled actions and these skills are responsible for the production of occupational behaviors and child include the necessary communication, process, and perceptual motor skills to interact effectively with their environment (Neville, Kielhofner, & Royeen, 1985).

**Communication skills** enable the child to interact with the human environment. When functional, the child can make his needs known and develop even further his verbal and nonverbal skills. A dysfunctional child may not develop enough communication skills to interact effectively with his environment.

**Process skills** afford the child the ability to plan courses of action and to use problem-solving strategies. The process skills incorporate judgment skills and abstract mental manipulations. When a child is functional, he demonstrates the ability to solve goal-oriented problems. A dysfunctional child may have difficulty in developing mental strategies, which may result in frustration or disinterest and feelings of helplessness.

**Perceptual motor skills** incorporate the neurological, musculoskeletal, and symbolic rule components. The processing and integration of information allow the child to react effectively to motor demands. A functional child processes sensory information efficiently and responds with appropriate motor output. Functional abilities in the performance subsystem may be seen in the developing child as he attains new and more sophisticated behavioral levels. This process takes into account maturation and internalization of sensory feedback from the muscles and joints as these data relate to gravity. The dysfunctional child cannot process sensory information adequately and responds with an unacceptable motor output.

*Age-Appropriate Skill*

| Age-Appropriate Skill | Inadequate Skill Development |
|---|---|
| FUNCTION: Adequate performance in communication, problem-solving, and perceptual motor abilities | DYSFUNCTION: Inadequate performance in communication, problem-solving, and perceptual motor abilities |
| BEHAVIORS INDICATIVE OF FUNCTION: | BEHAVIORS INDICATIVE OF DYSFUNCTION: |
| Age-appropriate communication and interaction abilities, both verbally and nonverbally | Difficulty communicating and interacting verbally or non verbally |
| Communicates effectively with peers | Difficulty in communicating with peers, and may be a bully, or class clown |
| Communicates effectively with adults | Difficulty in communicating with or responding to adults |
| Demonstrates ability to plan a course of action mentally | Unable to plan a course of action mentally; may need to talk through an activity to complete it |
| Uses problem solving strategies | Difficulties with problem solving abilities, cannot identify alternate strategies, and may not be able to think out solutions |
| Motor output behaviors indicate adequate perceptual motor processing | Poor motor output based on inadequate perceptual motor processing or poor sensory motor skill development |

As previously stated, all the subsystems are interrelated and interdependent (Kielhofner & Barris, 1985). Distinctions are made among the continua for each subsystem, but they are not mutually exclusive. In real life, it may be difficult to categorize the functions of one subsystem over another.

# Evaluation

As the therapist approaches assessment in the model of human occupation, it is imperative to address each subsystem within the hierarchy and its component parts. Assessment in this frame of reference encompasses not only the child's performance abilities but also his habits, roles, motivation, competence, and achievement behaviors. In addition, consideration is given to the interaction of the child with his environment (Keilhofner & Barris, 1985; Mailloux, Knox, Burke, & Clark, 1985). Through the inclusion of the subsystems and environment, the evaluation process attempts to capture a total picture of the child in relation to occupational function (Miller, 1988; Sholle-Martin & Alessi, 1990). In the infant and toddler, it is difficult to ascertain functioning in any of the subsystems, because the family often shapes many of these areas. As the child matures, however, function in each subsystem continues to develop and becomes easier to assess.

The therapist selects from a wide range of assessment tools to evaluate each subsystem effectively. The therapist usually begins by examining the lowest subsystem—that is, evaluating performance to identify skilled behaviors. The other subsystems should be addressed subsequently. A firm understanding of the environment also is important to the evaluation process (Mailloux, Knox, Burke, & Clark, 1985).

Assessment of the performance subsystem is the area that occupational therapists feel most comfortable addressing because they are used to identifying a child's skills in terms of sensory, motor, and cognitive function. These skill levels are evaluated in three areas: communication skills, process skills, and perceptual motor skills. The development of each skill level should be observed to note the child's development and possible delays, disruptions, or problems with skill modulations. The development and integration of skilled behaviors provide the basis for the child's occupational status (Mailloux, Knox, Burke, & Clark, 1985).

Communication skills are assessed by observing and interacting with the child. Sensory, motor, and cognitive abilities are taken into account in providing a foundation for communication abilities. During free play, communication can be observed as the child interacts with others, expressing his needs, frustrations, or actions. Specific communication skills may be evaluated through the use of the play scales (Knox, 1974; McCune-Nicolich, 1983).

Process skills, also referred to as problem-solving skills, are assessed by observation of and interaction with the child. During assessment of these skills, the occupational therapist focuses on how the child approaches a task and uses problem-solving techniques to act on and resolve that task. Activity analysis and task analysis assist the therapist to ascertain the degree and extent of problem-solving that a child engages in when participating in an activity.

Perceptual motor skills are assessed by evaluating performance in gross and fine motor areas, visual perceptual areas, and activities of daily living (ADL). The therapist notes how the child processes information through his nervous system, how effectively he responds to motor demands, and whether the child functions at an age-appropriate level. Within the context of this frame of reference, a therapist selects various tools to assess perceptual motor skills: these may include the Bayley Scales of Infant Development (Bayley, 1969); Test of Sensory Functions in Infants (De Gangi & Greenspan, 1989); Hawaii Early Learning Profile (HELP) (Furano, 1984); Developmental Programming for Infants and young Children (D'Eugenio & Moersch, 1977; Schafer & Moersch, 1977); Miller Assessment for Preschoolers (Miller, 1982); Erhardt Developmental Prehension Assessment (Erhardt, 1982); Developmental Test of Visual Motor Integration (Beery, 1967); Test of Visual Perceptual Skills (Gardner, 1988); and Bruininks-Oseretsky Test of Motor Proficiency (Bruininks, 1978). Perceptual motor skills also may be assessed through functional tasks, such as ADL assessments (Coley, 1978). Some of these tools require specific training and are not geared for entry-level therapists. Therapists are encouraged to research these tools and choose those that are most appropriate to the child and to the therapist's skill level. Many other tests are useful for assessing performance areas (Pratt, Allen, Carrasco, Clark, & Schanzenbacher, 1989; Pratt, Allen, Coley, Stephens, Schanzenbacher, & Carrasco, 1989).

Assessment of the habituation subsystem considers the child's roles and habits. Information about the child's roles, including role expectations within the environment, is obtained through observation and interview. Observations are conducted in various environments, such as in the child's home, at school, or on the playground. These environments should specifically include the child's interaction with his peers and family. Interviews should be conducted with the child and, if possible, with his parents, significant care providers, and teachers. The focus of the interviews is to acquire information about the various role expectations that the child may have and then to see how he functions in these roles. The therapist needs to assess how appropriate the role expectations are for this particular child and whether they are realistic within the environment. The therapist should consider the following questions:

- Are the child's role expectations in keeping with the environment?
- Are the role expectations age-appropriate?
- Are the role expectations consistent with the child's performance level?
- Does the child use various roles, specifically familial roles, educational roles, and social roles?

When assessing the child's habits, the therapist should explore routines related to occupational performance. This includes patterns of behavior, such as sleep patterns, eating habits, self-care routines, and other daily activities. Various evaluation tools exist to give the therapist information about the child's habits. These include (but are not limited to) the Neonatal Behavioral Assessment Scale (Brazelton, 1984); Carolina Record of Infant Behaviors (Simeonsson, 1980); Vineland Adaptive Behavior Scales (Sparrow, Balla, Cichetti, 1984); ADL assessments (Coley, 1978); and self-care inventories. Additional information may be obtained from checklists or through interviews (e.g., Pratt, Allen, Coley, Stephens, Schanzenbacher, & Carrasco, 1989). As with roles, the therapist should interview the child and, if possible, his parents, significant care providers, and teachers. The following questions may be useful:

- Would you describe the child's typical day?
- What are the child's typical routines?
- How does the child organize himself for his daily routines?
- How effective are the child's self-care habits?
- How does the child respond to school routines?
- Does the child's performance of routines meet environmental expectations?

The therapist's major concern in assessing habituation is whether the child adequately performs developmentally appropriate role behaviors within the context of his environment.

Assessment of the volition subsystem takes into account the child's effectiveness in his environment (personal causation) and his values and interests. Evaluation instruments may include: Neonatal Behavioral Assessment scale (Brazelton, 1984); the Bayley Scales of Infant Development (Bayley, 1969); Piers-Harris Self Concept Scale (Piers-Harris, 1969); Children's Self-Assessment of Occupational Functioning (Curtain & Baron, 1986); Temperament scales (Chess, 1967); play histories (Takata, 1969); and play scales (Pratt, Allen, Carrasco, Clark, & Schanzenbacher, 1989; Pratt, Allen, Coley, Stephens, Schanzenbacher, & Carrasco, 1989). In addition, the therapist may gain important information through observations and interviews.

When examining the child's effectiveness (personal causation) in his environment, the therapist should consider the following questions:

- Does the child explore his environment?
- Does the child feel competent and take pride in his skills?
- What is the child's image of himself and what effect does it have on his activities?
- Does the child take responsibility for his actions?
- Does the child demonstrate internal control of his behavior?

When examining the child's values and their congruency with the environment, the therapist should consider the following questions:

- Is the child aware of the rules in the environment and does he respond to them appropriately?
- Does the child vary his patterns of behavior consistent with feedback from the environment?
- Does the child's behavior demonstrate that he has internalized the values of his environment?
- Does the child accept responsibility for actions consistent with the standards of his environment?
- Does the child demonstrate self-discipline?

When examining the child's interests, the therapist should consider the following questions:

- Does the child pursue various interests?
- Does the child engage in various activities that reflect his interests?
- Are the child's interests age-appropriate?
- Are the child's interests accepted by and consistent with the environment?

Play is the major medium for intervention, therefore play skills should be assessed carefully, within the context of the child's occupational performance (Mailloux, Knox, Burke, & Clark, 1985; Reilly, 1974). Observation of play, both structured and unstructured, in various environments, has been included in the assessment of the subsystems of performance, habituation, and volition because it is important to the human occupation frame of reference. Furthermore, the therapist must evaluate each subsystem in relation to the child's environment to get a holistic picture of the child's ability to function in terms of occupational performance.

## Postulates Regarding Change

Postulates regarding change delineate the therapeutic environment that needs to be created and suggest appropriate methods to the therapist to facilitate change. In the human occupation frame of reference, the therapist is concerned with the child from a holistic perspective, considering all the subsystems and the environment. In this frame of reference, in which the child is viewed as an open system, one general postulate serves as an overall guide for intervention:

> If the therapist creates an environment that provides input to the child, then change will take place in the child through his subsystems and through his interaction with the environment.

For the human occupation frame of reference, thirteen (13) postulates have been identified. Six postulates are related to the volition subsystem; the first two relate to personal causation:

1. If a child experiences a function deficit in the volition subsystem, it can be addressed through the encouragement of play experience in which the child can acquire a sense of control over the environment.
2. If a child is provided with experiences that are challenging and require problem solving and risk taking, then he will develop the belief that he is empowered to influence his environment.

The next two postulates are related to values:

3. If the therapist confirms a child's positive values, then the child will develop a practical value system accepted by his cultural group.
4. If the therapist gives positive reinforcement to a child when he acts in a constructive manner, then socially acceptable behaviors will develop.

Finally, two postulates relate to interest within the volition subsystems:

5. If a child engages in tasks and activities that he finds to be satisfying, then he will tend to become interested in those types of tasks and activities.
6. If a child is given various experiences and encouraged to choose those that he enjoys, then he will develop a set of personal interests.

The primary objective of postulates regarding change in the habituation subsystem is to develop habits that support the child's roles as a family member, player, and student. This eventually leads to the development of a worker role. Five postulates relate to the habituation subsystem; the first three relate to the development of roles:

7. If the therapist collaborates with the child's family to provide an environment that fosters play and role modeling of appropriate family roles, then the child will develop an appropriate role within his family.
8. If a child is provided with structured and unstructured play sessions with peers, then he will develop appropriate player roles.
9. If a therapist provides the necessary support, as well as encourages and expects the child to engage in educational experiences, then the child will develop an appropriate student role.

The following two postulates relate to the development of habits:

10. If the therapist creates an environment in which a child is responsible, with assistance, for performing daily self-care tasks, then the child will develop appropriate activities of daily living habits.
11. If a child is provided with specific routines to follow, then he will develop appropriate daily habits.

The primary objective of postulates regarding change in the performance subsystem is to develop performance skills in relation to communication, problem solving, and perceptual motor areas. Two postulates relate to the performance subsystem:

12. If the therapist provides a child with activities that facilitate the development of his performance in communication, problem solving, and perceptual motor skills, then the child will show improvement in his general performance areas.
13. If a therapist selects and uses appropriate techniques from another frame of reference that address a child's specific performance deficits and these

techniques are consistent with the human occupation frame of reference, then the child's performance skills will develop.

# Application to Practice

The application of the human occupation frame of reference is holistic in nature, intending to deal with the total function of the child within his environment. Because the family provides the major environment for the child, this frame of reference lends itself to situations in which the therapist and family are collaborators in treatment. This mandates that the therapist develop effective communication with the parents or care providers, to understand the roles and expectations of the child within the family environment. Consideration must be given to the family, as well as to their values and beliefs about the child. The demands of other environments should also be taken into consideration when developing a plan for intervention. During the intervention process, the therapist should be responsive to the parent's views of and expectations for the child. The family's values and beliefs should impact on intervention. Together, the therapist and the parents should determine accurate goals and expectations for the child. The therapist should engage the parents or care providers in developing the plan for intervention, helping them to understand the areas of dysfunction, so that they can achieve a better understanding of the child's levels of function (Bazyk, 1989).

Consistent with the principles of general systems theory, the therapist creates an environment that provides input to the child, because input is viewed as one of the major means of change. This frame of reference does not incorporate specific details of physical or emotional dysfunction that may impact on occupational performance (Kielhofner & Burke, 1985; Mailloux, Knox, Burke, & Clark, 1985). According to this frame of reference, when dealing with such physical or emotional deficits, therapists should draw on other frames of reference for specific techniques.

## *Volition Subsystem*

If a child experiences a deficit in the volition subsystem in the area of personal causation, the therapist should encourage him to engage in play experiences that develop a sense of control over the environment. Play is the primary medium for intervention in this frame of reference. The play experiences should be consistent with the child's age and developmental level.

With a young child, the therapist would start by providing sensory experiences that serve as a foundation for later learning. As the child gets older, the therapist should provide a variety of appropriate activities so that the child has choices. When the child has alternatives, it allows him to feel greater control over his environment. This helps him to understand that he can have some effect on his environment, as well as to foster a sense of self.

When the therapist observes that the child is more comfortable in choosing a varied repertoire of activities, she presents play activities that are challenging and that involve problem solving and risk taking. For example, with a preschooler the therapist might use a variety of enjoyable puzzles to encourage goal-directed activity that not only places a demand on the child but also requires a solution. This gives the child an opportunity to develop his problem-solving abilities in a safe, structured environment.

In therapy sessions, the child should experience success and failure alike. The therapist should choose activities carefully that challenge the child and develop a sense of success. This helps the child to develop a feeling of mastery over the environment and a sense of personal adequacy. Once the child is successful with these activities and appears to feel more confident, higher level activities may be presented. These activities should be more challenging, and the child may not experience success immediately. Dealing with success and failure helps him to understand the real world and to gain a sense of his own strengths and limitations.

As the child accrues a sense of competency, the therapist's expectations of the child are increased so that the child's skills and abilities become refined. In addition to working directly with the child, the therapist should apprise the parents of developmentally appropriate play activities. Various activities may be suggested, and the parents and therapist should determine together which activities are culturally and socially appropriate for the child's current level. The activities selected should be chosen carefully to ensure some degree of success and to foster not only a positive self-image but also a sense of mastery over the environment.

It is important that the therapist understand the family's values and beliefs, because parental expectations and attitudes are significant in shaping the child. The therapist also needs to understand those values that are acceptable among the child's cultural group and peers. Fantasy play in early childhood often reflects the values and attitudes that the child has seen at home. In individualized treatment, the therapist should reinforce positive values displayed by the child, because values tend to shape behaviors. Group play situations provide an opportunity for the child to interact with peers and to experiment with behaviors to determine which are acceptable. The therapist can shape the group experience by reinforcing constructive behavior and by identifying behaviors that are unacceptable to the group. As the child gets older, with continued experiences, he begins to internalize the standards of his group and understands the relevance of standards of performance in school and, ultimately, in work settings.

The development of interests is related to the variety of experiences that the child encounters. The child must explore different types of play and activities to determine his personal interests. The therapist should provide numerous activities, so that the child can begin to identify which tasks are most satisfying. All tasks presented should be at developmentally appropriate levels. It should be noted that a child's interests are closely related to his developmental level and neuromuscular abilities. Children enjoy practicing skills and exploring their abilities. The therapist should select activities at the child's developmental level as well as ones acceptable to the child's sociocultural group.

Through experimentation with choices and selection of activities, the child can develop interests. As he matures, however, these interests tend to change. For example, the young child first starts out at a sensorimotor level, selecting toys that he can mouth, things that he can feel, and items that he can manipulate. As he develops, he moves onto a new level where he begins to influence his environment, such as when he first chooses to play in a sandbox in the playground and later, when he is older, chooses to climb a ladder and go down a slide. For the preschooler, the therapist also may use activities that encourage fantasy play to promote interest development.

The school-aged child's interests usually progress to tasks that require refined perceptual motor skills, such as throwing and kicking a ball, or matching shapes and sorting objects. Interest in communication skills becomes more apparent to the child, so that he can interact more effectively with his peers and make his needs and interests known to others. To foster this development, the therapist may encourage the child to participate in group activities in various settings to encourage this development. Such activities may include participation in group outings, scouting activities, team sports, or other social events.

With his expanding repertoire of skills, the child's interests tend to become more complex and, at times, more specific. The therapist should be sensitive to this and individualize treatment programs for the child's unique interests. For an older child who wants to make something, constructional tasks (building models) may be introduced. Interests developed at this level may determine occupational interests for later.

## Habituation Subsystem

Intervention in the habituation system relates to the development of roles and habits. The child has many roles—that of family member, player, and student. As an infant, the initial role is that of player, usually within the context of the family. Both the therapist and parents can foster the development of this role by providing objects for play and play experiences. There should be minimal expectations of the infant. The infant's role in the family is determined by his parent's attitudes, behaviors, beliefs, cultural expectations, and values.

As the child gets older, environmental expectations become greater, with the child assuming various roles, each with more complexity. Consistent with the therapist/parent relationship described in the volition subsystem, they should collaborate to foster the development of appropriate family roles for the child. Family roles can be facilitated both through play and role modeling. The therapist should consult the parent when choosing activities to ensure that what is chosen is socially and culturally acceptable.

Many ways exist to enhance family roles for children. The therapist may act as facilitator by presenting the game or by supplying the environment for the child to explore freely. At other times, she may be an active participant in play activities that explore roles with the child. Fantasy and dramatic play may be used as a way of experimenting with roles, such as when children "play house." One important aspect of playing house is the exploration of family role. The child imitates behaviors that he has observed or tries out roles other than "child." The therapist also can play an active part and model additional (other than familial) roles for the child to observe.

Family roles often entail family responsibilities. The family may have expectations of the child within the family system, which may involve specific chores or duties. Chores can be learned through fantasy or dramatic play, where the therapist demonstrates a particular chore to the child and later asks him to "perform" that chore. Similarly, the development of role responsibilities can be fostered through having the child help clean up after the therapy session.

The occupational therapist also is concerned with the child's refinement of his role as a player. The therapist can facilitate this continuing development through the gradation of play from individual, sensorimotor-oriented play through parallel play activities, to group play, depending on the child's developmental and skill levels. When the therapist provides various structured and unstructured group play sessions, she gives the child the opportunity to try out roles such as friend, follower, and leader. He gets feedback from his peers, and the therapist, and develops appropriate player roles. This exploration allows the child to experience and become comfortable with different roles. Beyond the therapeutic experience, the child should be encouraged to engage in spontaneous play groups and clubs to facilitate this development.

When it is socially and culturally appropriate, the child must learn the student role. The therapist may facilitate this scenario by encouraging the child to engage in educational play situations. The student role involves more than just to participation in the classroom. The therapist may select educational games and tasks that promote the child's success in the educational environment. The therapist can help to identify the child's individual needs during transition into the elementary school environment. With her awareness of the child's other roles, she is able to provide the appropriate support for the cultivation of the student role in the school environment. She also provides support for the child's involvement in various educational experiences.

The emergence of habits initially stems from biological needs and parental regulations. Inherent in habits is the development of appropriate routines. The establishment of these routines involves an understanding of environmental expectations. The therapist and parents, therefore, must work together to formulate a plan for the development of an appropriate routine by knowing what behaviors are expected in the environment and by deciding which routines the child can achieve based on his age and skill level.

Activities of daily living comprise one area of major concern in the development of habits. The parents may role model activities of daily living for the child, and the therapist also can teach the child specific self-care skills. This can serve as the basis for the development of self-care habits. During the treatment sessions, the therapist needs to offer the child opportunities to use these recently acquired skills. This is one way to transform the skill into a habit. The therapist then may need to work with the child to facilitate the understanding of how these habits can fit into the routine of daily life. As the child becomes ready, the therapist should encourage him to engage in regular self-care activities and then assist him toward independence in performing these tasks.

Recognizing the routines within the home and school environments constitute the first step toward developing a sense of temporal organization for the child. In collaboration with the parents, the therapist can work with the school-aged child to identify the routines followed at home. Once general home routines have been identified, the therapist and child then can delineate the personal routines expected of him within the home. Based on this information, during a treatment session, the child may be asked to develop a schedule for his personal home routines. This can be a way of exercising temporal organization and control over the environment. The same thing then can be done for the school environment.

## Performance Subsystem

Intervention in the performance subsystem is concerned with the development of age-appropriate performance skills in relation to communication, problem-solving, and perceptual motor areas. Through information obtained during the evaluation process, the therapist can come to understand the child's current level of performance. Occupational therapy intervention in this subsystem involves the selection and application of specific activities that facilitate the child's skill development in deficit areas. Ultimately, the therapist wants to improve the child's general performance areas. For example, a young child who has difficulty with skilled motor performance may be presented with a constructional activity (building blocks or Lego™ toys). The initial activity can be to build a simple tower, which then can be upgraded to building a simple house. This evolution involves problem-solving and perceptual motor skill. Furthermore, the therapist may engage the child in conversation, talking with him about the activity. In this way, the child also can work on communication skills. (With an older child, a puzzle might be a more appropriate activity for promoting problem-solving and perceptual motor skills). Should communication skills be impaired, however, the occupational therapist could work in conjunction with a speech pathologist.

Group activities also may be used to enhance development in the performance area. In a group situation, the child has an opportunity to observe and interact with his peers. He can see how they approach tasks. Through this, he may gain information on how they problem solve and negotiate a new activity or situation. Group activities provide opportunities for the child to try out what he has observed and to see if these strategies are useful. Communication skills are promoted naturally in group situations.

Within the human occupation frame of reference, the therapist can select and use appropriate techniques from other frames of reference that address the child's specific performance deficits (Kielhofner, 1985). The therapist should choose these techniques with care to ensure that they are consistent with the principles of this frame of reference. By using other appropriate interventions, the child's performance skills can be developed even more.

## *Environment*

Throughout the human occupation frame of reference, the child's environment is important. Because of this, the therapist should always keep all the child's environments in mind when planning an intervention. This includes the home, school, and any other areas important to the child. The therapist should know the child's cultural background and the expectations placed on him in the environment.

The home environment is always of primary concern to the occupational therapist. She should develop a good rapport and maintain a positive relationship with the parents, so that she can help them understand their child's strengths and deficits and then work with them actively in the intervention plan. This may require familiarizing the parents with the normal sequence of child development and helping them to become aware of age-appropriate expectations. It also may involve discussing the influence of the child's disabilities on his functional performance.

## Summary

The theoretical base of the model of human occupation is grounded in systems and occupational behavior theory. Important concepts include open systems, occupation, occupational behavior, play, work, motivation, competence, occupational role, environment, and the hierarchy of subsystems and their component parts. The child is viewed as an open system, and the laws of organization and hierarchy exist within the three subsystems (volition, habituation, and performance). **Volition** encompasses a child's personal causation, interests, values, and temporal adaptation. **Habituation** addresses roles and habit patterns. **Performance** looks at a child's behavior in terms of perceptual motor, process (problem-solving), and communication skills. The child's environment—physical and social—and his interaction with the environment are major points of concern in the human occupation frame of reference.

Six function/dysfunction continua are fundamental to this frame of reference, and they provide the basis for evaluation and intervention. These continua give the therapist criteria by which to determine the child's abilities and deficits.

Postulates regarding change outline the therapeutic environment that should be created to effect change. One general postulate focuses on working with the child as an open system within his environment, whereas 13 other postulates facilitate change in three subsystems.

Application of this frame of reference into practice incorporates an effective collaboration among the therapist, the child, parents, or care providers. Because the child generally is a family member, family attitudes and values affect the child's occupational behaviors. Entry-level therapists are encouraged to discuss implementation of this frame of reference with supervisors and the child's family members to ensure that the child's needs are met.

Intervention strategies may include the use of play and other occupational behaviors to develop the child's values, personal causation, interests, habits, roles, and skills. Functional abilities also are considered in various environments (home and school). Proficiency in activity analysis is important for the therapist so that appropriate activities are chosen to meet the child's needs and interests. The child should be encouraged to develop holistically in terms of occupational behavior and performance in the environment.

The therapist may choose to use other frames of reference to address specific areas in the performance subsystem. The therapist should be sure that any such additional frames of reference are consistent with the model of human occupation.

## OUTLINE OF THE MODEL OF HUMAN OCCUPATION FRAME OF REFERENCE

I. Historical perspective
  A. Occupational behavior theory
    1. Meyer's time binding model
    2. Slagle's human habit patterns
    3. Occupational behavior
      a. Play
      b. Occupational roles
      c. Work behaviors
      d. Hierarchical organization of routines
        1. Exploration
        2. Competency
        3. Achievement
      e. Occupational choices
  B. General systems theory
    1. Laws of hierarchy
    2. Open systems
      a. Homeostasis
      b. Laws of organization
      c. Environment

II. Theoretical base
    A. Occupational behavior within the context of systems theory
        1. Environment
            a. Physical
            b. Social settings
        2. Open system
            a. Intake
            b. Throughput
            c. Output
            d. Feedback
        3. Assumptions compatible with general systems theory
    B. Occupation
        1. Purposeful use of time
        2. Exploration and mastery
        3. Meeting personal needs and standards of a social group
        4. Continuum of play to work
    C. Occupational behavior
        1. Activities of work, play, and daily living
            a. Mastery of environment
                1. Competency
                2. Achievement
                3. Occupational role
            b. Motivation
        4. Play and work
            a. Characteristics and purposes of play
            b. Characteristics and purposes of child work
            c. Motivation
            d. Sense of competence and mastery
        5. Environment
        6. Hierarchy—three subsystems
            a. Volition
                1. Personal causation
                2. Interests
                3. Values
                4. Temporal orientation
            b. Habituation
                1. Roles
                2. Habits
            c. Performance
                1. Skills
            d. Assumptions

III. Function/dysfunction continua
    A. Self-image
    B. Personal values
    C. Age-appropriate interests
    D. Age-appropriate roles
    E. Age-appropriate habits
    F. Age-appropriate skill development

IV. Evaluation
    A. Overall assessment
    B. Assessment of performance subsystem
    C. Assessment of habituation subsystem
    D. Assessment of volition subsystem

V. Postulates regarding change
    A. Those that relate to use of the model of human occupation frame of reference
    B. Those that relate to the volition subsystem
    C. Those that relate to the habituation subsystem
    D. Those that relate to the performance subsystem

VI. Application to practice
    A. Volition subsystem
       1. Play experiences
       2. Activity selection and use
       3. Interests
    B. Habituation subsystem
       1. Roles
       2. Habits
       3. Sense of temporal organization
    C. Performance subsystem
       1. Skill development
       2. Group activities
       3. Use of appropriate techniques from other frames of reference
    D. Environment

### Acknowledgments

The author wishes to thank Karen Stern and Diane Reis-Braaten for their valuable feedback in the writing of this chapter.

### References

Barris, R. (1982). Environmental interactions: An extension of the model of occupation. *American Journal of Occupational Therapy, 36,* 637–644.

Barris, R., Kielhofner, G., Levine, R., & Neville, A. (1985). Occupation as interaction with the environment. In G. Kielhofner (Ed.). *A model of human occupation* (pp. 42–62). Baltimore, MD: Williams & Wilkins.

Bayley, N. (1969). *Bayley scales of infant development.* New York: The Psychological Corporation.

Bazyk, S. (1989). Changes in attitudes and beliefs regarding parent participation and home programs: An update. *American Journal of Occupational Therapy, 43,* 723–728.

Beery, K. (1967). *Development test of visual motor integration.* Chicago, IL: Follet.

Boulding, K. E. (1968). General Systems Theory—the skeleton of science. In: W. Buckley, (Ed.). *Modern systems research for the behavioral scientist,* (pp. 3–10). Chicago, IL: Aldine.

Brazelton, T. B. (1984). *Neonatal behavioral assessment Scale,* (2nd Ed.). Philadelphia, PA: J. B. Lippincott.

Bruininks, R. (1978). *Bruininks-Oseretsky test of motor proficiency.* Circle Pines, MN: American Guidance Service.

Bruner, J.S. (1970). The skill of relevance or the relevance of skills. *Saturday Review, 20,* 66–73.

Burke, J. P. (1983). Defining occupation: Importing and organizing interdisciplinary knowledge. In G. Kielhofner (Ed.). *Health through occupation: Theory and practice in occupational therapy* (pp. 125–138). Philadelphia, PA: F. A. Davis.

Chess, S. (1967). Temperament in the normal infant. In J. Hellmuth (Ed.). *Exceptional infant,* (Vol. I). New York, NY: Brunner and Mazel.

Coley, I. (1978). *Pediatrics assessment of self-care activities.* St. Louis, MO: C. V. Mosby.

Curtain, C., & Baron, K. B. (1986). *The child's self assessment of occupational functioning.* Chicago, IL: University of Illinois at Chicago, College of Associated Health Profession, Department of Occupational Therapy.

DeCharms, R. (1968) *Personal causation.* New York, NY: Academic Press.

DeGangi, C. A., & Greenspan, S. I. (1989). *Test of sensory functions in infants.* Los Angeles, CA: Western Psychological Services.

D'Eugenio, D. B., & Moersch, M. S. (1977). *Developmental Programming for infants and young children,* (vols. 4,5). Ann Arbor, MI: The University of Michigan Press.

Erhardt, R. (1982). *Developmental hand dysfunction: Theory, assessment, treatment.* Laurel, MD: RAMSCO Publishing.

Florey, L. (1969) An approach to play and play development. *American Journal of Occupational Therapy, 25,* 275–280.

Furano, S. (1984). *Hawaii early learning profile.* Palo Alto, CA: VORT Corporation.

Gardner, M. (1988). *Test of visual perceptual skills.* San Francisco, CA: Health Publishing.

Ginsberg, E. (1972). Toward a theory of occupational choice: A restatement. *Educational Guidance Quarterly, 20,* 169–172.

Kielhofner, G. (1978). General Systems Theory: Implications for theory and action in occupational therapy. *American Journal of Occupational Therapy, 32,* 637–645.

Kielhofner, G. (1980a). A model of human occupational. Part II. Ontogenesis from the perspective of temporal adaptation. *American Journal of Occupational Therapy, 34,* 657–666.

Kielhofner, G. (1980b). A model of human occupational. Part III. Benign and vicious cycles. *American Journal of Occupational Therapy, 34,* 731–737.

Kielhofner, G. (1983). *Health through occupation: theory and practice in occupational therapy.* Philadelphia, PA: F. A. Davis.

Kielhofner, G. (1985). Introduction. In G. Kielhofner (Ed.). *A model of human occupation* (pp. xvii–xx). Baltimore, MD: Williams & Wilkins.

Kielhofner, G., & Barris, R. (1985). The development of occupational behavior. In G. Kielhofner (Ed.). *A model of human occupation* (pp. 78–81). Baltimore, MD: Williams & Wilkins.

Kielhofner, G., & Burke, J. (1977). Occupational therapy after 60 years: An account of changing identity and knowledge. *American Journal of Occupational Therapy, 31,* 675–688.

Kielhofner, G., & Burke, J. (1980). A model of human occupation: Conceptual framework and content. *American Journal of Occupational Therapy, 34,* 572–581.

Kielhofner, G., & Burke, J. (1985). Components and determinants of human occupation. In G. Kielhofner (Ed.). *A model of human occupation* (pp. 12–36). Baltimore, MD: Williams & Wilkins.

Kielhofner, G., Burke, J., & Igi, C. (1980). A model of human occupation: Assessment and intervention. *American Journal of Occupational Therapy, 34,* 777–788.

Klavins, R. (1972). Work-play behavior: Cultural influences. *American Journal of Occupational Therapy, 26,* 176–179.

Knox, S. (1974). A play skills inventory. In M. Reilly (Ed.). *Play as exploratory learning: Studies in curiosity behavior,* (pp. 247–266). Beverly Hills, CA: Sage.

Mailloux, Z., Knox, S., Burke, J., Clark, F. (1985). Pediatric dysfunction. In G. Kielhofner (Ed.). *A model of human occupation* (pp. 306–351). Baltimore, MD: Williams & Wilkins.

McClelland, D. (1953). *The achievement motive.* New York, NY: Appleton-Century-Crofts.

McCune-Nicolich, L. (1983). *A manual for analyzing free play.* New Brunswick, NJ: Department of Educational Psychology, Rutgers University.

Meyer, A. (1922/1977). The philosophy of Occupational Therapy. *American Journal of Occupational Therapy, 31,* 639–642.

Miller, L. J. (1982). *Miller assessment for preschoolers.* Littleton, CO: The Foundation for Knowledge in Development.

Miller, R. J. (1988). Gary Kielhofner. In R. Miller, K. Sieg, F. Ludwig, S. Shortridge, & J. Van Deusen (Eds.). *Six perspectives on theory for the practice of occupational therapy* (pp. 169–203). Rockville, MD: Aspen.

Neff, W. S. (1968) *Work and human behavior.* New York, NY: Atherton.

Neville, P., Kielhofner, G., & Royeen, C. (1985). Childhood. In G. Kielhofner (Ed.). *A model of human occupation* (pp. 306–351). Baltimore, MD: Williams & Wilkins.

Piers, E., & Harris, D. (1969). *Piers-Harris children's self-concept scale.* Los Angeles, CA: Western Psychological Services.

Pratt, P., Allen, A., Carrasco, R., Clark, F., & Schanzenbacher, K. (1989). Instruments to evaluate component functions of behavior. In P. Pratt & A. Allen (eds.) *Occupational therapy for children* (2nd Ed.). (pp. 168-197). St. Louis, MO: C. V. Mosby.

Pratt, P., Allen, A., Coley, I., Stephens, L., Schanzenbacher, K., & Carrasco, R. (1989). Instruments to evaluate childhood performance skills. In P. Pratt & A. Allen (eds.) *Occupational therapy for children* (2nd Ed.). (pp. 198–217). St. Louis, MO: C. V. Mosby.

Reed, K. (1984). *Models of practice in occupational therapy.* Baltimore, MD: Williams and Wilkins.

Reilly, M. (1962). Occupational therapy can be one of the great ideas of the 20th century medicine. *American Journal of Occupational Therapy, 16,* 1–9.

Reilly, M. (1966). A psychiatric occupational therapy program as a teaching model. *American Journal of Occupational Therapy, 20,* 61–67.

Reilly, M. (1969). The education process. *American Journal of Occupational Therapy, 23,* 299–307.

Reilly, M. (1971). The modernization of occupational therapy. *American Journal of Occupational Therapy, 25,* 243–246.

Reilly, M. (1974). *Play as exploratory behavior.* Beverly Hills, CA: Sage.

Schafer, D. S., & Moersch, M. S. (1977). *Developmental programming for infants and young children,* (vol. 1–3). Ann Arbor, MI: The University of Michigan Press.

Shannon, P. (1970). The work-play model: a basis for occupational therapy program-ming in psychiatry. *American Journal of Occupational Therapy, 24,* 215–218.

Shannon, P. (1972). Work-play theory and the occupational therapy process. *American Journal of Occupational Therapy, 26,* 169–172.

Sholle-Martin, S. & Alessi, N. E. (1990). Formulating a role for occupational therapy in child psychiatry: A clinical application. *American Journal of Occupational Therapy, 44,* 871–882.

Simeonsson, R. J. (1980). *Carolina record of infant behavior.* Chapel Hill, NC: University of North Carolina.

Slagle, E. C. (1934). Occupational therapy: recent methods and advances in the United States. *Occupational Therapy and Rehabilitation, 13,* 289–298.

Slagle, E. C., & Robeson, H. A. (1941). *Syllabus for training of nurses in occupational therapy,* (2nd ed). Utica, NY: State Hospitals Press.

Sparrow, S. S., Balla, D. A., & Cicchetti, D. V. (1984). *Vineland adaptive behavior scales.* Circle Pines, MN: American Guidance Service.

Takata, N. (1969). Play history. *American Journal of Occupational Therapy, 23,* 314–318.

von Bertalanffy, L. (1968). General systems theory—a critical review. In W. Buckley, (Ed.). *Modern systems research for the behavioral scientist,* (pp. 11–30). Chicago, IL: Aldine.

White, R. W. (1959). Motivation reconsidered: The concept of competence. *Psychological Review, 66,* 297–333.

White, R. W. (1971). The urge toward competence. *American Journal of Occupational Therapy, 25,* 271–274.

Woodside, H. (1976). Dimensions of the occupational behaviour model. *Canadian Journal of Occupational Therapy, 43,* 11–14.

# 10

# Psychosocial Frame of Reference

LAURETTE OLSON

Children are referred for psychiatric evaluation because their behavior interferes with their ability to function in their normal roles and activities—that is, their behavior may be disruptive or disturbing at home, in school, or in their community. The child may exhibit impulsiveness; verbal or physical aggression toward others; ritualistic, bizarre, or phobic behavior; or withdrawal from daily activities or family members. Care providers may be overwhelmed with the exacerbation of behaviors that previously were difficult but nonetheless manageable; or they may be troubled by sudden negative shifts in behavior.

Environmental stressors may lead to negative behavioral changes. Such things include familial issues (parental discord or divorce), chronic physical or mental illness, physical abuse, neglect, or sexual abuse. New environments may make different or greater demands on the child's cognitive, social, and psychological skills. Stressors may be academic or school-related rather than familial. These include changes in setting or expectations, as well as, specific difficulties that may arise with educational performance. Innate vulnerabilities in the child (learning or language disabilities, a difficult temperament, developmental delays, autism or autistic-like features) may exacerbate even more the effects of the stressors.

## Theoretical Base

The theoretical base for the psychosocial frame of reference derives from various theories that address a child's emotional development. These theories consider innate temperament, attachment, peer interaction, play, ability to cope, and environmental interaction. The area of psychosocial dysfunction is complex, and this chapter describes only one frame of reference directed toward understanding and providing psychosocial intervention for children.

## *Innate Temperament*

Temperament is the inborn, inherited style with which a person approaches and responds to his environment. Specific behavior patterns are discernible even in the first days of life. Components of temperament include activity level, regularity of biological functions, approach/withdrawal tendencies for new situations, adaptability to change, sensory threshold, quality of mood, intensity of mood expression, distractibility, and persistence and attention span (Chess & Thomas, 1984). Temperament has a powerful effect on a person's interaction with his human *and* nonhuman environments.

Some infants are easy to please and adapt readily to their environments. They have regular eating and sleeping patterns and are generally attentive and cheerful with their care providers. Other infants may be similar in their reaction to consistency but may withdraw and become anxious when faced with change. Adaptation is slow. Still other infants are labeled **difficult,** meaning that they are less easy to please, have frequent and strong displays of negative moods, have irregular eating and sleeping patterns, and are less likely to respond to care providers in a warm, cuddly fashion. Some infants may demonstrate hyperactivity, hypersensitivity, distractibility, emotional lability, or insatiability. Care providers may find it difficult to respond to such a child in a soothing, consistent way.

**Compatibility** refers to the match between the temperaments of parent and child. This means that their temperaments may be similar, mesh easily, or that the parent can understand and empathize with the child's different temperament and yet nurture its adaptation to the world. A "good" match is important for the development of a positive, reciprocal relationship between care provider and child. The consistent response of the care provider to the child is necessary to calm the child and yet to foster the development of appropriate adaptive behavior (Chess & Thomas, 1984). When the temperaments of parent and child are not compatible, the relationship may not be positive, and interaction often becomes tense, negative, and unpleasant. Negative interaction cycles tend to become repetitive. This may result in a lack of development of appropriate adaptive behaviors for the child.

It is important to remember that although temperament is biologically determined and especially affects the child's first relationships, it can be modified by environmental influence. The structure of the environment and style that care providers use in relation to the child's temperament are crucial for functional development.

## *Attachment*

A stable and secure relationship with parents or care providers is essential for children to develop into happy, competent adults. Care providers are responsible for maintaining an environment in which the child's biological needs are met and in which he is protected from danger. This very special relationship between adult and child has been called **attachment relationship** (Bowlby, 1969). It is an enduring, emotional, discriminating bond that develops over time (Ainsworth, 1967). Ideally, its behavioral organization is flexible so that it promotes the child's development. As the child grows and becomes more autonomous and competent, he seeks out his care providers less frequently, in different ways, and for different reasons. Parents should continue to adapt their caregiving approach to the child's needs.

In examining this attachment, it is important to understand its components. The relationship is composed of a smooth, reciprocal interaction between the child's attachment and the care providers' responses. Attachment behaviors are those that children exhibit to attract parents or care providers; they are the signals that children emit to let their care providers know that they need stimulation, want to play, or are experiencing some degree of distress. In the latter case, a child might be hungry, cold, afraid, or in pain. Providing care includes all the behaviors exhibited in response to the child's attachment behavior. This process is based on an understanding of the child's verbal and nonverbal cues (Fig. 10.1).

The security of the attachment relationship is of particular concern to the therapist. It must be consistently nurturing so that the child knows what to expect. It is important that a child anticipate comfort, protection, and help as a matter of course. A child's degree of enthusiasm, resilience, willingness, and ability to engage in challenging tasks and his competence among peers have been correlated directly with the history of a secure attachment relationship (Arend, Gore, & Sroufe, 1979; Lieberman, 1977; Waters, Wittman, & Sroufe, 1979). The quality of early attachment relationships exerts powerful effects on a child's ability to establish and maintain relationships with peers and adults other than his parents.

Securely attached children perceive their parents and care providers as responsive and readily available. Children in these environments are reasonably confident that they can receive comfort, assistance, or encouragement when needed. Securely attached children can engage in play, seek out care

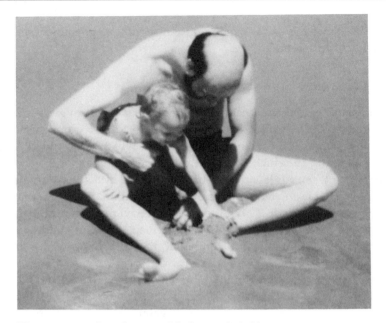

**Figure 10.1.**   Attachment of father and child.

providers for comfort, and then can reengage in play. When a secure attachment is developed in infancy, it is believed that the child demonstrates enthusiastic, persistent, and cooperative behavior during play. Secure children engage in problem-solving activities, and, when they become frustrated, they seek appropriate assistance from adults (Fig. 10.2).

Insecurely attached children are not certain of the extent to which they can rely on care providers. This insecurity may prevent these children from becoming involved in activities because they are never sure that a secure homebase will be available to them. They may engage in play but do not necessarily seek comfort when stressed. Anxiety caused by external pressure and challenges, therefore, may remain unsoothed. Other children may approach care providers for comfort, but, because of feelings of uncertainty about the adult's response, insecure children may not seek help rather than risk feelings of rejection. Children who have insecure attachment relationships are thought to be easily frustrated by challenges and, consequently, give up. Furthermore, they may demonstrate resistant and acting-out behaviors (Matas, Arend, & Sroufe, 1978). Children who have demonstrated insecure attachment behavior as infants may be more withdrawn socially and hesitate to interact with peers (Lieberman, 1977).

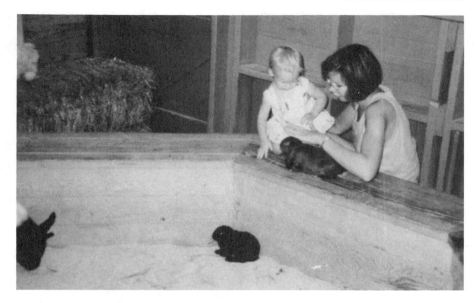

**Figure 10.2.**   Securely attached child playing with mother and pet.

In the past, mothers or maternal surrogates were responsible for helping children to form attachments. Economic and social changes in Western culture have altered this process of child rearing dramatically. Many mothers now work, even though their children are infants. More fathers are taking responsibility for the child's daily care. In addition, the role of professional child care has increased dramatically. Large numbers of infants and children spend more time per week with care providers who are not their parents.

## Peer Interactive Skills

Although adult/child relationships are different from child/child relationships, parent/child interaction serves as a catalyst for the development of peer interactive skills. The ability to make eye contact and to initiate and respond to playful overtures is reinforced by the resulting pleasure and comfort of parent/child relationships. The child is naturally interested in others, especially other children, and anticipates the same attentiveness and pleasure in play that he has experienced with adult care providers. He soon learns, however, that other children have their own wishes and are less accommodating than adult playmates. Other children are more like him in size, skill level, vigor, and interest, and, therefore, are much sought after. If peers are going

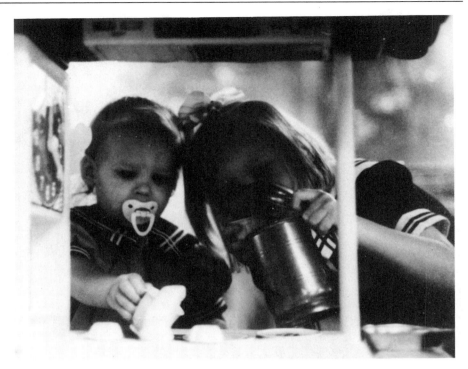

**Figure 10.3.**   Children playing house.

to play together, they must figure out whose wishes will direct the group. Adult/child relationships are asymmetrical; an adult can easily dominate. Parents frequently use control and constraint. If they have definitive ideas about an activity, children generally must accommodate. Among equals, no one point of view is automatically better than another. Each person is free to pursue his own point of view through various avenues. The result may be separate, solitary activity unless some form of negotiation occurs. Ideally, children first learn to take turns and then gradually learn the sophisticated skills of presenting ideas, listening to each other, and working out compromises. During the preschool years, children learn to take turns in some activities such as going down a slide; but, in other situations, they often remain content with parallel activities. Five- and six-year-old children explore the ideas of taking turns and compromising around play activities that require greater cooperation and organization. Examples are simple board games or playing house (Fig. 10.3).

During childhood, the depth and complexity of friendships develop. At the age of six years, particular activities interest the child and he will seek companionship accordingly. A friend is someone to play with and with whom he can share objects in a concrete, reciprocal fashion. Gradually, who the other child is becomes more important. Children learn that some peers are more compatible than others as a result of their particular interests, skill levels, and temperaments. By the age of nine years, friendship has a new and deeper meaning. Friends help each other and share secrets. By the age of eleven years, children are concerned with the welfare of their friends and seek secure relationships based on mutual trust. Shared interests and abilities form the foundation of long-term friendships.

Group interaction provides an effective way to promote change in children with psychosocial dysfunction. It is important for the pediatric occupational therapist to understand the activity group therapy process.

Behavioral difficulties often occur when assisting children with psychosocial dysfunction to develop play, task, and social skills. Although much of the activity group therapy literature refers to psychotherapeutic approaches, this information can be useful in developing occupational therapy groups (Redl & Wineman, 1952; Slavson & Schiffer, 1980). Skillful use of structured group play and activity engages such children in therapy. They learn that they can successfully and enjoyably participate in activities and play with peers. Activity groups become a place in which children feel secure; more open expression of feelings occurs behaviorally and verbally. With the mediation of the leaders, children begin to identify the feelings that they are expressing and learn ways to cope effectively with those feelings.

The purpose of activity group therapy is to provide children with kind, supportive relationships in a safe environment in which past experiences can be resolved in a positive, corrective way (Slavson & Schiffer, 1980). The goal is to provide a peer group experience supervised by quietly available adults. The activities that are used vary depending on purpose and the developmental needs of the children. For example, imaginary play or art may be used to allow expression or reenactment of traumatic situations and difficult interpersonal relationships through metaphor. Constructional activities and games can build ego strength by encouraging displacement and sublimation.

In the process of activity group therapy, the leaders interrupt activity when regression or aggression occurs. Clarification or interpretation of the group process may be required. This helps children to acquire a greater understanding of behavior. It also reduces their anxiety about feeling out of control. Activity can then be resumed. In addition, throughout the group, the leaders facilitate group problem solving, encourage helping behaviors, participate in activity, and provide concrete task assistance as needed. As a result of positive

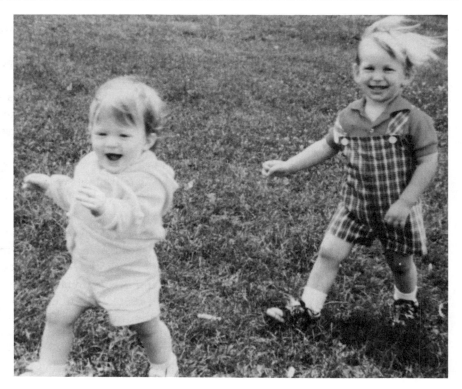

**Figure 10.4.** Spontaneous play.

participation in activity group therapy over a period of time, children become more secure, related, self-reliant, confident, and socially skilled; their behavioral symptoms that interfered with functioning decrease significantly.

## Play

*Play is activity for its own sake;* it is not a means to an end. It exists for the intrinsic pleasure of the moment and includes the exploration and recombination of sounds, movements, objects, and concepts (as in stories), all for the joy in the activity. A healthy child is invested and motivated for play. Without conscious effort, this process results in the development of physical, cognitive, psychological, and basic social skills. Play helps a child learn to manage the everyday stresses of life and to interact appropriately with family and peers (Fig. 10.4).

Play behaviors begin in early infancy and are encouraged by the parent/ child relationship. Parents or care providers and children engage each other because of their natural attraction. The mutually pleasurable experience that ideally occurs encourages and fosters the interaction and the probability that it may recur often and consistently. In a natural, healthy interaction, the care provider mirrors the child but also gradually elaborates on the child's response to make play challenging and interesting. The child, in return, also builds on the care provider's response and, in his own way, molds the parent's behavior and retains the adult's interest. This reciprocal engagement leads to the development of basic learning, interaction, problem solving, and coping skills.

As skills in peer interaction evolve, adequately developed play skills become increasingly important. Both sets of skills—play and interaction—are interdependent and reciprocal. Basic play skills are a prerequisite for engaging and communicating with other children. Children who get along with other children have greater opportunities to expand and elaborate on their play.

*Play is distinct from recreation.* In play, each player can be flexible in his approach to the activity; he has the power to engage or to change it. In group play, the rules and processes are developed through the interaction and negotiation that occur among the players. In organized recreational activities, the rules and processes of interaction are predetermined. Certain skills that have been developed previously through play and education generally are required for success.

The interests and skills of other children stimulate and challenge a child to expand his repertoire even more. Consider the child in the playground who is hesitant to climb or to do a flip on the monkey bars. As this child associates with other children who are competent in the activities, he can observe other children attempting these same activities. Because of the motivation to be liked and accepted by his peer group, the child most likely will attempt to join in the activity. It is rare that a child would experiment with "new" or difficult activities without the influence of the peer group.

All children have strengths and limitations that enhance or inhibit their abilities to engage with others. For example, children who have strong language skills can learn more quickly to communicate their needs and interact better verbally with other children. Children who have specific strengths, such as motor or verbal skills, may attract adults or other children to play with them. These children have an advantage in the development of play and adaptive skills.

### Types of Play

There are different types of play. Over time, many distinct types have been observed and consistently identified by developmental theorists, teachers, and therapists as being important for a child's development. These include sensorimotor, imaginary, constructional, and game play. Although each type play is specific, overlap occurs as children frequently combine forms of play. A nine-year-old child may build a boat and then use it in imaginary play. There is no right or wrong in play (as there is in recreational activities). During play, children discover the consequences of their actions and the types of reactions that may be provoked; some are more desirable than others. Children then build on what they have previously learned, using new experiences to elaborate and enhance their skills.

During the first two years of life, infants engage in **sensorimotor play.** They become aware of their bodies and acquire an understanding of their sensorimotor abilities. Children spend endless hours moving their bodies and limbs, experiencing different sensations. First, they gain the ability to move their trunk and limbs and then the entire body through space. This process makes them aware of how body parts feel, taste, look, and move, and they spontaneously integrate this knowledge to coordinate locomotion and intentional interaction with objects and people. The feel, reaction, and response of objects and other people are incorporated into the ever-expanding knowledge base of the physical world, resulting in the development of motor, perceptual, and cognitive skills (Fig. 10.5).

Through **imaginary play** and with increasing physical skill, children expand their play in ways that lead to a better understanding of the socialized world around them. Children learn about people and their characteristics and functions. Children use objects representationally to imitate the actions of the adults around them. Imaginary play grows in complexity and is used to gain a better understanding of societal roles. Social interactions are reenacted, and real experiences are modified to create a pretend world that can be controlled. Children make believe that they are other people, animals, or objects, and they reenact confusing or complex events. They may expand on these occurrences or change the outcomes. Through this process, important events, people, and the rules in their world are better understood. Anxiety and tension are reduced, and negative experiences can be resolved. Gradually, a child's internal control over his behavior grows as a result of this process (Fig. 10.6). An example of this is when a child imitates scenes in which the "baby" is bad and "mommy" gets mad and exacts punishment. Taking on the role of mommy helps the child identify with his real mother and helps him gain a better understanding of the antecedents of punishment and the process of reconciliation. Manipulating people and objects in fantasy is a prelude to dealing with a reality that cannot be so easily controlled.

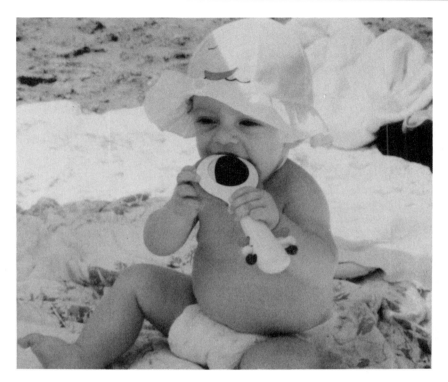

**Figure 10.5.**   Sensorimotor play.

Through **constructional play**—building and creating things—children naturally enhance the development of their fine motor and cognitive skills, as well as their confidence and ability to handle challenges. As children play with scrap materials and recombine them in various ways, they discover new uses for things. This creative process occurs spontaneously through play, not with a preconceived plan. The child is relaxed and allows himself to examine all possibilities. He often expresses surprise and pleasure with what he has created; what he first thought would be a building has turned into a car and then a space mobile. Problem-solving skills are developed in addition to a growing sense of mastery and self-efficacy (Fig. 10.7).

Through **game play,** children develop internal control and an understanding of rules. This occurs through the process of definition—that is, deciding what rules are important to maintain their interest, decrease frustration, and mediate the competing wishes of all players. The need for all players to agree mutually to contain personal impulses for the greater enjoyment of the group becomes apparent in game play. During games, young children change the

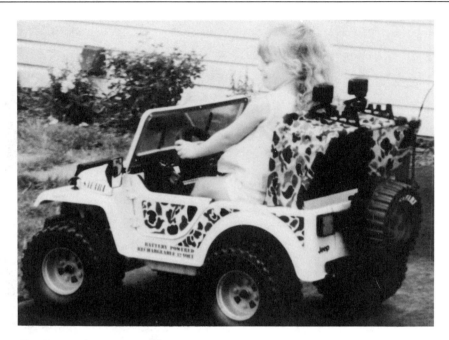

**Figure 10.6.**   Imaginary play.

rules frequently and haphazardly as they attempt to master the physical and cognitive skills necessary to play. Impulse control is not consistent (Fig. 10.8).

As they continue to learn, children begin to value challenge and coordinated interaction for added interest. Basic rules of reciprocal social interaction, such as turn taking, are applied to maintain the activity. As children mature to school age, rules become very important and are enforced heavily. Rules add meaning, organization, and challenge—these things make an activity "fair." Rules provide a way for all participants to play with some harmony and, ideally, to subordinate personal wishes and impulses in the interest of the "group." Children who break the "agreed-upon rules" are strongly censored by their peers. This has a powerful impact on socialization because there is a naturally strong desire to be accepted by peers.

The combination of peer interaction and play behaviors changes play groups into what is commonly referred to as **gangs** during preadolescence. This term is used specifically to mean groups of children of the same sex and not the common street meaning of "gangs" that has a distinctly different and negative connotation. Play in gangs is related to game play because, by its nature, it is based on the ability to follow rules. It is more complex, however,

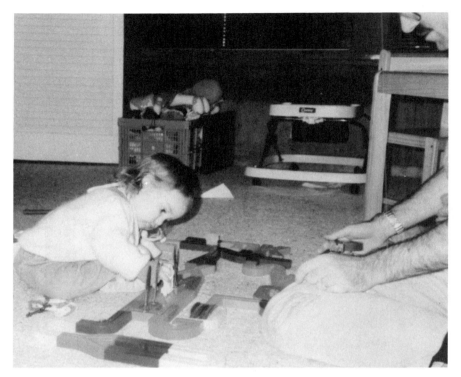

**Figure 10.7.**   Constructional play.

in that group rules affect interaction and behavior beyond a particular game. Adherence to agreed-upon rules and loyalty to group members are expected. Through a positive group alliance like this, children learn to function as members of a community. Cooperation and working together are facilitated within clearly defined group rules and expectations (Opies, 1969) (Fig. 10.9).

Play sets the stage for work (Erikson, 1959). Play is the major rehearsal area and practice arena for the development of occupational roles (Reed, 1984; Reilly, 1974). Through play, the child learns appropriate task skills and interactive behaviors. This becomes the foundation for the ability to engage later in work.

Concepts that lead to the capacity to perform work are competence, an ability to cope with the environment, ego strength, and an investment in life. Competence emerges out of the opportunity provided by activities to build skills toward workmanship. The ability to cope with the environment is learned through activity and relates to the management of anxiety. The assimilation of anxiety during activities allows the child to develop produc-

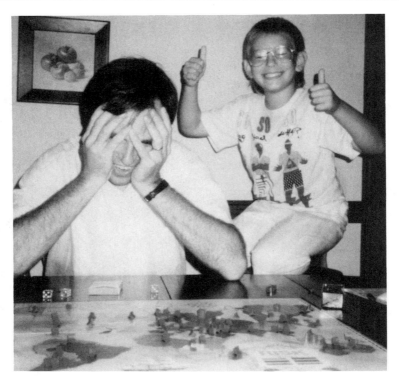

**Figure 10.8.**    Game play.

tive, active, and flexible behavioral strategies that are appropriate to his environment and that enhance his efforts to care for himself. Ego strength allows the child to integrate and express contradictory realities, emotions, and demands. The child begins to feel that he has some control over himself in his environment. He ritualizes, redirects, or channels aggression. This is a safety valve that spares the child conflict with real people in the environment, diminishes the impact of drives, and circumvents regression. An investment in life grows out of feelings of pleasure and competence. Pleasure in doing develops through activities (Cotton, 1984).

The experience of enjoying one's own efforts is the unique pleasure associated with play and work alike. The capacity to invest self is the internal link in the child's ability to use what he has and what he might develop (Cotton, 1984). Play behavior in children, therefore, is critically important to the development of adaptive life skills and behaviors. Through play, without being conscious of it, children gain basic skills for successful participation in activities. They develop physical skills, learn to cope with anxiety and

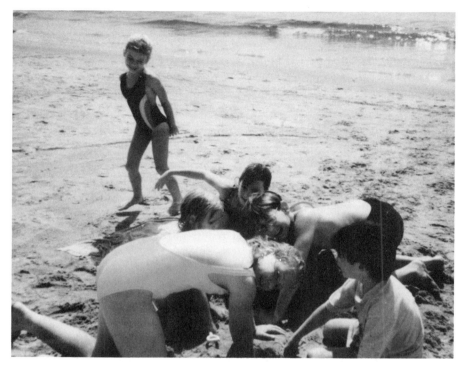

**Figure 10.9.**  Group play.

frustration, gain an understanding of social rules, and develop self-control. Children also learn to problem solve, to take reasonable risks, and to make appropriate decisions. Most importantly, through the intrinsic enjoyment of play, children develop an appreciation of interaction and a desire to invest and participate actively in life.

## Ability to Cope

Ability to cope is how children deal with new and difficult situations, and how they measure success in competence and mastery. Children develop the ability to cope based on their care providers' ability to facilitate coping methods compatible with personal temperament. Initially, children develop the ability to cope by sending signals about their emotional states to their care providers, both verbally and nonverbally. The care providers interpret those signals and attempt to manipulate the environment to promote the child's adaptation.

As children develop, they take increasing responsibility for regulating their own behavior through understanding these signals, using them to interpret their present internal and external situation, and then initiating an appropriate action or interaction. In response to the stimulation of a new situation, resilience allows the child to return to a state of equilibrium in a short time. This means that the child is emotionally calm and able to focus on play or on a required activity. At times, when uncertain or insecure, to regain equilibrium, a child might retreat into safety, take time out, or delay a response until the unfamiliar is more carefully examined. In the aftermath of stressful or overwhelming occurrences, this process also may involve self-comforting, playing out traumatic experiences, and using fantasy to transform reality temporarily (Anthony, 1987). This is important to withstand life pressures and to "bounce back" from the reduced function that occurs under stress.

A child's resilience is challenged in ordinary ways on a daily basis. For example, if a resilient child is rejected by his playmates, he needs to recognize his rejection, decide what led to it, and then respond in a way that produces acceptance or does not worsen the injury to his self-esteem. He may retreat to the safety of his home to talk to a parent, but he will "bounce back" by figuring out how to make amends, seek more compatible playmates, or find other interesting activities.

If a child has difficulty performing a construction task, he might change the building approach so that the chances of success become greater. The child might switch to another activity if overwhelmed, or he might seek help from an older child or adult. In any case, the child will find a way to confront the difficult situation in a positive way that relieves frustration and injury to his self-esteem. The child may withdraw but only for a brief time, to compose himself. The child who has developed the ability to cope is invested in his environment, as well as in the many types of play and activity available. The motivation to play and to be involved is, therefore, stronger than any impulses to give in to frustration.

## Environmental Interaction

The child's environment must be examined for its capacity to provide safety, support, space, and facilities for functional skill development. A safe environment has mechanisms to reduce the impact of any inherent or sudden risks. This may mean greater availability of family supports if a parent is chronically ill; safe community play space if a family lives in a cramped tenement; or additional educational supports for a child who exhibits learning deficits. Negative events that occur during human interaction should be neutralized by support and other positive opportunities that promote the child's feelings of self-efficacy and self-esteem.

The design of the environments and the requisite supplies available will change, depending on the culture. The primary environments for all children, however, are **home, school,** and **community.**

## Home

A good home environment has sufficient supplies to feed, clothe, and provide warmth and shelter for all family members. There is adequate security from danger by physical design or by the vigilance of the care providers. In addition, there are resources for play and for the transmission of cultural values, rituals, and life roles. The elaborateness of these resources differs depending on socioeconomic and cultural variables. For example, play things may be pots and pans or they may be expensive, crafted toys. The most important element in a good home environment is the availability of a consistent, caring adult, who provides structure and sets guidelines for the child so that he is socialized to function within his community. If a child is having difficulty, this adult pursues appropriate measures or gets outside help to foster the child's development. The adult is sensitive to the child's innate abilities, as well as his vulnerabilities. This helps the child minimize his weaknesses and capitalize on his strengths.

## School

It is important that the child be physically safe and have his basic biological needs met in the school setting. Space, supplies, and equipment are available to assist him to learn. On the most basic level, books, paper, and writing utensils must be available. The wealth of the school district determines what additional resources become mandatory. Of primary importance to the school environment is the availability of a caring teacher who provides the necessary structure and support so that a child can invest his attention on learning. Through educational activities, the teacher expands and adds to the child's

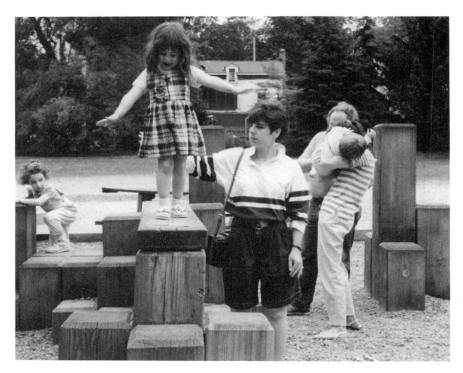

**Figure 10.10.**   Safe play in the community.

previously acquired living skills and offers new opportunities to develop innate abilities and to compensate for vulnerabilities. The teacher also structures group prework and leisure activities to promote the development of the social skills necessary for community living and working.

### Community

In his community, a child should be able to explore his physical environment safely. Within a well-structured community, peers and adult role models should be readily available. A community contains space, resources, and the freedom to engage in various play and community activities (Fig. 10.10).

## *Summary*

Each child is born with an innate temperament that may help or hinder him in establishing a secure attachment relationship with his care providers. Throughout childhood, it is important that his care providers understand his temperament and personal style and then interact with him in a way that facilitates his personal development. The quality of this primary relationship affects coping, play, and peer interaction skills in a major way. As a child grows, each skill area influences the others. Improvement in a child's ability to cope or to play is likely to lead to more positive family and peer relationships. This, in turn, fosters the desire to master developmental tasks. All of this is shaped and occurs within the context of home, school, and community. Although environments vary greatly, depending on culture and socioeconomic class, their adequacy to meet the basic needs of the child and family always should be examined.

# Function/Dysfunction Continua

Function/dysfunction continua provide therapists with descriptions of observable behaviors that are clinically relevant and that identify function and dysfunction in children.

## *Temperament*

Temperament is a person's spontaneous style and approach to deal with environments, events, and people. As a person is exposed to environments, experiences, and changes over time, daily functions become routinized, and temperament may not be so evident. During infancy, the child's temperament is very apparent. When a child's temperament is functional, he can adapt to family, school, and community demands effectively.

In the psychosocial frame of reference, when a child's temperament is dysfunctional, then he may have difficulty in regulating his activity level and attention span appropriately. Such a child may have difficulty in dealing with new situations or adapting to change. This may interfere with his ability to be accepted and to succeed in his environment. A child who shows dysfunctional temperament may not learn appropriately or effectively, may not respond appropriately to nurturing and guidance, or may not engage in appropriate peer play groups. When a child has a difficult temperament, he has trouble adapting to the demands of his environment. This may contribute to pervasive, negative effects on attachment relationships, coping, play, and peer interactive skills.

| Innate Adaptation | Inadequate Adaptation |
|---|---|
| FUNCTION: Ability to respond to the environment appropriately | DYSFUNCTION: Inability to respond to the environment appropriately |
| BEHAVIORS INDICATIVE OF FUNCTION: | BEHAVIORS INDICATIVE OF DYSFUNCTION: |
| Routinely meets biological needs | Biological schedule is erratic or inconsistent with environmental demands |
| Activity level is appropriate for situational expectations | Activity level is inappropriate for situation |
| Orients to relevant sensory input and is able to ignore environmental distractions | Responds to everyday sensory input with fear or irritation or cannot inhibit awareness of irrelevant sensory input |
| Mood is appropriate to situation | Mood is generally inappropriate to the situation; or may tend to be negative |
| Emotional response is appropriate to situation | Emotional expression is intense and poorly regulated |
| Attends to an activity for an appropriate length of time, given age and situation | Attention span is inappropriate given age and situation; it can be either too short or too long |
| Adapts appropriately to new situations | Adaptation to new situations is erratic; it may be characterized by disorganization or withdrawal |

## Attachment

Attachment is the special relationship between an adult and child required for positive growth and development. One aspect of attachment is the interaction between care provider and child, in which the care provider gives protection, meets biological needs, nurtures for emotional security, and teaches the basic life skills. Attachment involves initiation of and response to playful and affectionate interchanges. The responses of the child allow the care provider to feel effective in giving support, comfort, and protection. A child who is positively attached is also generally compliant to structure, rules, and limits provided by caring adults because he wants to gain acceptance. If the child receives consistent care from adults, he exhibits security in his attachment relationships. Usually, the child who has developed secure attachment relationships feels confident that he can count on adults.

The child who exhibits dysfunctional attachment behavior does not attract care providers successfully to get his needs met. In the literature, this is sometimes referred to as **insecure attachment.** This dysfunction may be the result of having experienced inconsistent, neglectful, or abusive parenting, or it also may be related to the child's innate deficits. The child with dysfunctional attachment may not develop positive interactions and relationships with care providers. Frequently, he may initiate negative interchanges. Passive, resistive, or aggressive behavior may be exhibited regularly in response to adult attempts to structure or support him. He does not expect or is uncertain about the likelihood of nurturance or good will from adults.

When parents (one or both) exhibit dysfunctional or inconsistent attachment behaviors, a child may demonstrate many functional behaviors with care providers outside his family. At times, these children form adequate attachments with others, or they are inconsistent in their ability to form any attachments. (This chapter not address function/dysfunction continua in relation to parenting skills.)

| Attachment | Insecure Attachment |
|---|---|
| FUNCTION: Ability to form adequate attachments with care providers | DYSFUNCTION: Inability to form adequate attachments with care providers |
| BEHAVIORS INDICATIVE OF FUNCTION: | BEHAVIORS INDICATIVE OF DYSFUNCTION: |
| Clearly signals care providers about concerns and needs | Inconsistent interactions about needs and concerns, including signals and responses |
| Engages in mutual pleasurable activity with care providers | Does not or rarely initiates or responds to playful interchanges |
| Initiates and responds to playful interchanges with care providers | Avoids or rejects care provider's assistance in challenging situations and activities even though behavior indicates distress |
| Generally responsive to structure and limits set by authority figures | Overly and indiscriminately dependent or does not seek help and support as needed |
| Seeks care providers for support, reassurance, and assistance in challenging situations and activities | Does not engage in mutual pleasurable activities with care providers |
| Accepts help and support as needed but seeks appropriate autonomy | Generally resistive to structure and limits from authority figures |

## *Peer Interaction*

Functional peer interaction is exhibited when a child is accepted in an age-appropriate and developmentally appropriate group. A child who can approach peers in a positive way to initiate play and who responds in kind to most overtures by peers demonstrates functional peer interaction. In the interest of becoming involved in group play, he takes turns and increasingly develops the skills of compromise, cooperation, and negotiation. He is responsive to the verbal and nonverbal cues his peers give to indicate their emotional states, as well as their reactions to him. His behavior supports his confidence in a situation, and it is also adaptive if he can change his approach to succeed in that situation. Willingness to help peers in play and to accept help are also skills that he exhibits. These behaviors facilitate closer bonds with peers and support the child's ability to cope, thereby encouraging peer acceptance.

The inability to respond to peers appropriately leads to rejection or limited acceptance gained only through physical force or threats. The child who exhibits poor peer interaction may not initiate play in a positive way. This child may attempt to bully peers or may be intrusive. Often, he is not aware of or is insensitive to social cues from others and, therefore, does not alter unsuccessful methods of engagement. Help from peers is not accepted because it is perceived as threatening to his self-esteem. Another child who exhibits poor peer interaction may be overly dependent and passive. He may not offer to help peers or may use inappropriate methods. The result of either behavior is a lack of true collaboration and friendship.

| Peer Interaction | Lack of Friendship and Collaboration with Peers |
|---|---|
| FUNCTION: Ability to interact successfully with peers | DYSFUNCTION: Inability to interact successfully with peers |
| BEHAVIORS INDICATIVE OF FUNCTION: | BEHAVIORS INDICATIVE OF DYSFUNCTION: |
| Approaches peers positively to initiate play | Avoids peers |
| Takes turns with peers | Approaches peers aggressively or intrusively |

—*continued*

| | |
|---|---|
| Responds to verbal and nonverbal social cues | Resistant to turn taking, even with adult intervention |
| Negotiates with peers | Exhibits little awareness of or response to verbal and nonverbal social cues |
| Compromises with peers in the interest of group play | Unable to negotiate with peers |
| Is willing to help and accept help from peers | Refuses to compromise with peers |
| | Uses aggression typically to reach his personal goals or withdraws from situation |
| | Unable to offer help or accept it |

## Play

Functional play is demonstrated when a child approaches all play activities with a willingness to experiment and explore. He spontaneously seeks out individual and group experiences. He engages with vigor and continuously elaborates on the activity to maintain its interest and vitality. Through this process, he develops basic skills for all occupational performance areas. He is drawn naturally to some activities over others because of personal interests and capabilities, although he may enjoy and learn spontaneously from all activities. Through sensorimotor play, he learns about and integrates the sensory and motor abilities and responses of his body. Imaginary play allows him to work through confusing or conflicting events, to allay anxiety, and to understand better the structure and rules of social living. Through constructional play, he develops visual perceptual, motor, and cognitive skills. Finally, through game play, he develops internal control—a necessary tool for successful group functioning.

A child who exhibits deficits in play skills does not participate actively in play activities. When he does participate, it is not with full investment and he does not build sufficiently on prior play experiences. Rigidity toward activities may limit his play potential. As a result, his underlying perceptual, motor, cognitive, emotional, and social skills do not develop adequately.

| Play Skills | Inadequate Play Skills |
|---|---|
| FUNCTION: Ability to engage successfully in individual and group play | DYSFUNCTION: Inability to engage successfully in individual and group play |
| BEHAVIORS INDICATIVE OF FUNCTION: | BEHAVIORS INDICATIVE OF DYSFUNCTION: |
| Approaches play with vigor and interest | Approach to play is tentative or avoidant |
| Fully explores and experiments in new play situation | Does not explore and experiment |
| Expands on prior play experiences | Narrow range of play interest |
| Flexible during play with peers | Rigid approach to play |
|  | Play is repetitive, fragmented, or child ceases involvement rapidly |
|  | Does not successfully initiate play with other children |
| Follows the sequence and structure of group play activities | Unable to follow the sequence of group play activity |
| Accepts rules in group play | Does not accept or follow group play |

## Ability to Cope

The child who has developed the ability to cope has a broad range of interests and resources that gratify him. These things provide him with a basis for success and skill; he feels confident. When challenged or overwhelmed, he engages in productive problem solving, based on self-esteem and previously developed skills. He is able to use various methods spontaneously to resolve problems so that a positive involvement in his environment is maintained. Ability to cope is closely related to the child's temperament and how he adjusts to changes in his environment. Security in his attachment relationships also influences the child's ability to cope. The child who is more secure in his attachment relationships usually is more adaptable and, thus, able to cope more effectively.

A child is dysfunctional when he does not expect to get pleasure from activity. He may avoid activities and tends not to be invested in them. Few activities provide gratification, therefore, the child has not developed a repertoire of skills and lacks a feeling of success. When challenged, he often gives up in frustration and avoids involvement. He may not engage in spontaneous problem-solving activities and may become bored and emotionally labile.

| Ability to Cope | Inability to Cope |
| --- | --- |
| FUNCTION: Ability to adapt to various situations | DYSFUNCTION: Inability to adapt to various situations |
| BEHAVIORS INDICATIVE OF FUNCTION: | BEHAVIORS INDICATIVE OF DYSFUNCTION: |
| Engages in new experiences | Avoids new experiences |
| Spontaneously attempts new experiences | Needs much encouragement to attempt new tasks |
| Is excited by new tasks | Expresses fear, reluctance, or withdrawal when faced with new tasks |
| When challenged in play, seeks solutions to master the activity or finds a satisfactory substitute activity | When challenged in play, will withdraw or revert to more infantile behaviors |
| Returns to a state of equilibrium after stress | Takes an extended period of time to recover from stress |

## Environmental Interaction

The theoretical base for the psychosocial frame of reference addresses the importance of environment in the provision of safety, support, and facilities for functional skill development. The child's three primary environments are the home, school, and community. It is impossible to present all function/ dysfunction continua relative to environmental interaction that encompass the varied situations and experiences to which children currently are exposed; therefore, function/dysfunction continua are not presented in this section. Therapists should consider the child's environments in their practice and determine what indicates function or dysfunction in these situations.

# Evaluation

The major concern of the occupational therapist who uses the psychosocial frame of reference for assessment is how the child functions in his daily life. The purposes of an occupational therapy evaluation of the child are (1) to identify those activities in which the child is functional; (2) to determine the child's skills, abilities, and strengths; and, (3) to determine whether the child's environment is stable and appropriately structured to encourage use of his skills. During assessment, occupational therapists should determine the specific skills and deficits that a child exhibits. Then, the therapist must ascertain how these strengths and limitations affect the child's ability to participate in activities. In this frame of reference, the psychosocial implications of the activities are of primary concern to the therapist.

Consistent with the theoretical base, the six major sections of this evaluation include **innate temperament, attachment, peer interaction, play, ability to cope,** and **environmental interaction.** The order of the evaluation is designed to minimize any anxiety of the child and his family, and to help the therapist gain as much information as possible. (This assessment does not follow the specific order of the six major sections of the psychosocial frame of reference.).

The occupational therapy evaluation begins with a review of the historical material available on the child and his family. Background material may include school and medical reports, psychological evaluations, and summaries of past treatments. These data assist the occupational therapist to determine relevant areas for assessment and how to best proceed with a formal evaluation. The data also give the therapist a general idea of the child's temperament, attachment relationships, ability to cope, level of play and peer interaction skills, and environments, as perceived by the parents and other professionals. Specific areas relevant to occupational therapy may need a more detailed assessment.

It is important to get the child's perception, if possible, of his relationships with his care providers, his play skills, peer relationships, ability to cope, and comfort in and satisfaction with his environments. This is crucial to understand what areas concern the child most; these areas should have priority in the assessment and treatment.

It is often easier and more productive to gather information about the child's major concerns when the child is engaged in a simple, nonstressful, enjoyable play activity. The child most likely will relax and be able to talk more easily with the therapist as he plays. The therapist should be organized in her approach and direct and honest with the child about her desire to understand better how he plays and gets along at home, in school, and in his neighborhood. It is equally important that the therapist be sensitive to the child's cues about his ability to tolerate this verbal interchange. At times, conversation is interspersed with periods of reciprocal play between the therapist and the child. This is important, because some information can be expressed only nonverbally, through behavior and play.

At the end of the play interview, the therapist should have information about the following topics:

- Play activities that the child enjoys when he is alone, with peers, and with his family;
- Activities that bore and frustrate the child or are too hard for him; and his perception of why;
- Activities in which the child would like to improve;
- The child's school experiences, his academic performance, relationships with his teachers and peers, and special likes and dislikes;
- Jobs that interest the child; what he wants to be; jobs held by those adults in his life;
- What an average day in his home and community is like; (this may include an activity configuration dictated to the therapist, written or drawn by the child);
- The child's relationship with different family members (who he feels that he gets along with best); and,
- The child's understanding of friendship (who his friends are, what are they like, and how they treat him).

When play deficits are suggested by the child's history or the child's self-report, screening competency in play should be the next step in the occupational therapy psychosocial assessment. Often, deficits in basic play skills make participation in play with peers or family members difficult, or even impossible. The child may be emotionally labile, act out, or refuse to participate because the challenges presented by the play activities are beyond his capabilities. Other children may exclude or ostracize him because he cannot play as skillfully as others in his age group. Although it is difficult for the therapist at times, it is important to make distinctions among deficits in basic play skills, coping skills, and social skills.

To complete this aspect of the assessment, the therapist should observe the child in a play activity appropriate for his age and environment. This includes sensorimotor, imaginary, constructional, and gross and fine motor game play. No formal assessment tools are available to explore play at this level, so the therapist must choose appropriate activities based on her understanding of child development and the activities common in the child's environment.

Sensory, motor, or neurological deficits may be causative factors in play deficit. Standardized tools are available to assess these areas, such as the Bruininks-Oseretsky Test of Motor Proficiency (Bruininks, 1978) and the Sensory Integration and Praxis Tests (Ayres, 1989). Because they are time-consuming to administer, they are used most often in a child psychiatry setting once play deficits are identified, or if there is a strong suspicion of contributing underlying deficits. Data gained from these assessments may be useful to determine whether another frame of reference is necessary for intervention.

The therapist should also observe social skills in a structured group activity, as well as in free play. With age-appropriate expectations in mind, the following should be noted:

- Initiations and responses with peers;
- Turntaking, compromising, and negotiating in activities;
- Aggression toward and from peers;
- Incidences of helping and being helped by peers.

The opportunity to observe parent/child interaction in the context of an activity is also very useful. It can provide many insights into the family's adaptation to or difficulty with the child's psychiatric dysfunction. The quality and process of the occurrence, or lack of same should be noted along the following lines:

- Engagement in mutual or parallel activity;
- Enjoyment expressed verbally or nonverbally;
- Communication of needs and desires during the activity, and the subsequent response;
- Structure set by the parent and the child's response to it;
- Level of involvement between parent and child;
- Resolution of frustrations and problems during the activity to everyone's satisfaction.

When feasible, a play history interview should be conducted with the primary care provider. This allows for a deeper understanding of the child's development to his current interests and level of functioning. Specific questions should relate to the types of play and specific activities that the child enjoys or resists. This interview may also include the child's reactions to his care providers, siblings, and peers, his temperament and coping styles, and response to school and particular academic subjects. The data can help put the parent/child interaction into perspective.

The Coping Inventory, devised by Zeitlin (1985) helps to analyze how adaptively the child copes in caring for himself and how he responds to environmental demands. Both coping areas are explored in ranges: active to passive; productive to nonproductive; and flexible to rigid. This helps the therapist identify specifically how the child manages everyday challenges and stressors; the way in which he responds to stressors and challenges; and the effects that the environment may have on his responses. Many children, even those who have overall deficits in their ability to cope, are likely to have some assets in one or more areas that can be used to foster adaptation in daily activities.

After gathering these data, the therapist must integrate and interpret them into an overall picture of the child's functional assets and deficits in meeting the challenges of his developmental tasks. It is critical to identify the areas which should be addressed in the intervention process. From a functional perspective, it can be anticipated that if intervention is directed toward the appropriate areas, then problematic behavior will decrease and the child will experience greater success in his daily activities.

As it has been described here, a full psychosocial occupational therapy assessment is difficult to complete unless the child is in a therapeutic milieu. Such settings allow the therapist to observe the child in various group activities over a period of time, as well as the time to do an individual assessment. A complete assessment is the ideal; however, in many settings, it is not possible, and the therapist must use her judgment to decide which sections of the suggested assessment are necessary and viable in the particular setting.

# Postulates Regarding Change

It is believed that a child is born with innate temperament (Chess & Thomas, 1984). Although temperament is inborn, this does not preclude change through environmental influence. When a child displays a difficult temperament, the environment, and the approach of his care providers are critically important for his adaptation. Without proper support, he is vulnerable to psychosocial dysfunction:

1. If the therapist assists a child's care providers in establishing a routine for activities that are difficult or disorganizing for the child, then the child will become calmer, more cooperative, and organized around that daily activity.
2. If the therapist assists care providers to understand the discomfort of a child with a difficult temperament and how to manage it in the child's and the family's best interest, then the care providers and child will have more positive interactions.
3. If the therapist helps the child develop cognitive strategies to confront activities that produce overwhelming anxiety, then the child will more likely be able to approach and participate in these activities.

To increase the likelihood of a parent providing the necessary physical and emotional support, it is important for the parent/child interaction to be viewed as primarily positive or rewarding. The child also requires a sense of security to grow into a healthy, functioning adult. He needs to expect comfort and assistance when stressed or overwhelmed. When this is not the case in his home, then the therapist should provide a secure and rewarding opportunity for the child to experience mutual interaction with another adult. Four postulates regarding change are concerned with building a positive relationship between children and care providers.

4.  If a therapist provides an environment in which parent and child can enjoy mutual play, this then will promote positive engagement between parent and child.
5.  If a therapist demonstrates ways that care providers can facilitate a child's functioning and then provides an activity in which this can be practiced, then a parent or care provider will be more likely to respond similarly in the future.
6.  If a therapist assists care providers in experiencing comfort and competence in activities with their children, then they more likely will relax and see positive behavior in their child's play.
7.  If the therapist can assist the child in clearly stating or showing his parents or care providers what his needs are in relation to an activity, then it is more likely that his parents or care providers will respond to those needs.

With peer interaction, the meaning of the situation is decided through the natural negotiation that occurs between children. The development of effective interaction skills is a step-by-step process. First, children need to be able to approach peers positively to initiate an interaction. They then have to be able to respond reciprocally, be supportive, and help each other, when appropriate. Finally, children need to be able to have realistic expectations for the particular situation. Five postulates regarding change are concerned with peer interactions:

8.  In a safe and accepting environment, if a child sees the opportunity to do an enjoyable and extrinsically rewarding activity, then the child will more likely attempt to cooperate with peers in a group activity.
9.  If a child learns to help another successfully and to accept help, then the child will be more likely to seek out others for mutual activity.
10. If a child learns the basic social skills needed to play with other children, this will likely increase their peer interaction. Therefore, the child's interests and activity skills expand.
11. If a therapist guides a group of children through the process of imaginary or game play activities, then the children will gain an understanding and

acceptance of the structure, sequence, and rules innate in satisfactory and enjoyable group play. The children will be more motivated to follow the rules, to censor each other, and be less impulsive.

12. If a therapist assists a child in identifying with other children the rules necessary for group play, then the child is more likely to accept rules and limits. Furthermore, the child will be more likely to censor himself and others within such a group.

Play involves exploration, experimentation, and imitation for the sake of pleasure and serves as the basis for specific aspects of learning as well as for the development of many skills. When engaged in play, children develop physical, cognitive, psychological, and social skills without conscious effort. The following four postulates regarding change apply to play:

13. In a safe environment, if a therapist provides the child with a play activity that is intrinsically motivating, the child will then invest time and energy in that activity.

14. If a therapist provides a child with a sensorimotor activity that is pleasurable to the senses, the child will then initiate and engage in that play activity.

15. If a therapist "guides" the child's play, the child then will elaborate on that play and maintain interest in that activity. Consequently, the child will be more likely to seek out similar play activities independently.

16. If a therapist introduces an activity that has properties similar to those of an activity that the child enjoys, then the child will most likely approach the new activity.

The ability to cope means that a child can deal with new and difficult situations. Five postulates regarding change are concerned with the child's developing the ability to cope.

17. If a therapist assists a child to approach a new activity in a way that decreases fear, then the child will be more likely to participate in that activity.

18. If a therapist gradually introduces opportunities to explore risktaking in activities, then the child will more likely tolerate the activity.

19. If a therapist introduces strategies to cope with a challenge within an activity, then a child will more likely attempt to use one of the strategies to meet the challenge.

20. If the therapist provides firm limits and a safe and quiet place for the child to regain control during an activity within the child's capabilities,

then a child will use these external mechanisms gradually, to maintain emotional control.

21. If the therapist assists the child in noting the signs of his increasing frustration and anxiety during challenges in activities, then the child will begin to note his own signals.

To promote change in a child's mental health, the child's environments (home, school, and community) must provide safety and support as well as space and facilities for functional skill development. Five postulates regarding change are concerned with the child's interactions within his environment:

22. If the therapist assists a care provider in increasing the safety of the home environment for play, then the child will have more opportunity for secure exploration and will be more likely to engage in productive play.

23. If the therapist assists the care provider in creating and organizing an appropriate play space, then the child will be more likely to be engaged positively and to be more focused in activities at home.

24. If the therapist assists the care provider in identifying and implementing ways to monitor and supervise the child's community based play successfully, then the care provider will be more successful in managing the child's behavior.

25. If the therapist helps the care provider involve the child in positive community based activities, then the child will be more likely to develop positive role models.

26. If the therapist helps the care provider to increase the opportunities for learning and involvement in appropriate activities, then the impact of negative elements in the child's environment will be reduced significantly.

## Application to Practice

Learning to help and to accept help have been identified as the most important psychological skills for promoting for mental health in children. Experiences that facilitate the development of these skills are those in which the child is a helper, those in which he is helped, and those in which the child has an opportunity to observe caring between two other people. It is believed that the central theme of helpfulness and caring is related to considerable skill development (Strayhorn, 1988). These two elements—helpfulness and caring—are, therefore, integrated into all therapeutic interventions in this frame of reference. Although temperament, attachment, peer interaction, play, the ability to cope, and environmental interaction all have been identified specifically in the theoretical base, the application to practice for these areas is not as specific. Intervention in the areas of temperament, attachment, and environmental interaction, particularly with regard to the home and community, focuses on the relationship between the child and parent or care providers. Intervention in the areas of peer interaction, play, and the ability to cope focuses on the child's ability to function in a group situation with his peers. When dysfunction severely interferes with the child's overall ability to function, it usually encompasses more than one function/dysfunction continuum. In such cases, intervention usually takes place in a therapeutic milieu in which the treatment can be comprehensive. In general, specific occupational therapy intervention within this frame of reference usually is provided in a group setting.

## Settings for Practice

It is important to have a general understanding of the settings in which the children who exhibit psychosocial dysfunction may be seen. The setting for service delivery or the type of help offered depends on the circumstances of the referral, the degree of dysfunction, and specific types of behavior disturbance. The most common settings for intervention are special education classes, outpatient child psychiatric clinics, pediatric day hospitals, pediatric inpatient units, and residential treatment facilities.

Children who cannot participate successfully in regular classes because of their behavior or learning problems secondary to emotional stressors may require special education. A major educational objective is to promote the child's ability to learn and participate in the classroom. As part of a comprehensive special education program, children may receive counseling or occupational therapy services. When occupational therapy services are provided within the educational setting, goals must be related to the child's educational needs. Issues that may not affect the child's school functioning are not within the realm of intervention in the special education classroom.

Children may be seen in an outpatient child psychiatric clinic when their problems cannot be dealt with sufficiently in school, or when the problems are not educationally related. Individual, group, or family services may be offered by the occupational therapist. In some cases, children are seen in outpatient clinics when their specific problems are not severe enough to warrant a special class placement (but still interfere with their ability to function).

Some children may need more structure and therapeutic intervention than can be provided in an educational setting or an outpatient child psychiatry clinic. A day hospital program provides a full day's program that includes both educational and mental health services. Classes usually are smaller in this setting, and a wider variety of professional staff are regularly available to the children. Occupational therapy services usually are integrated into this setting.

Children are admitted to a child inpatient unit because they require intensive intervention and their behavior often is perceived as being harmful to themselves or others. Typical things that lead to hospitalization are the child's threatening behaviors or attempts to hurt or kill himself, violent behavior in school or at home, or excessive withdrawal. Occupational therapy services frequently are an essential part of the services offered in this setting. A child's stay in an inpatient unit usually is relatively short and is followed up with other services frequently provided by an outpatient clinic, day hospital, or residential treatment center.

When children cannot be maintained in their communities or need more long-term intervention, they may be referred to a residential treatment facility, in which a 24-hour structured living situation is provided. The children live in small groups with supervising counsellors. Usually, a strong behavioral program is used so that privileges are earned. Special education and activity services are provided, and occupational therapy services may be part of such a program.

### Therapeutic Milieus

A pediatric inpatient unit, a day hospital, or a residential treatment facility is often referred to as a **therapeutic milieu.** When an occupational therapist works in such settings, her role should be defined within the goals of the milieu. The milieu provides a comprehensive daily living environment. It can be an effective intervention that provides reinforcement of mutually established goals among various therapies for children who demonstrate severe dysfunction. Usually, nursing or child care workers carry out most of the actual interaction with the children, but other disciplines, including occupational therapy, can play a major role in establishing a milieu structure that reinforces growth and development.

The therapeutic milieu should incorporate elements important for an ideal home and community for a child. This should be set up collaboratively among all disciplines involved. The establishment of an ideal milieu may be limited because of institutional philosophy. Important elements in a therapeutic milieu are daily structure, rules that ensure safety for all, a forum for open dialogue about issues that concern members, responsibilities for community members, and opportunities for spontaneous play.

Rituals are an important part of the daily, weekly, seasonal, and yearly life of all humans. They provide organization and structure, mark the passage of time, and help people deal with transitions, such as seasonal or life changes. Rituals bind families and communities together, mark important events in a culture or among groups of people, and give continuity between the past and future. Within each day, a healthy child has routines or rituals. With some flexibility, self-care, meals, work, and preparation for bed all occur within a general order and time frame. Within a school program, certain activities mark the beginning of the day, with other activities that regularly follow, and other activities signal the end of the day. This routine gives order and is calming. Without it, life might be chaotic, and children would tend to be anxious because they could not anticipate a sequence of events.

In a therapeutic milieu, it is important to develop routines and rituals. Daily routines, such as a time for self-care in the morning and evening, and established meal and snack times provide structure for the child who has more serious dysfunction. Weekly rituals might include a community meal, community meetings, or a unit-wide activity. Such routines and rituals tend to provide order and comfort, thereby lessening anxiety and giving the child some idea of what to expect.

Rules and structure that provide safety for all participants in any activity are important in the therapeutic milieu. Certain rules are common to any school or community group, such as listening to authority, following the implicit and explicit structure and rules within the activity, not hitting others, and so forth. Children who exhibit psychosocial dysfunction often require additional structure. Very explicit rules, with immediate and clear consequences for breaking them, are needed to help these children manage their impulses and respond to social cues.

A therapeutic milieu, like a healthy home situation, must give children formal and informal forums to air their concerns and wishes. This also allows children to digest past and present events, as well as to prepare for future circumstances. Frequently, in psychiatric settings, children initially need adults to help them verbalize their concerns. Poor impulse control, inability to express oneself clearly through language, limited trust in adults because of past negative experience, and limited behavioral or cognitive organization often interfere with the child's ability or willingness to articulate his thoughts. Children require nurturing and support from adults to feel free enough to express their concerns. Often, adults need to offer safety and possible strategies for solving issues before children express any troubling concerns. Sometimes, a child's behavior or play expresses his thoughts, and the therapist must address this verbally. For example, the therapist may raise a concern that one child in the milieu appears to be threatening others covertly. The child who feels threatened may appear so anxious that he cannot play or participate in daily activities, or he may become aggressive. By stating her concerns, the therapist provides the opportunity for the anxious child to express himself. The opportunity to express concerns verbally and through play and then to work through coping strategies and receive support and attention from caring adults can dramatically help a child express emotion appropriately. This assists the child to understand, separate, and modulate his emotions. In addition, the child can come to understand his feelings consciously.

Issues arise in formal meetings, groups, and individual sessions, as well as in informal gatherings in the milieu. Children need to be able to deal with their concerns in some way when they arise. Unlike adults, children cannot hold onto an issue long enough to wait for a formal meeting. Frequently, they need help to understand the situation at the time it arises so that their anxiety is lessened and does not affect their behavior. Sometimes, "stop-gap" procedures can help them wait for a more proper time or a more appropriate setting (a community meeting or an individual session with the therapist) to express their concerns.

In most family situations, children have age-appropriate responsibilities. This is an important aspect of development, promoting the child's ability to live and to work with others and to participate in the maintenance of his community. Responsibilities in a child's daily life in the therapeutic milieu may include self-care, care of personal possessions, maintenance of a common play space, organization of toys and games, decoration of the milieu for special events and holidays, and setting up and cleaning up after community events.

In a therapeutic milieu, it is easy to provide too much structure in the interest of maintaining order. Play time is important, and structured, group play is necessary for the development of age-appropriate socialization skills. Free play periods facilitate the child's application of what he has learned in therapy to community living. It also fosters the generalization of socialized skills. Spontaneous play allows the child to "practice" independent and self-directed play and gives him the opportunity to explore his own inner world without intrusion or to initiate or respond to the play of others without the direction or coaxing of adults.

## Temperament, Attachment and Environmental Interaction

When dysfunction is evident in temperament, attachment, and environmental interaction, the role of the therapist is to facilitate the relationship between the child and his parents or care providers. The therapist acts as a role model and advisor to parents and care providers alike. As an advisor, she can make suggestions regarding the structure of daily routines and can clarify the demands and situations in the home. She can help the parents to define goals clearly for the child and can help the family to establish priorities. The therapist can assist the parents in offering support to the child and in presenting reasonable alternatives to actions and behaviors. This can be particularly useful for a parent who must deal with a child who displays a difficult temperament. It helps the parent to provide a secure atmosphere with appropriate and consistent expectations that then provide organization for such a child.

In specific interactions, the therapist may serve as a role model, demonstrating effective ways of dealing with difficult behaviors. The therapist might subtly assist the parent and child in an individual or group activity, so that the parent then can take on that role and instruct the child. In this case, the therapist does not direct the situation actively and, therefore, avoids becoming an authority figure. She might gently point out the parents' strengths in a particular activity as they fit into the group process. In this way, the therapist gives the parent authority, promoting the child's confidence in the parent. The child sees his parent as competent and someone to rely on. This is believed to strengthen the parent/child attachment. The goal is to promote a more harmonious relationship through a benign, supportive, and structured environment in which the child can respond more calmly and cooperatively, and to make it easier for the parent to function effectively with the child.

When the therapist serves as a role model, she can foster positive parenting. The therapist sets up a reciprocal interaction in which the child learns that he can share concretely his interest in activity and depend on care providers for help and praise. The therapist can demonstrate an active respect for the child's feelings and growing autonomy. Through whatever activity is chosen, the therapist can provide gentle but firm behavioral limitations and positive reinforcement for appropriate behavior. This shows the parents how to accentuate the positive aspects of their child without focusing excessively on the negative. The child begins to understand that cooperation is expected and rewarded.

Occupational therapy can play a vital role in implementing change in the parent/child relationship by fostering productive and pleasurable interaction through play and activity. This can be accomplished by working with individual families or leading a group of multiple parent/child pairs or trios. The former is most likely to occur when difficulties in interaction are severe and are not likely to be resolved without the intensive teaching of skills; when a family identifies a specific problem that they wish to focus on solely; or when a group is not available or desirable to the parents. Using a group format is helpful in a school setting, in a hospital, or in a residential treatment center. In these environments, many families share similar concerns or difficulties and they provide a strong support network for each other in that they are open to suggestions or ideas from one another. These characteristics all are important curative elements found in successful therapeutic groups.

Particular methods for the parent/child activity group have been described by Olson, Heaney, and Soppas-Hoffman (1989). The theories of attachment, coping, and play that were previously described in this chapter form the basis for the rationale, structure, and methods used in successful parent/child therapy. Two distinct play periods are used. In the first, parents assist children in constructional play. This activity is used because the materials presented are structured, familiar items such as boxes, paper, and tape. The activity can be enjoyed at different skill levels, and the range of complexity and variety is great. In initial attempts at mutual activity, parents and children may struggle to come up with ideas or figure out ways to build what the child imagines. By observing other families work through this process, as well as by problem solving with the therapist, these sessions promote greater and more productive interactions. Ability to cope with the challenges presented in the activity is increased, resulting in the experience of pleasure and pride that is gained in mutual accomplishment.

In the free play period that follows, parents and children have the opportunity to choose their own activities. Many tabletop and gross motor activities are available. The task is to choose an activity that is both enjoyable and promotes growth for the child but is also one that the parent can tolerate and enjoy. Listening to one another and making decisions based on the child's interest, along with the parent's understanding of what presently is best for the family, are some of the skills that are the focus of this part of the group. The therapist can observe first hand how a child participates in his favorite activities with his parents. Because these activities are likely to occur in the home or community, the goal at this level is to enhance pleasure and organization through the same activity. Throughout the course of this group intervention, a family's investment in mutual play grows, resulting in more complex play and a stronger parent/child relationship. The child becomes more attentive and receptive to his parent's initiatives and requests. Care providers come to understand their children better and exhibit greater confidence, skill, and pleasure in guiding the child's development.

## Peer Interaction, Play, and Ability to Cope

Intervention with children who experience dysfunction in peer interaction, play, and the ability to cope frequently is accomplished through activity groups with peers. Activities provide the means for interaction among the children. The activity may be a structured project introduced by the therapist, or it may involve more spontaneous play.

Activity groups work on the premise that the child is intrinsically interested in both play and peer acceptance. Unless a child is severely withdrawn or extremely hyperactive or aggressive, he will be drawn into many activities if peers are involved. His desire to be included in a peer group forces him to focus on the goals of others and often results in behavior modification. The child generally is open to cooperation and negotiation in an activity if they are necessary to promote involvement with peers. The therapist provides a benign and supportive group environment in which children feel safe enough to explore interaction with other children in the context of an activity. Children referred for group treatment often have experienced multiple failures and rejections from others, despite their intrinsic interest. This may be the result of deficient play, social, or coping skills. The therapist needs to provide the appropriate structure and adaptations to support each child so that he may increase his skills in deficit areas. Grading the activity, facilitating "helping" behaviors among the children, and encouraging group problem solving are some of the methods that might be used.

As stated previously in the theoretical base, the therapist should have a thorough understanding of the development of play skills. She should be familiar with all types of play so that she can promote the development of these skills and assist children to develop elaboration and flexibility in their play. The book, *Children's Games in Street and Playground* (Opies, I., & Opie, P., 1969) can be helpful in the understanding of games in particular. Play groups should be geared toward the participants' levels of developmental play involved, and the specific play skills that the therapist wants to facilitate. The therapist also can provide different amounts of structure. For example, when engaging a group in constructional play, it is important for the therapist to guide the children through the exploration of materials, ideas, and approaches, but she should avoid giving specific instructions. Specific instructions may limit exploration and discourage problem solving, although it temporarily may lessen the group leader's anxiety.

Many resources are available on age-appropriate activities for children, and they may provide helpful ideas and direction, especially for the beginning therapist. The therapist should be careful, however, to avoid presenting an activity as a lesson or to give an excessive amount of structure because this will limit the emergence of natural play and the development of interactive patterns.

Regardless of the activity, the therapist should start by observing how children organize themselves, the situation, and the rules, and how these things change as play evolves. Then she may become more active, structuring the play situation somewhat, providing feedback, and making specific suggestions.

Redl and Wineman (1952) have described techniques that address the development of the ability to cope in group play. The following are things that are basic and applicable to any activity group that includes emotionally disturbed children. When children have few internal resource to maintain control, the therapist needs to grade the amount of frustration inherent in the activity. This has been referred to as **budgeting frustration.** When an outburst or conflict occurs, a problem-oriented discussion helps the children learn to identify their own emotional signals and then learn to resolve the situation adaptively. For example, if one child becomes angry during play, he may need to learn to remove himself from the game to regain emotional control before he can discuss his differences with his peers. The length of the group and the point at which the therapist intervenes in the process of play should be considered carefully so that the group can refocus or the play can end before the children's behaviors deteriorate to either regression or aggression. To encourage the development of **depersonalized controls** helps gain compliance in a group code of behavior. This means that the rules are based on successful and pleasurable group play as opposed to rules imposed by an authority figure. Participative planning of the group rules, structure, and activity is the process through which this can be achieved. Over time, as the children have pleasurable experiences in the group, these positive memories are used as an internal resource to work out challenging or frustrating situations in daily life. The therapist also should be skilled in the cultivation of **interest contagion**—that is, spreading the enthusiasm for particular activities from one or a few children to the whole group. Additional techniques are described in detail in the works of Redl and Wineman (1952).

Activity interview group therapy is sometimes suggested for children who present with intense fears and anxieties, hyperactivity, or aggression (Slavson & Schiffer, 1980). For this group, play materials are chosen that facilitate the child's reenactment in play of traumatic situations and difficult interpersonal relationships. The therapist acts as interpreter for the feelings expressed through play. Group discussion frequently is interspersed with play to allow greater understanding of problems and to relieve any intense anxiety that the children experience. This type group combines activity therapy and psychotherapy, and an occupational therapist might be coleader, along with a psychiatrist or psychologist, that she might contribute her unique understanding of and ability to engage children in play. Modified approaches to activity group therapy have been suggested for children who exhibit different types of psychosocial dysfunction (Schamess, 1976).

Some emotionally disturbed children do not play, use minimal language to communicate, and initiate minimal interaction with others. Their activity focuses around basic needs, self-stimulation, or exploration of the environment that is disorganized and does not lead to effective adaptation. They might destroy things, disrupt others, or put themselves in danger. When others attempt to limit their activity, they might be physically aggressive. Often, these children benefit from a play approach that uses sensory and motor activities. The therapist initiates and structures activities at first using sensory and motor input to engage the child and to promote purposeful play. If sensations are pleasurable, then the child attends and seeks to continue the activity. The therapist has successfully involved the child in purposeful and organized play in this way.

# Summary

This chapter presents a wealth of theoretical information based predominantly on developmental psychology and organizes it into a framework for occupational therapy practice in pediatric psychosocial settings. Temperament, attachment, peer interactions, play, and the ability to cope are the central issues in the development of good mental health and in the functional interventions that deal with pediatric psychosocial disorders.

Throughout childhood, the development of play, peer interaction, and the ability to cope are strongly related to the adaptation of the child's temperament to his environment, to the security of his attachment relationships, and to the adequacy of his environments. Each of these areas is defined specifically with regard to function and dysfunction, specific methods of evaluation, and postulates regarding change. Because all these facets are interconnected in a growing child, and because they facilitate or hinder overall developmental progress reciprocally, they cannot be separated out in practice.

The discussion of application to practice focuses on addressing these complex issues in an integrated way. When the therapist attempts to improve parent/child activity interaction, she must consider the parent's understanding of the child's temperament and the adequacy of their mutual environments. The therapist may use play as one method to facilitate positive interaction, with the hope that this fosters more adaptive coping behaviors as a response to the challenges confronted in the activity. Overall, the therapist's intervention influences the child's total psychosocial functioning.

### Outline of Psychosocial Frame of Reference

I. Theoretical base
   A. Innate temperament
   B. Attachment
   C. Peer interactive skills
   D. Play
      1. Parent-child
      2. Peer interaction
      3. Types of play
         a. Sensorimotor
         b. Imaginary
         c. Construction
         d. Game play
      4. Peer interaction and play
   E. Development of occupational roles
   F. Ability to cope
   G. Environmental interaction
      1. Home
      2. School
      3. Community

II. Function/dysfunction continua
   A. Temperament
   B. Attachment
   C. Peer interaction
   D. Play skills
   E. Ability to cope

III. Evaluation
   A. Historical review
   B. Play
   C. Standardized assessment

   D. Socials skills assessment
   E. Observation of parent/child interaction
   F. Parent interview
   G. Coping skills inventory

IV. Postulates regarding change
   A. Those that relate to temperament
   B. Those that relate to building a positive relationship between the child and care providers
   C. Those that relate to peer interactions
   D. Those that relate to play
   E. Those that relate to developing the child's ability to cope
   F. Those that relate to the child's interactions within his environments

V. Application to practice
   A. Learning to help
   B. Accepting help
   C. Helpfulness and caring
   D. Settings for practice
      1. Special education
      2. Outpatient psychiatric clinic
      3. Day hospital
      4. Inpatient unit
      5. Residential treatment facility
   E. Therapeutic milieu
      1. Rituals
      2. Rules and structure
      3. Healthy home situation
      4. Play
   F. Intervention related to temperament, attachment and environmental interaction
      1. Role model
      2. Advisor
      3. Individual activity
      4. Group activity
   G. Intervention related to peer interaction, play, and ability to cope
      1. Activity groups with peers
      2. Play
      3. Activity interview group therapy
      4. Using sensory and motor activities

### References

Ainsworth, M. (1967). Object relations, dependency and attachment: A theoretical review of the infant-mother relationship. *Child Development, 40,* 969–1020.
Anthony, E. J. (1987). Risk, vulnerability and resilience: An overview. In E. J. Anthony, & B. J. Cohler, (Eds.). *The invulnerable child.* New York, NY: Guilford Press

Arend, R., Gore, F. L., & Sroufe, L. A. (1979). Continuity of individual -adaptation from infancy to kindergarten: A predictive study of ego resilience and curiosity in pre- schoolers. *Child Development, 50,* 950–957.

Arnold, E. (Ed.). (1978). *Helping parents help their children.* New York: Brunner/Mazel, Inc.

Ayres, A. J. (1979). *Sensory integration & the child.* Los Angeles, CA: Western Psychological Services.

Ayres, A. J. (1989). *Sensory integration and praxis tests.* Los Angeles, CA: Western Psychological Services.

Bowlby, J. (1969). *Attachment and loss* (Vol. 1). New York: Basic Books, Inc.

Bruininks, R. (1978). *Bruininks-Oseretsky test of motor proficiency.* Circle Pines, MN: American Guidance Service.

Chess, S. & Thomas, A. (1984). *Origins and evolutions of behavior disorders: from infancy to early adult life.* New York, NY: Brunner and Mazel.

Cotton, N. (1984). Childhood play as an analog to adult capacity to work. *Child Psychology and Human Development, 14*(31), 135–144.

Erikson, E. (1959). Identity and the life cycle. *Psychological Issues, 1,* 1–171.

Lieberman, A. F. (1977). Pre-schoolers' competence with a peer: Influence of attachment and social experience. *Child Development, 48,* 1277–1287.

Matas, L., Arend, R., & Sroufe, L. A. (1978). Continuity- of adaptation in the second year: The relationship of the quality of attachment later competence. *Child Development, 24,* 65–81.

Olson, L., Heaney, C., & Soppas-Hoffman, B. (1989). Parent-child activity group treatment in preventive psychiatry. *Occupational Therapy in Health Care, 6*(1), 29–43.

Opie, I., & Opie, P. (1969) *Children's games in street and playground.* Oxford: Clarendon Press.

Reed, K. (1984). *Models of practice in occupational therapy.* Baltimore: Williams and Wilkins.

Redl, F., & Wineman, D. (1952). *Controls from within: Techniques for the treatment of the aggressive child.* New York: The Free Press.

Reilly, M. (1974). *Play as exploratory learning.* Beverly Hills: Sage Publications.

Schamess, G. (1976). Group treatment modalities for latency-age children. *International Journal of Group Psychotherapy, 26,* 455–474.

Slavson, S. R., & Schiffer, M. (1975). *Group psychotherapy for children.* New York: International Universities Press.

Strayhorn, J. (1988). *The competent child: An approach to psychotherapy and preventive mental health.* New York: The Guilford Press.

Waters, E., Wittman, J., & Sroufe, L. A. (1979). Attachment, positive affect and competence in the peer group: Two studies in construct validation. *Child Development, 50,* 821–829.

Zeitlin, S. (1985). *Coping inventory.* Bensonville, IL: Scholastic Testing Service.

# 11

# Coping Frame of Reference

G. GORDON WILLIAMSON / MARGERY SZCZEPANSKI /

SHIRLEY ZEITLIN

Coping is a major component of the adaptive process that occupational therapists address in promoting optimal function (Fine, 1991). Coping is the integration and application of developmental skills for functional living. The more effectively a child copes, the more effectively a child learns (Garmezy & Rutter, 1983; Larson, 1984). Effective coping is positively correlated to academic achievement, self-esteem, and a sense of personal mastery (Di-Buono, 1982; Kennedy, 1984; Zeitlin, 1985).

The coping frame of reference is based on a theoretical model. It emphasizes the development and use of coping resources that enable the child to deal with current and future challenges and opportunities. A key feature is its positive orientation, which focuses on healthy adaptation rather than on pathology. The coping frame of reference is targeted to the improvement of the child's ability to cope when engaged in all areas of occupational performance. Application of this frame of reference can be tailored to children and adolescents who have a wide range of special needs and who come from varied sociocultural backgrounds.

The coping frame of reference is somewhat different from the other frames of reference presented in this textbook because, typically, it is used in conjunction with them. It can be applied readily in most occupational therapy programs. Because the outcome of any intervention is influenced by the child's coping competence, this approach should be incorporated into any intervention plan when it has been determined that a child has limited coping abilities.

# Theoretical Base

This coping frame of reference organizes theoretical concepts related to stress and coping in children into a unique set of guidelines for occupational therapy practice. Numerous experts in the field of child development have studied aspects of coping in children related to their coping resources, vulnerabilities, and behavioral responses to stressful events (Compas, 1987; Garmezy & Rutter, 1983; Murphy, 1976; Werner & Smith, 1982).

*Coping is the process of making adaptations to meet personal needs and to respond to the demands of the environment.* A child copes with self when managing thoughts, feelings, and preferences. A child copes with the environment when managing the social and physical worlds. The goal of coping is to maintain or enhance feelings of well-being—that is, children cope with circumstances and situations to feel good about themselves and their place in the world. A child's coping competence is determined by the match between needs or demands and the availability of resources for managing them. Effective coping reflects sufficient resources for handling the demands of daily life. Long-term outcomes of effective coping are the acquisition of a positive identity and the capacity for intimate social relationships (Shahmoon, 1990).

Coping is an essential component of the broader concept of adaptation. The process of coping is directed toward the generation of effortful and purposeful actions. It does not include reflexes or automatic habitual behaviors that are so well established that they no longer require active effort. Within the context of this frame of reference, such automatic or well-established behaviors are not addressed. Although this distinction is not always clear, it avoids a global definition of coping that encompasses all the child's interactions with the environment (Compas, 1987).

Basic assumptions for this frame of reference are that the coping process is transactional and that coping strategies are learned. Coping transactions occur in the context of the social and physical surroundings and in sequential, cyclical interactions with them. The environment has an ongoing, ever-present influence on the coping process. Through transactions with the environment, children try out, practice, and integrate coping strategies into their behavioral repertoire. Coping strategies that have been acquired previously are modified in response to changing demands and environmental expectations. This frame of reference, therefore, can be considered **acquisitional in nature** because it assumes that one can learn to cope more effectively.

The coping process is generated by personal needs or environmental demands that result in stress. **Stress is tension** that is experienced physically, cognitively, or emotionally in response to an event perceived as threatening or harmful to a person's feelings of well-being or to an event perceived as challenging (Lazarus & Folkman, 1984; Zeitlin, Williamson, & Rosenblatt, 1987). Within this theoretical base, coping with stress is defined broadly and not restricted to the child managing adverse circumstances. Stress interpreted by the child as potentially harmful or threatening tends to have a negative inference. Stress interpreted as a challenge often is associated with positive, energizing emotions. *A developmentally appropriate level of stress, different for each child, facilitates motivation, learning, and mastery.*

Stress can evoke positive or negative feelings of tension based on the child's unique perception of the situation. The varied responses of children escorted to a therapy session demonstrate this point. One child may enter the therapy room, glance at toys enticingly displayed on a table, and then run from his mother's side to play with them. This child interprets the situation as a challenge. Another child, on entering the same therapy room and glancing at the same toys, remembers that it is time to leave his mother's side. This child perceives the situation as threatening and begins to cry. Still another child may view the situation initially with caution and spends a few minutes at his parent's side. With the therapist's encouragement, this child is able to approach the toys comfortably.

Although stress is a reaction, **stressors** are the actual internal or external events that elicit the reaction. Internal stressors include thoughts, feelings, interests, motivations, physical sensations, and the presence of a handicapping condition. External stressors are the demands of the environment, which can include negotiation of physical surroundings, management of objects, and interaction with people. External stressors can range in intensity from minor upsets in daily routines to major events, such as a change of residence or domestic discord. Because children frequently experience stress in relation to internal or external demands and expectations, these terms are used in this chapter in reference to stressors. The way children manage stress can be appreciated only by observing their coping transactions. Observation of transactions is the vehicle for understanding how a child's adaptation—that is, **the coping process**—is expressed in daily life.

## The Coping Process

Various researchers have described the coping process (Antonovsky, 1979; Haan, 1977; Lazarus & Folkman, 1984; Moos & Billings, 1982; Zeitlin, Williamson, & Rosenblatt, 1987). Drawing from their work, the authors developed a coping model designed to be clinically useful. It provides a structure for observing, understanding, and analyzing the coping process in children.

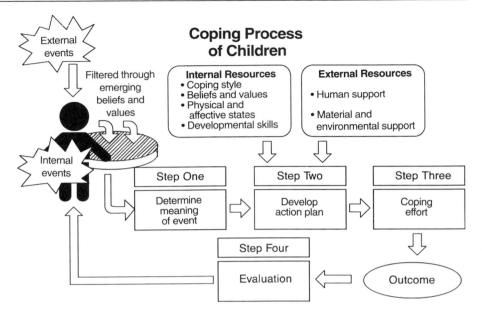

**Figure 11.1.** Coping process of children

The model is presented from a cognitive-behavioral orientation, but it should be noted that the mental processes in children are not so clearly delineated. In the earliest years, coping is primarily emotionally driven. In the older child, the cognitive contribution becomes more influential in each step of the process.

The coping process occurs in the context of **coping transactions.** A coping transaction, which is a sequence of interactions between the child and the environment, consists of elements related to both the child and the environment. All of these elements contribute to the outcome of the coping process. When observing coping transactions, then, it is important to appreciate the contributions of the environment and the steps of the process experienced by the child. From the child's perspective, this transactional model views coping as a four-step, interrelated process (Fig. 11.1). The four steps include:

1. Determine the meaning of an event;
2. Develop an action plan;
3. Implement a coping effort; and
4. Evaluate its effectiveness.

The environmental contributions to coping transactions include the creation of external demands on the child that frequently initiate the coping process and the environment's response to the child's coping effort. This environmental feedback influences how the child perceives the effectiveness of the coping effort—that is, it contributes to the child's evaluation of how effectively the situation was managed. Using this model, analysis of coping transactions helps the therapist understand how the child functions on a daily basis.

**Step 1. Determine the Meaning of an Event.**   The coping process is initiated by the child's experience of an internal or external event perceived as a demand or expectation. The stress of internal demands and expectations in young children can be inferred only through their actions. Older children may be able to express internal demands verbally. Examples of these inner demands include the child's personal goals, preferences, concerns, expectations for success or failure, physical sensations, and the broad range of emotions experienced by the child.

In a child's early years, external demands and expectations are made primarily by family members and other caregivers and then later by teachers and the community. Most adults have a unique set of demands and expectations for a child's social behavior, performance, and management of daily activity that creates stress. When demands and expectations match the child's coping resources, they provide an appropriate level of stress. When they are too high or too low, effective coping and development are hindered. Sample external demands and expectations particularly relevant for children include goals for developmental or academic achievement, independence in self-care, and participation in social and community activities. In addition, the physical environment imposes a unique set of external spatial and temporal demands for the child to negotiate, such as maneuvering in crowded surroundings, reacting to moving objects, and obtaining toys in inaccessible settings.

Cognitive and emotional processes are used to appraise events as they are filtered through the child's emerging beliefs and values. The meaning of the event may be interpreted as threatening, harmful, or challenging to the child's sense of well-being. When the event is identified by the child as a stressor, the next step is to decide a course of action.

**Step 2. Develop an Action Plan.**   A child's decision about how to manage a stressor depends in large part on the availability of resources on which the child can draw to deal with the situation. A child's decision-making skills develop over time and become more sophisticated as abstract thinking emerges. The young child who has limited cognitive skills tends to develop an action plan based on emotions, immediate personal needs, and an evolving awareness of cause-and-effect relationships, whereas the older child may be able to think through alternatives and choices to manage the situation. The ability to predict the logical consequences of one's actions increasingly mediates the decision-making process.

Coping resources are aspects of the self and the environment that influence the child's determination of an action plan. They can be classified as internal (within the child) or external (in the environment). The major internal resources are the child's coping style, beliefs and values, physical and affective states, and developmental skills. External resources include human supports as well as material and environmental supports. The critical importance of these resources is discussed later in a separate section.

**Step 3. Implement a Coping Effort.** The third step of the coping process involves making a coping effort in response to the demand or expectation. A coping effort is what the child actually does to manage stress. In a coping effort, cognitive or behavioral coping strategies are used to handle the situation. One coping strategy may be used in isolation, or several strategies may be used simultaneously. Coping efforts are usually directed toward dealing with the stressor, managing the emotions associated with the stressor, or modifying related physical tension.

Action-oriented coping efforts are specifically directed toward the stressor (demand). For instance, a child who cannot complete homework may choose to review the textbook, request parental help, or call a classmate to clarify the assignment. Coping efforts to manage emotions associated with the stressor are geared toward helping the child feel better. A child who experiences frustration may choose to withdraw from the situation that generates it, may seek comfort from others, or may use defense mechanisms to counteract or deny the feelings. Coping efforts used to manage emotions also are used frequently to modify associated physical tension. For example, a child who experiences fatigue may choose to take a break, change the activity to one that is less demanding, or persist in the activity regardless of the fatigue.

The child's coping effort produces an outcome that elicits the next important element of the coping transaction—the response of the environment to the child's coping effort. The child experiences feedback from both the physical and social environments. For example, a child making efforts in learning to ride a bicycle may receive feedback from the actual movements of the bicycle or from an adult's verbal comments.

**Step 4. Evaluate Effectiveness.** The fourth step in the coping process involves the child's evaluation of the outcome of the coping effort and its resulting feedback. The evaluation includes a cognitive appreciation of the results of the coping effort as well as the personal meaning that these results have for the child. From the child's perspective, coping efforts result in a range of positive and negative feelings about self and the environment. If the child's coping effort is effective, stress is managed either by its reduction or elimination. The child feels better emotionally, and a sense of well-being is enhanced or restored, and the coping cycle is completed until the next tension-generating event. When a coping effort is not effective, stress continues and another coping cycle is generated in which similar or new strategies may be tried. A child who has a history of unsuccessful coping may gradually develop a negative self-concept and an expectation of failure.

The child's feelings about the effectiveness of coping are internalized and then influence a sense of personal adequacy and subsequent coping efforts. Therapists must be sensitive to the child's perception of coping competence and the varying moods and emotions that result from different coping transactions. Over time, this internalization plays a critical role in determining the nature of the child's identity and capacity to develop intimate relationships.

An adult's view of the goals and effectiveness of coping efforts may not be the same as the child's. Many coping efforts cannot be readily interpreted from an adult's success-or-failure paradigm; instead, the child's evaluation reflects personal thoughts and feelings. Because children have idiosyncratic views of the world, they often change the goals of their activities and are fluid in shifting their expectations for outcome. For example, an adult may interpret a child's difficulty in completing a puzzle as a lack of success that will lead to frustration, whereas the child may be perfectly happy with an outcome that involves looking at the shapes and colors of the pieces. Likewise, an adult may request an action from a child that appears simple. Although complying to the request, the child may not feel that the situation was managed effectively.

Coping with daily living is ongoing and continuous. A child may cope simultaneously with several stressors of varying intensity or may cope with a long-term stressor over time. The following vignette depicts the four steps of the coping process in a child who has to manage the daily impact of a motor handicap.

> Timmy, a five-year-old child who attends kindergarten, is faced with playground time. He hates playing outdoors because he is slow and clumsy and cannot keep up with the other children. When the teacher tells the class to go outside, he perceives the situation as threatening and experiences *stress*. Timmy then determines an ***action plan.*** Based on past experience, he decides to linger in the classroom to avoid the situation. He slowly puts his toys away despite encouragement

to hurry and then goes to the bathroom, making another stop at the water fountain. By the time Timmy is finally coaxed outdoors, the class is lining up to come inside for lunch. He feels relieved that the worst part of his day is over.

Although Timmy managed the situation for the moment, his pattern of avoidance may have undesirable consequences if used habitually. The reality is that participation in physical activity is an ongoing demand during the school-age years. Continuation of avoidance strategies perpetuates Timmy's stress, isolates him socially from his peers, and prevents him from learning and enjoying gross motor activities. His coping efforts, therefore, have a detrimental impact over the long run.

## Coping Resources

Specific resources—internal and external—assist in the process of coping. The internal resources include coping style, beliefs and values, physical and affective states, and developmental skills. The external coping resources include human supports as well as material and environmental supports. Familiarity with these resources is critical to the understanding of how a child copes and to the application of this frame of reference in intervention. Adequate coping resources positively influence the child's ability to manage demands, whereas inadequate resources result in ineffective coping or a vulnerability to stress.

### Internal Coping Resources

**Coping Style.**    Coping style refers to the child's characteristic way of behaving in situations that require coping efforts. The coping styles of infants and toddlers can be described by the unique patterns of their sensorimotor organization, reactivity, and self-initiation (Zeitlin, Williamson, Szczepanski, 1988). These coping characteristics are demonstrated by the integrated use of developmental skills to produce goal-directed coping efforts.

**Sensorimotor organization** refers to the child's regulation of psychophysiological functions and to the integration of the sensory and motor systems, including responses to auditory, visual, tactile, proprioceptive, and vestibular sensations. Representative attributes in the category of sensorimotor organization are the child's ability to self-comfort, to organize information from the different senses simultaneously for a response, to adapt to being moved by others during caregiving, to maintain an appropriate activity level, and to demonstrate visual attention.

The category of **reactivity** addresses the actions used by the child in response to the demands of the physical and social environments. Attributes that typify this category are the ability to respond to vocal or gestural direction, to react to the feelings and moods of others, to adjust to daily routines, to accommodate to changes in the surroundings, and to bounce back after stressful situations. In general, this type of coping behavior is elicited by external events.

**Self-initiation** refers to autonomously generated actions of the child that meet personal needs to interact with objects and people. Such coping behavior is intrinsically motivated and is not linked directly to environmental cues. Sample attributes are the child's ability to explore objects independently using a variety of strategies, to initiate interactions with others, to apply previously learned behaviors to new situations, to demonstrate persistence during activities, and to anticipate events.

Coping styles of preschool and school-aged children and adolescents can be described by the characteristic patterns used to cope with the environment and cope with self (Zeitlin, 1985). Relevant coping attributes include task-oriented behaviors such as staying with an activity until it is completed; interactive behaviors such as reacting to social cues in the environment, emotionally-based behaviors such as being able to express anger or love; and psychologically based behaviors such as reappraising a situation that initially was perceived as threatening. Table 11.1 presents **sample coping attributes** relevant to preschool and older children.

**Beliefs and Values.**    Beliefs are the ideas held as true about the self and the world. In the young child, emerging beliefs relevant to coping are related to an evolving sense of efficacy—the perceived ability to produce an effect, control events, and trust others to be responsive to needs. These beliefs usually are reflected in the child's self-esteem and can be inferred from behavior. Examples of beliefs in the older child are illustrated by such statements as "I can do it;" "I am a good person;" "My parents always will be there when I need them;" and "I am the clumsiest kid in my school."

Values reflect a child's desires or preferences. They contribute to the personal goals and serve to motivate commitments to their attainment. A value system eventually influences the child's views about what is important in life. Values in children are demonstrated in behaviors related to such issues as adult approval, academic achievement, task mastery, and preferences in play and leisure.

Beliefs and values are shaped and strongly influenced by familial and social experiences as well as by cultural background. They influence coping

*Table 11.1*   Sample Coping Attributes in Children Over Three Years of Age

## Coping with Self

Frustration tolerance
Expression of personal needs and feelings
Initiation of action to meet needs
Ability to request help when needed
Balance independence with dependence
Acceptance of substitutes
Flexibility in changing plans and behavior to achieve a goal
Task persistence
Demonstration of pleasure in successful accomplishment of activities

## Coping with the Environment

Curiosity
Socialization with others
Adaptation to daily routines
Ability to follow instructions
Awareness of others' feelings
Acceptance of warmth and support from others
Resiliency following disappointment
Ability to become actively involved in situations
Awareness of and response to social expectations
Response to new and difficult situations

in two ways: First, they contribute to perceptions of events and the determination of whether an event is threatening, harmful, or challenging; and second, they serve as a motivating force for determining the initiation or avoidance of specific actions (Bandura, 1977).

**Physical and Affective States.**   **Physical state** refers to general health and physiological condition, such as endurance and wellness. **Affective state** reflects characteristic moods and emotions. Every coping transaction occurs in the context of variations in the child's physical and affective states, which can enhance coping effectiveness or create a vulnerability to stress. Chronic illness, repeated hospitalizations, a handicapping condition, emotional instability, and depression influence physical and affective states and may result in ongoing stress for the child.

**Developmental Skills.**   The child's levels of developmental competence and skill acquisition contribute to the range of behaviors available for coping efforts. The child's skills in the cognitive, psychosocial, communicative, and motor domains provide a basis for learning coping strategies. As the child matures, coping strategies become increasingly more complex, depending on previously acquired developmental skills. Coping with the sensation of hunger serves as an example: A six-month-old infant may fuss and cry to obtain the caregiver's attention; a twelve-month-old child may crawl to the mother and protest verbally; a two-year-old toddler may request "Mommy, cookie," whereas a four-year-old child may go to the cupboard and find something to eat independently.

### External Coping Resources

**Human Supports.**   Persons in the environment who influence the child's coping efforts are considered **human supports.** They include parents, siblings, extended family members, peers, teachers, health professionals, and members of the community. Parents and other primary caregivers are perhaps the most significant external resources for coping in the child's early years. Parent/child interactions serve as the milieu in which coping efforts are initiated, practiced, and reinforced. Through the normal course of childrearing, caregivers influence coping transactions by buffering the child's exposure to stress, making demands, modeling coping strategies, encouraging and assisting the child in coping efforts, and giving contingent feedback. A number of factors influence the adequacy of human support, such as the quality of social interaction, nurturance, consistency, and limit setting.

**Material and Environmental Supports.**   **Material supports** are items and services that money can buy. A family's material resources include the ability to provide sufficient food, clothing, shelter, and medical services as well as to provide motivational toys and activities for the child. **Environmental supports** are the conditions of the physical surroundings such as air quality, organization of space, levels of noise and light, and opportunity for safe exploration. Environments that are chaotic, unpredictable, or overstimulating or that lack adequate stimulation may undermine the child's development and ability to cope.

## Coping in Children who have Special Needs

Research indicates that preschool and school-aged children who have disabilities are less effective as a group in their coping behavior than their nondisabled peers (Kennedy, 1984; Lorch, 1981; Yeargan, 1982). In these studies, children who have disabilities were found to be more inconsistent or inflexible in their adaptive functioning. The literature also suggests that children who live in poverty tend to cope less successfully than their more affluent peers (Brooks-Gunn & Furstenberg, 1987; Murphy & Moriarty, 1976).

Few studies examine the coping styles of infants and toddlers who have special needs. The available research generally addresses a discrete component of coping, such as social interaction (Ramey, Beckman-Bell, & Gowen, 1980), environmental exploration (MacTurk, Vietze, McCarthy, McQuiston, & Yarrow, 1985), or self-generated problem solving (Brinker & Lewis, 1982). These investigations suggest that very young children who have disabilities are less competent in these coping-related domains.

The authors conducted studies that were specifically designed to compare the coping styles of the two groups of children (Williamson, Zeitlin, & Szczepanski, 1989; Zeitlin & Williamson, 1990). They found that infants and toddlers who have developmental disabilities tended to have minimally to situationally effective coping styles, whereas the nondisabled young children coped effectively more often than not. The most significant difference between the groups occurred in self-initiation. It is important to realize, however, that individual children in both groups demonstrated the entire range of coping effectiveness. This finding confirms that the presence of a handicapping condition does not necessarily imply that a child will have an ineffective coping style. Instead, it suggests that a child who has special needs may be more vulnerable to the stress of daily living.

Children who have disabilities may have fewer resources to support adaptive coping efforts. A neuromotor, cognitive, or communication handicap can interfere with the acquisition of developmental skills and, thereby, restrict the variety and sophistication of available coping strategies. Parents may be less accessible as a supportive external resource if they also are experiencing psychological distress or physical exhaustion from the requirements of daily caregiving (Turnbull & Turnbull, 1990). In addition, children who have disabilities often have to manage atypical stressors such as treatment regimes, hospitalization, restrictions in activity, and disruptions in daily routines (Drotar, Crawford, & Ganofsky, 1984). They tend, therefore, to face a greater number of stressors with a limited repertoire of coping resources. This vulnerability accentuates how important it is for occupational therapists to assess the coping efforts of each child.

# Function/Dysfunction Continua

Coping function and dysfunction can be described best as one broad, general continuum of effectiveness that reflects the child's ability to use internal and external resources to manage demands and expectations encountered on a daily basis. The continuum ranges from effective coping at the functional end to ineffective coping at the dysfunctional end. Function or dysfunction is determined by the **goodness of fit** between demands and expectations and the child's available coping resources. Effective coping reflects sufficient resources to meet demands of daily living, whereas ineffective coping reflects inadequate resources or excessive demands.

The broad, general function/dysfunction continuum is discussed next. It is followed by specific function/dysfunction continua that stem from the general continuum.

| Effective Coping | Ineffective Coping |
|---|---|
| FUNCTION: Sufficient internal and external resources to meet demands of daily life. Demands are within the child's ability to manage | DYSFUNCTION: Insufficient resources to meet the demands of daily life, or demands inappropriately exceed child's ability to manage |
| BEHAVIORS INDICATIVE OF FUNCTION: | BEHAVIORS INDICATIVE OF DYSFUNCTION: |
| Variety of available resources used appropriately in a wide range of situations that require coping efforts | Lacks necessary internal and external resources to manage routines, opportunities, challenges, and frustrations in daily life |
| Able to meet personal needs and interact productively with people and objects | Unable to meet personal needs nd interact productively with people and objects |
| Healthy sense of well-being and drive toward task mastery | Negative sense of self; expectation of failure |
| Consistently effective coping style | Minimally effective coping style; may present a unique pattern of ineffective or maladaptive coping behavior |

Because coping effectiveness is dependent on the match between demands and coping resources, it is clinically useful to have additional function/dysfunction continua that address each of the resources. Intervention focuses in large part on these more specific continua that are related to coping style, beliefs and values, physical and affective states, developmental skills, human supports, material and environmental supports, and demands and expectations. These continua should be interpreted in a fluid manner. Given the complexity of daily living, the adequacy of a child's coping resources can vary, and demands can change, depending on environmental contexts.

## Coping Style

**Coping style** refers to the way in which a child typically selects certain strategies over others to manage situations perceived as threatening, harmful, or challenging. This continuum ranges from a coping style that is consistently effective at the functional end to one that is minimally effective at the dysfunctional end. Three major coping styles are represented in this continuum: consistently effective, situationally effective, and minimally effective. Effectiveness means coping efforts are (1) appropriate for situations, (2) appropriate for the child's developmental age, and (3) used successfully to achieve desired results.

At the functional end of this continuum, the child who displays a consistently effective coping style demonstrates coping efforts that meet the above-mentioned criteria. This child has a repertoire of coping attributes that can be drawn on to produce positive outcomes. Strategies are generalized in a flexible way to unique environmental contexts. This child copes successfully with self and the environment most of the time.

The child who demonstrates a situationally effective coping style falls in the midrange of the continuum and has some coping competence. This child has coping attributes that support the effective use of strategies in some situations but cannot generalize them to other types of situations. For example, in a therapy session the child may be able to manage when the parent is present but cannot manage independently with the clinician; or, the child can manage gross motor but not fine motor tasks. Thus the ability to use coping strategies depends on environmental circumstances, such as the presence or absence of human support, the type of activity, or the physical demands of the surroundings. In general, the child whose coping effectiveness is situationally determined is very dependent on external resources to support coping efforts.

The child who displays a minimally effective coping style is at the dysfunctional end of the continuum and has a limited repertoire of effective coping strategies. Three characteristic patterns may be observed:

1. Coping behaviors are inconsistent and unpredictable. There is an erratic, trial-and-error quality to the child's performance.
2. Coping behaviors are rigidly repetitious in that the child continually repeats the same behavior regardless of the circumstance and fails to achieve successful results. The child cannot alter or change behavior based on the demands of the setting.
3. Coping behaviors reduce immediate stress but generate negative outcomes over time. For example, habitual use of temper tantrums may help the child to avoid or diffuse stressful events, but they have undesirable long-term consequences for learning and development.

Examples of maladaptive coping efforts include stereotypic body movements, persistent denial or avoidance, verbal abuse, nail biting, and overactive or distractible behavior.

It is important to keep in mind that a child may exhibit variations in effectiveness according to particular categories of coping attributes. For example, differences may be evident between coping with self and coping with the environment or between reactivity and self-initiation. In addition, the child may differ in the use of specific coping attributes (as depicted in the sample list of behaviors indicative of function and dysfunction related to coping style).

| Consistently Effective Coping Style | Situationally Effective Coping Style | Minimally Effective Coping Style |
| --- | --- | --- |
| FUNCTION: Coping strategies are used effectively in a wide variety of situations. Coping efforts are appropriate for the child's developmental age and successfully achieve desired results. | SITUATIONAL FUNCTION: Coping strategies used effectively in one situation are not generalized to other situations. Coping efforts are variable in their appropriateness to the situation and their success. | DYSFUNCTION: Coping strategies are erratic and unpredictable, or are rigidly repetitious, or reduce immediate stress but tend to generate negative outcomes over time. Coping efforts are inappropriate and usually unsuccessful. |
| BEHAVIORS INDICATIVE OF FUNCTION: | BEHAVIORS INDICATIVE OF SITUATIONAL FUNCTION: | BEHAVIORS INDICATIVE OF DYSFUNCTION: |
| Organizes information from the different senses for a response | Organizes certain types of sensory information but not others | Unable to tolerate sensory input |
| Self-regulates activity level | Variable regulation of activity level | Poor regulation of activity level |
| Coordinates movement as required by the activity | Coordination of movement varies with type of activity | Uncoordinated movement that fails to meet task demands |

—continued

| FUNCTION: | SITUATIONAL FUNCTION: | DYSFUNCTION: |
|---|---|---|
| Adapts to daily routines and changes in schedule | Adapts to daily routines but does not tolerate change | Unable to adjust to daily routines and changes |
| Engages in reciprocal social interactions | Interacts socially with some people but not with others | Unresponsive to social interaction |
| Solves problems independently | Solves problems with adult support and guidance | Unable to solve problems even with assistance |
| Generalizes learning to new situations | Applies acquired learning only in certain contexts | Unable to generalize learning |

The continuum related to coping style was discussed in detail because of its importance to this frame of reference. The following additional continua are presented in shorter form to clarify the nature of other coping resources (as well as demands and expectations). Attention to the sample behaviors indicative of function and dysfunction assists the therapist in recognizing how these resources are demonstrated concretely in the child's life.

## Beliefs and Values

| Beliefs and Values Support Effective Coping | Beliefs and Values Interfere With Coping |
|---|---|
| FUNCTION: Beliefs and values support coping to meet personal needs and demands of the environment | DYSFUNCTION: Beliefs and values interfere with coping to meet personal needs and demands of the environment |
| BEHAVIORS INDICATIVE OF FUNCTION: | BEHAVIORS INDICATIVE OF DYSFUNCTION: |
| Trusts that personal needs will be met | Believes that the world is uncaring and unresponsive |
| Expects success | Anticipates failure |
| Demonstrates high self-esteem | Demonstrates low self-esteem |

## *Physical and Affective States*

| Physical and Affective States Support Effective Coping | Physical and Affective States Interfere with Coping |
|---|---|
| FUNCTION: Physical and affective states support coping to meet personal needs and demands of the environment | DYSFUNCTION: Physical and affective states interfere with coping to meet personal needs and demands of the environment |
| BEHAVIORS INDICATIVE OF FUNCTION: | BEHAVIORS INDICATIVE OF DYSFUNCTION: |
| Experiences emotional well-being | Experiences overwhelming or persistent anxiety, fear, or insecurity |
| Possesses adequate physical endurance | Lacks physical endurance for age-appropriate tasks |
| Regulates mood effectively | Demonstrates erratic mood swings or depression |

## *Developmental Skills*

| Developmental Skills Support Effective Coping | Developmental Skills Do Not Support Coping |
|---|---|
| FUNCTION: Developmental skills support coping to meet personal needs and demands of the environment | DYSFUNCTION: Developmental skills are absent or not used effectively in coping efforts |
| BEHAVIORS INDICATIVE OF FUNCTION: | BEHAVIORS INDICATIVE OF DYSFUNCTION: |
| Demonstrates a range and variety of skills appropriate to age level | Demonstrates limited skills for age |
| Applies skills spontaneously in daily functioning | Cannot generalize skills in daily functioning |
| Acquires skills through experience and various instructional methods | Acquires skills only through highly individualized, repetitive instruction |

## *Human Supports*

| Human Supports Foster Effective Coping | Human Supports Do Not Foster Coping |
|---|---|
| FUNCTION: Human supports foster coping to meet personal needs and demands of the environment | DYSFUNCTION: Human supports are not available or interfere with coping |
| BEHAVIORS INDICATIVE OF FUNCTION: | BEHAVIORS INDICATIVE OF DYSFUNCTION: |
| Adults are nurturing and responsive to the child | Adults are unavailable or negative toward the child |
| Adults serve as role models for appropriate behavior | Adults model and reinforce maladaptive behavior |
| Feedback regarding coping efforts is accurate, timely, and contingent | Feedback is inaccurate, absent, or noncontingent |

## *Material and Environmental Supports*

| Material and Environmental Supports Foster Effective Coping | Material and Environmental Supports Interfere with Coping |
|---|---|
| FUNCTION: Material and environmental supports foster coping to meet personal needs and external demands | DYSFUNCTION: Material and environmental supports are limited or interfere with coping to meet personal needs and external demands |
| BEHAVIORS INDICATIVE OF FUNCTION: | BEHAVIORS INDICATIVE OF DYSFUNCTION: |
| Adequate food, clothing, shelter, and activities to support growth and development | Basic needs not adequately met, thereby contributing to poor health and compromised developmental competence |
| Visual and auditory stimuli appropriately regulated to foster attending behavior | Overstimulating environment results in short attention span and high level of distractibility |
| Organization of physical environment maximizes independence | Physical barriers impede independence causing child to be overly dependent on others |

## *Demands and Expectations*

| Demands and Expectations Are Appropriate | Demands and Expectations Are Inappropriate |
|---|---|
| FUNCTION: Demands and expectations by the social and physical environment produce developmentally appropriate stress. The child's demands and expectations are manageable. | DYSFUNCTION: Internal or external demands and expectations produce developmentally inappropriate stress (e.g., too high, too low, or inconsistent). |
| BEHAVIORS INDICATIVE OF FUNCTION: | BEHAVIORS INDICATIVE OF DYSFUNCTION: |
| Activities presented to child at home and in school are consistent with the child's cognitive and functional abilities | Activities presented to child are too easy or too hard given child's competence |
| Child is provided support and guidance as needed in new and threatening situations | Child is expected to manage all situations independently or is repeatedly placed in threatening situations without regard for coping capacity |
| Child's personal expectations for performance are realistic | Child's personal expectations for achievement are so high they result in a persistent sense of failure or so low they impede motivation |

# Coping Assessment

A comprehensive assessment identifies the child's level of coping competence and factors that influence adaptive functioning. The assessment focuses on the nature of the child's coping transactions as well as on internal and external coping resources. This section provides considerations for addressing each of these factors. A coping-related assessment can be incorporated readily in the context of a regular occupational therapy evaluation. In addition, the therapist may draw on evaluation data obtained from other professionals. An in-depth assessment is indicated when the child has problems with coping.

## *Assessment of Coping Transactions*

The coping process, as previously described in the theoretical base, can be observed only in the context of coping transactions. To assess these transactions the practitioner needs to observe the child in various situations over time. Multiple observations in different contexts give the clinician a better sense of the ways in which elements of coping transactions facilitate or interfere with effective coping. The therapist needs to identify the demands and expectations (stressors) experienced by the child, the coping efforts that the child uses to manage demands, and the feedback that the child receives from the physical and social environments.

In assessing demands and expectations, it is necessary first to identify them and then to determine their developmental appropriateness. Demands and expectations of others can be identified through interviewing adult care-givers or through observing social interactions. Demands of the physical environment are best delineated through direct observation of the child in typical surroundings. Assessment of the child's coping efforts in response to external demands and expectations must consider (1) the repertoire of available coping strategies, (2) flexibility in their use, (3) circumstances under which they are applied, and (4) their success in managing specific stressors. In assessing the nature of the feedback in coping transactions, the therapist must appreciate how it is provided (e.g., physically, verbally); whether it gives accurate information regarding the child's performance; and whether it is offered in a timely and contingent manner.

In addition to direct observation of the child's coping transactions, information about the child's past coping experiences can be gathered through parent interview. Older children and adolescents can be asked directly about their history of coping transactions. Guiding questions to the parent may include the following:

- Are any particular situations stressful for your child?
- What does your child do in these situations? What do you do under these circumstances?
- How does your child respond to change?
- Does your child like to explore and try new things?

The assessment of coping transactions helps the occupational therapist understand how the child manages specific situations. To gain further information needed for intervention planning, it is also useful to assess the child's unique internal and external coping resources.

### Assessing Coping Resources

**Coping Style.**   To assess coping style, it is necessary to consider the overall effectiveness of the child's coping competence as well as to identify the most and least adaptive coping attributes. It is important to observe the child in various situations to obtain a representative sample of the child's coping efforts and the degree of their effectiveness in managing demands and expectations. The following criteria are useful in making these clinical judgments: (1) appropriateness of the coping efforts to various situations; (2) appropriateness of the coping efforts for the child's developmental age; and (3) extent to which the efforts successfully achieve desired outcomes.

There are a number of instruments that address certain aspects of coping such as temperament, social skills, locus of control, and personality traits. Two observation instruments are recommended, however, because they specifically assess the child's coping style. These are the *Early Coping Inventory* (Zeitlin, Williamson, & Szczepanski, 1988) and the *Coping Inventory* (Zeitlin, 1985). The *Early Coping Inventory* is designed for children aged 4 to 36 months or for older children who have special needs who function within this developmental range. The *Coping Inventory* is intended for children aged 3 to 16 years.

Items in these instruments target coping attributes that have been documented in the professional literature as being associated with adaptive functioning in children. A five-point scale is used to rate each item, ranging from ineffective to consistently effective across situations. The results of the inventories yield an overall level of coping effectiveness and identify coping style. Comparisons can be made among the different categories of the instruments. In addition, the child's most and least adaptive coping attributes are delineated. The instruments are uniquely structured to help the clinician interpret findings and plan intervention.

Several issues need to be highlighted when assessing coping style:

1. To what extent does the child engage in self-initiated behaviors and are these coping behaviors productive?
2. Is the child able to use coping strategies flexibly across various situations?
3. Is there a difference between how the child copes with self and how the child copes with environmental demands?
4. How does the child evaluate the effectiveness of coping efforts?

This last issue is critical because the child's interpretation strongly influences the development of self-esteem.

**Beliefs and Values.**  Emerging or existing beliefs and values are evaluated through observation and interaction with the child. Inferences about the child's self-esteem can be made during play and purposeful, goal-directed activity. The following behaviors reflect the child's feelings about the ability to influence the environment: willingness to engage in activities, to create or accept challenges, to make efforts to complete tasks, and to respond to frustration and success. This information is critical in the selection and grading of activities that foster personalized intervention. In addition, formal instruments can be useful in assessing self-esteem in school-aged children. One of these instruments is the *Piers-Harris Children's Self-Concept Inventory* (Piers & Harris, 1969), which can be administered by the advanced therapist or by other team members. Also, play and activity histories obtained from the parent or child generate information that reflects the child's preferences.

With verbal, older children, the clinician can explore beliefs and values directly through informal interview. Issues that can be addressed include: what the child likes to do now and wants to do in the future; what is important to the child; what ideas the child has about any present handicapping condition and about disability in general; and how the child is the same or different from other people.

Because beliefs and values are influenced strongly by the family, a parent interview can be useful in obtaining additional information. This interview may address such factors as the parents' perception of the child and the child's behavior, goals and expectations for the child's future, and approaches to managing behavior at home. For example, a high parental value on educational achievement may result in punishment for academic failure. Likewise, parental value for socially acceptable behavior may result in a developmentally inappropriate concern about a toddler's inability to share, take turns, and get along with others.

**Physical and Affective States.** A medical history and health examination by professionals in other disciplines can contribute information about the child's physical status. Additional relevant information is obtained directly by the occupational therapist during a developmental and sensorimotor assessment (e.g., joint range of motion, muscle strength and coordination, sensory processing, functional mobility, and manipulative skills). The assessment of affective status includes observation of the appropriateness of affect and mood, range of emotional expression, and feelings of well-being. The occupational therapist provides a unique contribution to the interdisciplinary team by observing the emotional responses of the child to a variety of purposeful activities and performance demands.

**Developmental Skills.** To assess developmental skills as a coping resource, the therapist must be familiar with the standard practices described in this book for evaluating various developmental domains. In determining adaptive competence, the child's strengths and vulnerabilities are identified in all areas, including cognitive, psychosocial, communicative, and motor development. Because the acquisition of developmental skills does not lead automatically to effective coping, assessment focuses not only on what the child can do but also on how well the child applies skills as integrated coping efforts within situations. Direct observation of the child in the natural contexts of activities of daily living, school, and play is critical for collecting data relevant to coping. A process-oriented, coping-related approach to developmental assessment includes identification of the circumstances in which skills are demonstrated, the degree to which the child uses skills in a self-initiated manner, the approach to and organization of structured and unstructured tasks, and the ability to solve problems. Play assessments used by occupational therapists also guide observation of the child's spontaneous use of developmental skills in a functional context.

**Human Supports.**    Availability and quality of human supports are identified as they relate to the child's coping. During home and clinic visits, parents and other caregivers are observed in their roles as primary facilitators of development and mediators between the child and the environment. Observations of parent-child-environment interactions are made to delineate the demands and expectations created by caregivers, their role in facilitating or interfering with the child's coping efforts, and the feedback given to the child. This information contributes not only to the assessment of the social resources available to the child but also to the assessment of the caregiver's needs in relation to parenting.

As the child enters school and participates in community activities, human supports beyond the family unit are examined increasingly. For example, observation in the classroom and playground enables the therapist to appreciate how teachers and peers influence the child's coping at school. It also is helpful to assess the potential for expanding the range of human supports available to the child. With proper guidance, previously uninvolved older siblings, grandparents, or neighbors may be recruited to assist the child.

**Material and Environmental Supports.**    A child's needs relative to material and environmental supports vary based on age, developmental capability, and the presence of a handicapping condition. The therapist determines whether the surroundings are organized, accessible, and offer various developmentally appropriate toys. When the child has a disability, it is essential to examine the material supports that the child requires to function optimally. These supports may include mobility and positioning equipment, adaptive toys, communication aids, and architectural modifications. The *Home Observation for Measurement of the Environment* (Caldwell & Bradley, 1979) is one instru-

ment that can be used by occupational therapists to assess the external resources of young children and their general responses to the social and
physical environments.

### Linking Assessment to Intervention Planning

After the assessment data pertinent to the child's coping transactions and
resources have been collected, the information needs to be analyzed so that
the findings can be translated into an intervention plan. The following decision-making questions can be useful when designing intervention to increase
coping effectiveness:

---

- How and under what circumstances does the child cope effectively? Ineffectively?
- What factors facilitate effective coping and what factors interfere?
- Of the factors that interfere with effective coping, what can be changed (e.g.,
  demands and expectations, coping resources, the environment's response to the
  child's coping efforts)?
- What changes will make the most difference in facilitating the child's coping competence?

---

Table 11.2 summarizes the material gained from the comprehensive assessment of the coping resources of Carol, a 15-month-old girl referred to occupational therapy because of parental concerns about her developmental delays.
The discussion that follows exemplifies how the four decision-making questions were used to make clinical decisions necessary for planning intervention

1. How and under what circumstances does the child cope effectively? Ineffectively? In transactions during evaluation sessions, Carol responded in
   some ways to the demands of the occupational therapist. She was able to
   listen, make eye contact, imitate simple actions, and play with toys when
   given emotional and verbal encouragement. In contrast, coping transactions in the family were characterized by few demands for Carol to interact
   with people and objects, as well as a lack of reinforcement on those
   occasions when she demonstrated purposeful activity. Her behavior at
   home was, therefore, extremely passive. She waited for everything to be
   done for her and seldom indicated her needs to others. Carol had a minimally effective coping style; however, her reactive behaviors were rela-

*Table 11.2*  Assessment Summary of Carol's Coping Resources

<u>Internal Resources</u>

Coping Style
- Minimally effective with relative strength in sensorimotor organization; reactive behaviors slightly more effective than self-initiated coping behaviors

Beliefs and Values
- No obvious activity preferences
- Limited awareness of ability to impact on environment

Physical and Affective States
- Healthy; normal neurological status
- Low activity level
- Depression and flat affect

Developmental Capabilities
- Developmental skills at a 9-12 month level
- Failure to play spontaneously
- Limited social interaction

<u>External Resources</u>

Human Supports
- Genuine parental concern for child's welfare
- Low familial demands and expectations

Material and Environmental Supports
- Adequate food, clothing, and shelter
- Understimulating physical environment

---

tively more effective than her self-initiated behaviors. She rarely used acquired developmental skills to generate coping efforts.

2. What factors facilitate effective coping and what factors interfere? Carol's facilitative coping resources included her general health, neurological status, and the parents' concern for her welfare. Her developmental skills were a potentially positive resource if she could learn to apply them in coping efforts. The major interfering factor was the lack of understanding by Carol's parents about the physical and social environments needed to foster their daughter's development. This circumstance resulted in her marked passivity and limited self-initiation. Carol appeared depressed because of lack of nurturance and, she was developing a belief that the world was uninteresting and unresponsive. Consequently, Carol's emotional state was a significant vulnerability.

3. Of the factors that interfered with effective coping, what can be changed? Because Carol's parents were deeply concerned, they could be assisted to understand her needs more fully. Her emotional and developmental status could be influenced by providing a nurturing social environment that

fostered interaction, offered suitable challenge, and encouraged self-directed exploration.

4. What changes will make the most difference in facilitating the child's coping competence? The goal for Carol was to be emotionally involved in her surroundings. The therapeutic approach focused on supporting mutually satisfying parent/child interaction. This orientation helped her parents establish appropriate expectations, provide stimulating toys and activities, and respond to her in a contingent way. In addition to the occupational therapist's work with the family, direct services were needed for the child. The clinician focused on increasing Carol's developmental skills, modeled their use in coping efforts, and modified the environment to provide opportunities for self-initiated play. Emphasis was placed on the therapeutic relationship as a catalyst for enriching emotional development.

## Postulates Regarding Change

A primary goal of intervention is to promote a goodness of fit or *congruence between the child's coping resources and environmental demands and expectations.* When an appropriate match occurs, learning and development are fostered, and the child experiences a sense of mastery and well-being. Intervention is designed to establish a proper fit between the child and the environment so that previously acquired coping strategies can be modified and new ones can be learned to meet current and future demands. The postulates regarding change are based on the transactional nature of the coping process and how it can be influenced. These postulates address factors that influence coping and that are amenable to change, including (1) the demands of specific situations, (2) the child's coping resources for managing these demands, and (3) the environment's response to those efforts. The postulates that follow guide intervention. Although they are presented separately, these postulates usually are addressed simultaneously during therapy:

- Effective coping is facilitated by modification of environmental demands so that they are congruent with the child's capabilities.

- Effective coping is enhanced by expansion of internal and external coping resources.

- Effective coping is encouraged by appropriate, contingent responses to the child's coping efforts.

## *Modifying Demands*

The first postulate to facilitate effective coping involves the grading of environmental demands so that they are congruent with the child's coping capabilities. Therapists and parents must have a thorough understanding of the child's level of functioning so that appropriate goals and expectations can be established. A slight imbalance between demands and the child's functional competence is sought, so that demands provide the challenge necessary to foster motivation and learning. The adult can grade demands and expectations for the child in numerous ways, such as increasing or decreasing of complexity of the demand; modifying the way in which demands are presented to the child; and providing necessary assistance or supervision for the child to be successful.

Characteristics of both the physical and social environments place demands on children and influence their behavior. Therapists, therefore, must consider both environments when grading demands in intervention or adapting the home and school settings. The following examples illustrate the varied nature of demands and the ways in which they can be modified: (1) giving directions based on the child's language comprehension; (2) positioning the child physically so that toys are accessible; (3) grading sensory experiences according to the child's tolerance; (4) providing verbal guidance in anticipation of changes in activity; and (5) adapting the pace of intervention to accommodate the child's attention span and energy level.

A careful activity analysis helps the occupational therapist grade the type and sequence of intervention so that demands are appropriate. Activities therefore can be selected that are developmentally relevant and that create the proper level of challenge. The case of Jenny, a child with mental retardation, demonstrates the importance of grading demands. Jenny stubbornly refused to participate in any self-dressing activity. The therapist worked closely with the parent to devise a dressing program that was personalized to foster success and motivation. Initially, it was decided to simplify the endeavor by focusing solely on upper extremity dressing. Demands were introduced at contextually meaningful times when Jenny was motivated to accomplish the task. She enjoyed going to school and taking a bath but usually resisted going to bed. Therefore, putting on her shirt and coat before school and taking off the shirt before her bath were emphasized at home. Managing pajama tops was deferred to a later date. Likewise, donning and doffing a smock were encouraged during therapy sessions when she was to be engaged in a favorite messy activity like finger painting.

In addition, the therapist taught the parent an instructional procedure that divided the task into component parts that required Jenny to participate gradually in an increasing number of steps over time. Using a "backward-chaining" technique, the child was expected to perform only the last step, then the last two steps, then the last three steps, and so forth until the task was learned. Through these methods, demands were modified so that Jenny could acquire increased independence in dressing without eliciting resistant, maladaptive behavior.

It is important that the therapist works with parents, teachers, and other significant adults to ensure that everyone has mutually shared and consistent demands and expectations for the child. This collaboration is essential to avoid confusing the child with divergent messages that can interfere with learning new coping behaviors. Likewise, it prevents the child from being overwhelmed by unrealistic demands.

## Enhancing Coping Resources

The second postulate on which intervention is based involves enhancing the child's internal and external coping resources. These resources include coping style, beliefs and values, physical and affective states, developmental skills, human supports, and material and environmental supports. Many of the customary practices of occupational therapists are designed to expand these coping resources. Implementation of this postulate involves intervention to remediate or compensate for deficits in performance components (e.g., sensory processing, neuromuscular control) and to teach competencies in areas of occupational performance (e.g., play, activities of daily living). Each frame of reference described in this book contributes to helping the child acquire skills that can be applied in particular situations to cope. When a child has limited coping resources, the clinician usually draws on additional frames of reference to address the child's specific needs. For example, if a sensory processing deficit interferes with effective coping, then the sensory integrative frame of reference would be applied to remediate this vulnerability. The discussion that follows provides general guidelines to enhance specific coping resources.

**Coping Style.**    The coping behaviors of many special children are erratic, inconsistent, or limited in range. Based on an assessment of the strengths and vulnerabilities of a child's coping style, intervention can be targeted to expand coping behaviors related to such attributes as self-initiation, reactivity, flexibility, activity level, and self-regulation. Coping with emotions illustrates this point. Therapy can be tailored to assist the child to control and express anger in effective ways. The therapist can (1) label the emotion as the child begins to experience the feeling, (2) model appropriate verbal expressions, (3) teach cognitive/behavioral techniques for reducing affective tension (e.g., deep breathing, counting to ten), and (4) clarify what constitutes acceptable and unacceptable behavior (e.g., "toys are for playing, not throwing").

Specific goals, objectives, and activities of intervention are founded on a knowledge of the child's most and least effective coping attributes. As discussed previously, these attributes may be delineated through assessment instruments, observation, or parent interview. A list of least effective coping attributes identifies the major factors that interfere with learning and development. This list may be reviewed to determine which of these attributes realistically can be changed. Although most behaviors have a potential for change, some coping behaviors can be influenced more readily than others. For instance, it is basically easier to teach a child to accept help when necessary than to develop a vigorous energy level.

The coping attributes receptive to change are formulated into goals for intervention. A goal can be directed to change a specific behavior (e.g., to increase the child's persistence during play with familiar toys), or it can be written in broader terms (e.g., to expand the child's flexibility). Priorities in setting goals are established by determining which changes will make the greatest difference in fostering more effective coping. To determine specific objectives for intervention, the occupational therapist must consider what behavioral competencies the child has to learn (and in what sequence) to achieve the proscribed goals.

A list of most effective coping attributes identifies the factors that facilitate the child's performance. These coping attributes are essential to determine therapeutic strategies and activities. They are used to design intervention that builds on the child's strengths. For example, if a child's most effective coping behavior is the ability to coordinate and adapt movements to specific situations, then a therapeutic strategy to decrease passivity would emphasize motor activities. If all goes well, pleasure in successful motor performance will enhance the child's self-generated, active involvement.

It often is necessary to teach the child the specific coping strategies required to manage concrete circumstances. The child in a wheelchair can be taught ways to negotiate the hectic environments of the school and shopping center. The child who has a learning disability can be given methods to compensate in the classroom for perceptual deficits or poor handwriting. A fearful child can learn to ride comfortably on the school bus by sitting next to a friend in a seat near the driver. The child who demonstrates limited interpersonal skills can receive instruction on how to make friends or settle arguments (i.e., coping in a social context with peers).

As previously described, children can be classified according to their coping style—that is, as minimally effective, situationally effective, or consistently effective. The nature of intervention varies for each child. Treatment guidelines based on the adequacy of the child's coping style are presented later in this chapter.

**Beliefs and Values.** Coping is supported when beliefs and values contribute to a positive sense of self and facilitate the child's ability to implement effective coping efforts. A child's beliefs and values may create vulnerability to stress when they result in negative self-esteem or emotional responses that interfere with daily coping. The therapist can influence beliefs and values indirectly by providing experiences that foster a positive sense of self and competence in daily activities. For example, a child who has a physical disability may have a negative perception of self as a result of dependence on others. The child may develop a stronger sense of personal efficacy if activities are modified for more independent, self-initiated participation. For older children who are able to express their thoughts and feelings, intervention can focus on clarifying and altering their beliefs and values. It may be helpful to conduct discussions related to issues such as: "What is good about me?"; "What goals do I have for myself?"; and "How can I get there from here?".

When the family's beliefs and values have a negative impact on the child's coping, family-based intervention may be indicated. Parents can be assisted in recognizing their own beliefs and how they are reflected in child management, and how they influence their child's behavior.

**Physical and Affective States.** Many standard practices in occupational therapy influence the child's physical status. Activities can be designed to develop endurance, increase strength, and improve motor control. The child's unique physical characteristics may necessitate monitoring the daily schedule to prevent fatigue, modifying the environment to maximize function, and teaching alternative methods to compensate for disabilities. Therapy to influence affective state addresses the child's moods and psychological dynamics. Intervention is graded to support an appropriate level of self-control, emotional stability, and an awake-alert state needed for effective transactions. Sample treatment strategies include careful selection of activities, behavior management techniques, and therapeutic use of self. For example, a depressed child's mood may be altered by a warm, supportive therapeutic approach and the use of a favorite activity that invites active participation.

**Developmental Skills.** Because developmental skills provide a foundation for coping efforts, adaptive functioning can be facilitated by expanding the child's repertoire of available developmental competencies and by remediating performance deficits. The challenge, however, is to structure the therapeutic program so that acquisition of developmental skills is closely linked to outcomes related to coping. The child then has the opportunity to integrate and apply the skills in a functional, coping context. It is helpful to make this link by writing treatment goals that use phrases such as "in order to." For example, Pedro will improve his bilateral coordination *in order to* expand his play schemes, increase his self-initiated problem solving, or communicate his wants through gestures.

In some cases, intervention may focus on teaching prerequisite developmental skills that prepare a child to cope. To enhance self-initiation, a child who is physically challenged may need therapy to develop coordination of the upper extremities, instruction in operating assistive devices, or training to use eye gaze to indicate choices. It also is important that treatment objectives emphasize mastery and generalization of skills. Ample time in therapy needs to be committed to the practice of new behaviors under a variety and complexity of conditions. Therefore a level of mastery is achieved to ensure that skills are truly available under the stresses of daily living.

**Human Supports.** Because families serve as a major external resource to support the child's coping, occupational therapists must frequently develop a collaborative relationship with parents to plan and provide relevant intervention. How parents cope with the demands of raising a special child influences overall family health and the child's life outcome (Barber, Turnbull, Behr, & Kerns, 1988; Olsen & McCubbin, 1983; Williamson, 1987; Zeitlin & Williamson, 1988). Services are thus structured to be responsive to family concerns and can take many forms. In strengthening the child's human supports, the practitioner may address issues related to caregiving, parent/child interaction, behavior management, parental role development, and informational needs regarding community resources. Through these efforts, parents expand their abilities to facilitate the child's emerging competence. The therapist also serves as an important source of human support during ongoing treatment. This support can be extended by working with the child's teacher so that the classroom setting serves as a positive, external resource that promotes adaptive functioning.

**Material and Environmental Supports.** Occupational therapists are specialists in adapting the physical environment to foster successful coping in the home, school, and community. For instance, the therapist may modify lighting to maximize functional vision for a child who has an ocular deficit, may provide adapted seating for a child who has motor involvement, may regulate environmental stimulation for a hyperactive child, or may recommend materials and activities that are developmentally challenging. At times, intervention may involve temporary modifications to help a child manage a transitional period of stress. For example, after surgery the therapist may help the child who is immobilized in a cast handle self-care tasks. The practitioner also may work with the family to access needed community resources, such as daycare or afterschool programs, and social services related to housing, economic assistance, and primary health care.

## Providing Contingent Feedback

The third postulate is that effective coping is encouraged by providing appropriate, contingent responses to the child's coping efforts. Appropriate feedback can reinforce desired or newly acquired coping strategies, whereas inappropriate feedback can perpetuate ineffective or maladaptive coping behavior. When feedback is timely, positive, clear, and accurate in response to productive coping efforts, the child experiences a sense of mastery that contributes over time to a belief system that addresses personal worth and autonomy. Meaningful social feedback is not just verbal but can be expressed affectively through smiles, frowns, and looks of admiration or consternation. The nature of the feedback needs to be selected carefully to promote efficient learning of coping behaviors.

In considering the use of feedback, it is important to accentuate the development of self-directed, purposeful behavior. Such an approach focuses on the therapist responding contingently to the child's self-generated action. The emphasis is on a therapeutic environment that supports child-initiated activity and provides feedback that encourages the extension and elaboration of demonstrated, emerging skills. In this context, the child has the freedom to explore, solve problems, and experiment with alternative coping strategies. Attention also is required to ensure that a balanced turntaking occurs between child and therapist, with ample opportunity for the child to lead the interaction within socially appropriate limits.

Research suggests that children who have handicaps tend to assume passive, respondent roles rather than active, autonomous ones (Brinker & Lewis, 1982; Zeitlin & Williamson, 1990). This behavioral pattern can be reinforced unintentionally by parents and professionals. When a child has a disability, parents may tend to develop a strongly dominant interactional style (Barrera & Vella, 1987; Hanzlik, 1989; Rosenberg & Robinson, 1988). Likewise, professionals may tend to implement intervention that is highly structured and adult-directed with an emphasis on eliciting responses from the child that then are reinforced by the therapist (Dunst, Cushing, & Vance, 1985). In both cases, the child has little opportunity to learn that intrinsically motivated behavior can be used successfully to achieve personal needs.

# Application to Practice

In treatment planning to implement the postulates, it is useful to divide intervention strategies into two categories—direct and indirect. According to Hildebrand (1975), direct strategies influence the child's behavior through specific interaction with the adult. Traditional teaching techniques and procedures for behavior modification exemplify direct strategies. Some examples include: (1) verbal guidance to help the child solve a task; (2) the modeling of desired behaviors for the child to imitate; (3) physical prompting to assist performance of an activity; and (4) feedback through specific reinforcement schedules.

In contrast, indirect intervention strategies influence the child's behavior through management of space, materials, equipment, and other persons in the surroundings. These strategies "set the stage" for learning by modifying the environment. Sample indirect strategies include: (1) adapting the size and type of play materials; (2) eliminating distractions for the impulsive child; (3) grouping children together to foster social interaction; (4) providing a predictable sequence of activities during therapy for the child who has difficulty adjusting to change; and (5) using splints, adaptive devices, or special positioning equipment for children who have physical disabilities.

Typically, a combination of direct and indirect intervention strategies is necessary to facilitate skill acquisition and coping. Care is taken to avoid overreliance on direct guidance in therapy because this tends to reinforce reactive, dependent coping styles. Frequently, indirect approaches through environmental modification result in the child producing the desired behavior in a self-initiated manner. Jeremy, for instance, was a toddler who had a hemiplegic type of cerebral palsy and who resisted using his affected extremity. The therapist observed, however, that he would incorporate the arm spontaneously into tasks that required the use of two hands. Bilateral activities were then introduced as an indirect intervention strategy to foster self-generated hand use (e.g., playing with a large ball, pushing a toy lawnmower, riding a rocking horse).

## Intervention Based on Levels of Coping Effectiveness

The level of effectiveness of a child's coping style influences the selection of intervention strategies and the intensity of the therapeutic program. The discussion that follows provides guidelines for addressing the unique needs of children who have minimally effective, situationally effective, and consistently effective coping styles.

**Minimally Effective Coping Style.**   A child who displays a minimally effective coping style requires intensive intervention that consists of direct teaching of developmental skills and coping behaviors. This child's coping efforts are inconsistent, or rigidly repetitious, or reduce the stress of the moment but generate negative outcomes over time (e.g., habitual withdrawal or temper tantrums). It appears that a child continues to use ineffective coping behaviors either to avoid or gain control over stressful situations or because of a restricted repertoire of alternative coping strategies (Schaffer & Schaffer, 1982). The minimally effective child usually has limited developmental, behavioral, or environmental resources to draw on for coping efforts or is unable, for whatever reason, to adapt available resources to the situation. Therapy focuses on expanding the child's resources while grading environmental demands to decrease the need to use ineffective stereotypic behaviors.

Successful coping requires the integration of various developmental skills to produce functional, goal-directed coping efforts. Initially, intervention emphasizes expansion of developmental capabilities to achieve greater competence in postural control, mobility, object manipulation, cognitive processing, social interaction, and communication. In addition, treatment is designed to teach desired coping behaviors and to modify the environment to reduce opportunities for the reinforcement of maladaptive patterns. Consistency is necessary in the choice and presentation of activities, and practice is emphasized. Because the minimally effective child often is incapable of applying learned behaviors independently to new contexts, the therapist gradually introduces new activities in a variety of situations as the child's coping ability increases.

The parents and therapist need to establish priorities for intervention because it is unrealistic to address all developmental and coping-related problems at once. Likewise, it is important to determine appropriate expectations for the child's progress. A consistent and shared approach to behavior management is necessary to extinguish negative behaviors and to encourage emerging skills.

**Situationally Effective Coping Style.**   A child who demonstrates a situationally effective coping style has some adaptive competence. Coping efforts used effectively in one situation, however, are not generalized to other situations. Intervention is geared to help this child learn to generalize the use of effective coping strategies to settings and circumstances in which the child is currently less successful. Particular emphasis is placed on indirect intervention strategies because they foster self-initiation.

To plan a treatment program, the occupational therapist must identify the nature of the situations and environments in which the child demonstrates effective coping. Sample contextual variables to consider may include (1) the presence or absence of a caregiver; (2) the degree of structure; (3) solitary or group settings; (4) the time of day when demands are presented; (5) the child's preference for certain types of sensory input; or (6) the availability of adaptive equipment for a child with a physical disability. A major therapeutic strategy is to modify the environmental characteristics of situations in which the child copes ineffectively to resemble more closely the environmental characteristics of successful coping experiences. For instance, Sean was active and flexible in routine settings but became anxious in new surroundings. His parents were taught various techniques for making novel situations more familiar and less intimidating for their son. These strategies included previewing what to expect so that he could anticipate events, having him carry a tote bag that was a comforting object, and allowing time for him to warm-up and acclimate to situations. Under these conditions, Sean was able to generalize his adaptive behaviors comfortably to new environments.

**Consistently Effective Coping Style.** A child who displays a consistently effective coping style uses coping efforts that are appropriate more often than not. This child is able to generalize coping strategies across a variety of situations. No child copes successfully under every circumstance, but this child has sufficient resources to modify behavior and adapt to new demands. The child who has an effective coping style may receive occupational therapy to address other therapeutic needs; therefore, coping-related intervention becomes preventive and supportive in nature. The therapist monitors the balance between environmental demands and the child's coping resources and may use indirect intervention strategies to maintain and promote productive coping efforts. Attention is also targeted toward preventing deterioration in effectiveness during stressful life events. Activities of a preventive nature can support the child and family during situations that are predictably demanding—such as hospitalization, modifications in the child's current program, birth of a sibling, or changes in residency.

## Integrating Coping into Treatment

For some children, the primary therapeutic concern may be maladaptive behavior. In such cases, intervention may be based solely on a coping frame of reference. For most children, however, this frame of reference is used in conjunction with others to ensure that therapy is linked closely to adaptive functioning. For example, it helps the therapist to provide neurodevelopmental treatment in a way that strengthens the child's ability to meet personal needs and to respond to the demands of the environment. The following vignettes illustrate ways that coping goals were integrated into the ongoing treatment process.

---

- To encourage bilateral hand use and self-initiated problem solving in an infant who has hemiplegia, toys were hung from his highchair on strings of yarn. Through trial and error the child learned to pull up on the yarn with both hands to attain the toys. In the process he expanded his ability to change strategies when necessary to achieve a goal.

- A seven-year-old child had great difficulty separating from his mother during therapy sessions. The coping postulates regarding change were applied systematically to manage this situation. Demands were modified by grading the mother's presence over time (e.g., active involvement to an observational role to brief periods of absence). The child's coping efforts were supported by having him play with highly motivating, favorite toys during the mother's absence and using a timer to indicate when the mother would return to the room. Positive feedback and assurance were provided to reinforce the child's developing independence.

- A group of elementary-aged children who exhibited poor motor planning and interpersonal skills were engaged in making a collage to foster their sensorimotor development and cooperative play. The following therapeutic methods were used to structure the activity: (1) group determination of a common theme and title for the collage; (2) provision of diverse materials that required cutting, tearing, and other emerging manipulative skills; (3) limited supplies, which necessitated sharing; and (4) positioning of the canvas vertically on a wall, which required the children to press hard against the materials as the glue dried (i.e., proprioceptive input in antigravity holding patterns). This activity targeted not only sensorimotor goals but also treatment objectives related to coping with peers (e.g., responding to the feelings of others, accepting substitute ideas, sharing, taking turns, and accepting and giving praise).

---

Two sample case are presented to illustrate how this frame of reference can be applied to enhance occupational performance and coping effectiveness in daily life.

## Case 1

Edith was a 26-month-old child diagnosed as having spina bifida. Her parents were particularly concerned that she was growing increasingly frustrated by the limitations imposed on her by the physical handicap. Results of the developmental assessment indicated that her major strengths were her skills in cognition and communication. She understood simple sentences and used words and gestures during interactions. Edith had significant delays, however, in gross and fine motor skills. Although she could move about by pulling with her arms, this form of locomotion required excessive energy. Efficient use of the hands for manipulative play was restricted by the lack of postural control, requiring her to use one or both arms to support her in a sitting position. Motor limitations appeared to be interfering with her development of self-esteem and autonomy.

Edith's coping style was situationally effective. Her motivation to explore and interact with the environment was undermined by her restricted motor skills. The effectiveness of many coping efforts depended on proper physical positioning by an adult and structuring of the setting so that play materials were within reach. Edith's most effective coping attributes were related to her social competence. She was able to accept warmth and affection, was responsive to the feelings and moods of others, engaged in reciprocal social interactions, and had keen visual and auditory interests in her surroundings.

Her least effective coping attributes were strongly influenced by her physical involvement. She had poor control of her posture and minimal ability to adapt movements to meet the requirements of specific situations. As a result, she frustrated easily and lacked persistence during play. Edith attempted tasks but tended to give up quickly if her actions failed to achieve desired results. When frustrated, she typically arched into an extensor posture. Her motor difficulties hindered the development of independence in play. For example, skills that she demonstrated when supported on her father's lap could not be applied successfully when left on her own.

Major treatment priorities were to improve Edith's postural control, mobility, and manipulation. Her coping effectiveness was enhanced substantially by decreasing the impact of her physical disability on her performance. Stress related to motor demands was reduced and graded. Edith's ability to generalize coping strategies expanded as she developed motor skills. Gradually, she was able to persist with a task for a longer time and experienced less frustration.

Numerous intervention strategies were used to facilitate Edith's success in goal-directed activity during play. An adapted seat for use on the floor or in a regular chair provided the external support required for manipulation of toys (an indirect intervention strategy). Likewise, a small hand-propelled cart was used to allow independent mobility. At the same time, therapy focused on strengthening the muscles that Edith needed for postural stability and ambulation with braces.

Edith was taught to change her behavior to solve a problem before getting frustrated. When initial attempts to do something resulted in failure, her parents and the occupational therapist demonstrated alternative ways for Edith to move herself or the toy to achieve success (a direct intervention strategy). In addition, she was encouraged to use her social and communicative skills to obtain assistance rather than to arch into extension. Through activities, she was taught to be aware of when and how to request adult help by pointing and vocalizing. Edith's successful use of these coping efforts and developmental skills reinforced an emerging belief in her competence and resulted in more independent play.

## Case 2

Joe was an 11-year-old boy of normal intelligence who had poor impulse control and specific learning disabilities related to reading and mathematics. His primary academic placement was in a self-contained special education class, but he was mainstreamed for music and physical education. Joe was referred to occupational therapy by his teacher because of behavior problems in the classroom. The teacher complained that he had marked mood swings—compliant behavior alternated with episodes of acting out.

The occupational therapy assessment identified some sensory integrative deficits that possibly could be contributing to his erratic behavior. However, his behavior problems appeared to be most related to a minimally effective coping style. Joe had a great fear of failure that made him averse to any academic or social situation that he interpreted as difficult. Under these conditions, he tended to react explosively. It became clear that his compliant periods occurred under circumstances in which he was left alone to play or day dream. His least effective coping attributes were the inability to manage new or demanding situations and the inability to handle the associated anxiety. In contrast, his most effective coping occurred in low-demand, structured settings that were familiar and provided support and encouragement.

In consultation with the teacher, a three-pronged intervention approach was implemented in the school. First, Joe received individual occupational therapy to ascertain whether this would improve his sensorimotor organization and sense of empowerment. Second, the teacher was helped to adapt the classroom to be less threatening. For example, (1) the class schedule was made more routine and predictable; (2) Joe's desk was placed at the end of a row next to a friend who could serve as a peer helper; (3) Joe was asked to repeat directions to ensure that he comprehended the task; and (4) reading and math lessons were graded more carefully to promote success and were conducted in shorter periods throughout the day instead of being concentrated in the morning.

Finally, Joe participated in a small group conducted by the occupational therapist that concentrated on teaching cognitive-behavioral strategies to develop self-control and problem solving. Joe learned to identify and analyze difficult situations, to consider alternative actions and their consequences, and to plan steps for reaching desired goals. For instance, in stressful situations, he was taught to use a cognitive technique referred to as **STOP** (i.e., **S**top what I am doing, **T**ake a look back to see what has happened, look at my **O**ptions, and **P**lay back a different way of behaving). Over time, Joe was able to regulate his emotional reactions and resultant behavior more effectively.

# Summary

This chapter presents a frame of reference to increase the children's coping effectiveness. The transactional model of the coping process serves as a framework for the postulates regarding change—modification of environmental demands and expectations, enhancement of coping resources, and provision of contingent feedback. Direct and indirect intervention strategies are applied selectively to implement these postulates. Occupational therapy has a unique commitment to human adaptation and function that defines the very nature of effective coping. It is the intent of the authors that this frame of reference, in collaboration with others, will empower children to cope successfully with their own personal needs and environmental demands so that they can be productive in daily life.

**Outline for the Coping Frame of Reference**

  I. Theoretical base
    A. The coping process
      1. Coping transactions
      2. Environmental contributions to coping transactions
      3. Transactional model
        a. Determine meaning of an event
        b. Develop an action plan
        c. Implement a coping effort
        d. Evaluate effectiveness
    B. Coping resources
      1. Internal coping resources
        a. Coping style
        b. Beliefs and values

    c. Physical and affective states

    d. Developmental skills

  2. External coping resources

    a. Human supports

    b. Material and environmental supports

 C. Coping in children with special needs

II. Function/dysfunction continua

 A. Effective coping

 B. Coping style

 C. Beliefs and values

 D. Physical and affective states

 E. Developmental skills

 F. Human supports

 G. Material and environmental supports

 H. Demands and expectations

IV. Coping assessment

 A. Assessing coping transactions

 B. Assessing coping resources

  1. Coping style

  2. Beliefs and values

  3. Physical and affective states

  4. Developmental skills

  5. Human supports

  6. Material and environmental supports

 C. Linking assessment to intervention planning

IV. Postulates regarding change

 A. Those that relate to environmental demands

 B. Those that relate to internal and external coping resources

 C. Those that relate to appropriate responses to the child's coping efforts

V. Application to practice

 A. Intervention according to levels of coping effectiveness

  1. Minimally effective coping style

  2. Situationally effective coping style

  3. Consistently effective coping style

  4. Integrating coping into treatment

 B. Case examples

### References

Antonovsky, A. (1979). *Health, stress, and coping.* San Francisco, CA: Jossey-Bass.

Bandura, A. (1977). Self efficacy: Toward a unifying theory of behavior change. *Psychological Review, 84,* 191–215.

Barber, P. A., Turnbull, A. P., Behr, S. K., & Kerns, G. M. (1988). A family systems perspective on early childhood special education. In: S. L. Odom, M. B. Karnes

(Eds.). *Early intervention for infants and children with handicaps* (179–198). Baltimore, MD: Paul H Brookes.

Barrera, M. E., & Vella, D. M. (1987). Disabled and nondisabled infants' interactions with their mothers. *American Journal of Occupational Therapy, 41,* 168–172.

Brinker, R. P., & Lewis, M. (1982). Discovering the competent handicapped infant: A process approach to assessment and intervention. *Topics in Early Childhood Special Education, 2*(2), 1–16.

Brooks-Gunn, J, & Furstenberg, F. F. (1987). Continuity and change in the context of poverty: Adolescent mothers and their children. In: J. J. Gallagher, & C. T. Ramey (Eds.). *The malleability of children* (171–188). Baltimore, MD: Paul H Brookes.

Caldwell, B. M., & Bradley, R. H. (1979). *Home observation for measurement of the environment.* Little Rock, Arkansas: Center for Child Development and Education, University of Arkansas at Little Rock.

Compas, B. E. (1987). Coping with stress during childhood and adolescence. *Psychological Bulletin, 101,* 393–403.

DiBuono E. (1982). A comparison of the self-concept and coping skills of learning disabled and nonhandicapped pupils in self-contained classes, resource rooms and regular classes [Dissertation]. West Covina, CA: Walden University.

Drotar, D., Crawford, P., & Ganofsky, M. A. (1984). Prevention with chronically ill children. In: M. C. Roberts, & L. Peterson (Eds.). *Prevention of problems in children* (232–265). New York, NY: John Wiley & Sons.

Dunst, C. J., Cushing, P. J., & Vance, S. D. (1985). Response-contingent learning in profoundly handicapped infants: A social systems perspective. *Analysis and Intervention in Developmental Disabilities, 5,* 33–47.

Fine S. B. (1991). Resilience and human adaptability: Who rises above adversity? *American Journal of Occupational Therapy, 45,* 493–503.

Garmezy N. & Rutter M., (Eds.). (1983). *Stress, coping, and development in children.* New York, NY: McGraw-Hill.

Haan, N. (1977). Coping and defending: *Processes of self-environment organization.* New York, NY: Academic Press.

Hanzlik, J. R. (1989). Interactions between mothers and their infants with developmental disabilities: Analysis and review. *Physical and Occupational Therapy in Pediatrics, 9*(4), 33–47.

Hildebrand, V. (1975). *Guiding young children.* New York, NY: Macmillan.

Kennedy B. (1984). The relationship of coping behaviors and attribution of success to effort and school achievement of elementary school children [Dissertation]. Albany, New York, NY: State University of New York.

Larson J. G. (1984). Relationship between coping behavior and academic achievement in kindergarten children [Dissertation]. Teaneck, NJ: Fairleigh Dickinson University.

Lazarus R. S., & Folkman, S. (1984). *Stress, appraisal and coping.* New York, NY: Springer Publishing.

Lorch, N. (1981). Coping behavior in preschool children with cerebral palsy [Dissertation]. Hempstead, NY: Hofstra University.

MacTurk, R. H., Vietze, P. M., McCarthy, M. E., McQuiston, S., & Yarrow, L. J. (1985). The organization of exploratory behavior in Down syndrome and nondelayed infants. *Child Development, 56,* 573–581.

Moos, R. H., & Billings, A. G. (1982). Conceptualizing and measuring coping resources and processes. In: L. Goldberger, & S. Breznitz (Eds.). *Handbook of stress: Theoretical and clinical aspects.* (pp. 212–230). New York, NY: Free Press.

Murphy L. B., & Moriarty, A. E. (1976). *Vulnerability, coping, and growth.* New Haven, CT: Yale University Press.

Olsen, D., & McCubbin, H. (1983). *Families: What makes them work.* Beverly Hills, CA: Sage Publications.

Piers, E., & Harris, D. (1969). *The Piers-Harris children's self-concept inventory.* Nashville, TN: Counselor Recordings and Tests, 1969.

Ramey, C. T., Beckman-Bell, P., & Gowen, J. W. (1980). Infant characteristics and infant caregiver interactions. In: J. J. Gallagher (Ed.). *Parents and families of handicapped children. New directions for exceptional children.* Vol. 4 (pp.59–83). San Francisco, CA: Jossey-Bass.

Rosenberg, S. A, & Robinson, C. C. (1988). Interactions of parents with their young handicapped children. In: S. L. Odom, M. B. Karnes (Eds.) *Early intervention for infants and children with handicaps* (159–177). Baltimore, MD: Paul H. Brookes.

Schaffer, M. P., & Schaffer, S. J. (1982). Stress related to organically-based learning disabilities. In: A. S. McNamee (Ed.) *Children and stress: Helping children cope* (pp. 8–18). Washington, DC: Association for Childhood Education International.

Shahmoon, S. R. (1990). Parenthood: A process marking identity and intimacy capacities. *Zero to Three, 11*(2), 1–9.

Turnbull, A. P., & Turnbull, H. R. (1990). *Families, professionals, and exceptionality: A special partnership* (2nd ed.). Columbus, OH: Merrill Publishing.

Werner, E. E., & Smith, R. S. (1982). *Vulnerable but invincible: A study of resilient children.* New York, NY: McGraw-Hill.

Williamson, G. G. (Ed.) (1987). *Children with spina bifida: Early intervention and preschool programming.* Baltimore, MD: Paul H. Brookes.

Williamson, G. G., Zeitlin, S., & Szczepanski, M. (1989). Coping behavior: Implications for disabled infants and toddlers. *Infant Mental Health Journal, 10,* 3–13.

Yeargan, D. R. (1982). A factor-analytic study of adaptive behavior and intellectual functioning in learning disabled children [Dissertation]. Denton, TX: North Texas State University.

Zeitlin S. (1985). *Coping inventory.* Bensenville, IL: Scholastic Testing Service.

Zeitlin, S., & Williamson, G. G. (1988). Developing family resources for adaptive coping. *Journal of the Division for Early Childhood, 12,* 137–146.

Zeitlin, S., & Williamson, G. G. (1990). Coping characteristics of disabled and nondisabled young children. *American Journal of Orthopsychiatry, 60,* 404–411.

Zeitlin, S., Williamson, G. G., & Rosenblatt, W. P. (1987). The coping with stress model: A counseling approach for families with a handicapped child. *Journal of Counseling and Development, 65,* 443–446.

Zeitlin, S., Williamson, G. G., & Szczepanski, M. (1988). *Early coping inventory.* Bensenville, IL: Scholastic Testing Service.

# PRACTICE APPLICATION

# 12

# From Frames of Reference to Actual Intervention

JIM HINOJOSA / PAULA KRAMER

This chapter discusses the importance of appropriate use of frames of reference in practice. The first section focuses on the importance of understanding the frame of reference so that the therapist can articulate it clearly when treating a child. The second section focuses on the art of practice with children, with emphasis on the therapeutic relationship.

## Articulating the Frame of Reference

When students and entry-level occupational therapists are asked to explain what they are doing with a child, or why they are doing a particular activity, some common responses are "I'm not sure"; "It was just intuition"; "I know why, but I just can't put it into words"; "I saw another therapist do it and it worked well"; or "I was taught this in school, and my instructor said it works well." It is uncomfortable to be put on the spot and often difficult to respond quickly to such a complex question. As professionals, however, therapists are obliged to understand what they are doing and why they are doing it. They also need to be able to explain the rationale for what they are doing and why they are doing it to observers, especially to parents and other professionals.

In a recent clinical experience, a fieldwork student was asked to explain what she would do during a treatment session. She stated that she intended to play with the child, because the child would benefit from all types of stimulation. This response indicated a lack of understanding about the child's individual needs and a lack of clearly articulated goals. Furthermore, this suggests that the intervention was not well thought out or theoretically based. Any response or reaction from the child in this treatment situation, therefore, could not be explained from a theoretical perspective.

In this example, the student's apparent lack of understanding or inability to articulate a rationale for intervention may have resulted from a theoretical perspective that had not been identified clearly. This student has predetermined that the child will benefit from any sensory stimulation but has not stated specific problem areas or expected responses from the child based on the intervention. Intervention cannot be viewed in such a simplistic way. It is a step-by-step approach that is geared towards identifying problem areas, and providing a well-thought-out intervention designed to bring about change. As already mentioned, the structure for developing this organized systematic approach to intervention is the frame of reference.

Returning to the example, the student may have had a clear idea of what her goals were with the child, but without the structure of the frame of reference, her intervention appears to have no theoretical rationale for treatment. Furthermore, based on her intervention, she would have difficulty measuring change without this theoretical structure.

In another example, a student was asked to explain why she placed a child who had cerebral palsy in a prone position on an adapted scooter board. She responded that it seemed like the appropriate position for the child. When the instructor explored this further, asking for additional clarification of what theoretical framework the student was using, the student was able to explain that this developmentally appropriate position facilitated the child's exploration of the environment and that she was using the **biomechanical frame of reference** to allow the child to interact with and learn from his environment. Although the first response indicated her initial intuition, when pressed for details, the student was able to demonstrate a theoretical understanding of the intervention. Student intuition often is really knowledge based.

When students or therapists respond that their actions are based on intuition, they are not recognizing their knowledge base. At times, students and therapists do not appreciate what they have learned during their professional education, so they see their actions as being intuitive. In actuality, their decisions are knowledge based, but for some reason, it is difficult at that moment to articulate the theoretical rationale for the actions. Identification of the frame of reference, which is grounded in theory, again allows the therapist to cite clearly her knowledge base and rationale for treatment.

In addition, therapists sometimes undermine their interventions when they give simplistic rationales for what they do with a child. Much of occupational therapy looks like play to the casual observer. When the therapist says that she is playing with the child to provide stimulation, the response of the casual observer might be that anyone can play with a child and provide stimulation in that way. When the therapist acknowledges that she is working from a theoretical base, however, she can demonstrate that play designed to provide specific stimulation really is a highly skilled and well-thought-out intervention plan designed to bring about specific responses. **The purpose of the frame of reference is to provide this blueprint for practice.**

When therapists are asked what their frame of reference is, they may respond, "I'm eclectic." In some cases, the therapist has not identified the various frames of reference on which her interventions are based. When this is the situation, the therapist may not have a clearly thought-out intervention plan. She may not be using a frame of reference or may not have a clear understanding of the theoretical rationale for the intervention. At other times, a therapist may label her approach as eclectic, because she bases her interventions on various sources without synthesizing them into a clearly articulated frame of reference. Again, therapeutic interventions should be based on clearly articulated frames of reference that include well-delineated theoretical bases. If the therapist picks and chooses concepts, postulates, and techniques from various approaches without concern for the consistency of the theories on which they are based, then specific outcomes cannot be anticipated. The theoretical base of a frame of reference is built on theories that agree with each other and that present a unified approach to the change process (**consistency**). When the therapist uses various approaches without concern for consistency, change cannot be explained theoretically. **The frame of reference delineates what outcomes can be expected from each specified intervention.** The statement, "I'm eclectic," tends to indicate a lack of theory based intervention.

Just as a physician should not prescribe medication without knowing its consequences, so should a therapist not use a procedure without understanding its consequences. The therapist selects a frame of reference based on the child's presenting problems and on the specified changes or outcomes that she would like to promote. Techniques or procedures not derived from a frame of reference usually do not lead to organized change in a way that can be explained. At times, a misunderstood procedure can have consequences similar to a misused medication, such as when a neurophysiological technique like **vestibular stimulation** is used without a clear rationale for an expected response. To use vestibular stimulation without an understanding of the sensory integration frame of reference may result in an inappropriate behavioral response or a more severe central nervous system reaction.

Finally, because occupational therapy is concerned with and uses routine daily activities as the focus for intervention, it may appear to lack the scientific, empirical base of procedures used by other professions that are labeled **therapeutic.** Because occupational therapy with children is activity oriented and often uses play, it is crucial that the therapeutic value of chosen activities be readily explainable. The frame of reference provides the scientific, theoretical basis that explains the complexity of the activities used in the intervention process. What appears to be simple usually has complex theoretical underpinnings that are clarified for the therapist through the frame of reference, which brings the theories to a level at which they can be applied.

# The Art of Practice with Children

Previous chapters in this book presented specific frames of reference that are important to current pediatric practice. Working with children effectively involves more than knowing about and understanding frames of reference; it also requires an understanding of how to put them into practice effectively. Other occupational therapists have discussed and highlighted the art of practice in a global way as it applies to the whole profession of occupational therapy (Crepeau, 1991; Gilfoyle, 1980; Mosey, 1981a, 1981b; Peloquin, 1989, 1990). For example, Mosey presents the art of practice in a broad perspective, as part of the philosophical origins of the profession (1981a). The authors in this chapter intend to discuss the art of practice in much more specific ways, as it relates to children and as it relates to the implementation of the frames of reference.

Now that specific frames of reference have been presented in previous chapters, the art of working with children needs to be addressed. Working with children presents interesting challenges that are different from working with adults. **Children are not just miniature adults and they need to be approached in a way that is meaningful to them.** Just like adults, children have thoughts and feelings that must be taken into consideration, even though they may not be able to express them.

The therapeutic relationship is an interactive process between therapist and child. The goal is to assist effectively the promotion of positive change within the child. It does not necessarily involve equal participation of therapist and child. It is the therapist's responsibility to establish the tone of the relationship. The therapist guides the relationship, to some extent manipulating it to the child's benefit. Initially, it is important to engage the child, to get to know him, and to involve him in the intervention process. The therapist often acts as a stimulator and cheerleader—that is, a provoker of responses. At other times, the therapist must be more relaxed and give comfort.

To engage the child in effective intervention is the essence of artful practice for an occupational therapist. Unlike most adults, children may not necessarily see therapy as beneficial. The art of occupational therapy involves captivating the child through toys, objects, and games, or through the therapist's own actions so that the child becomes involved in the therapeutic process. This art is almost intangible and, therefore, difficult to describe. It is more than a skill, it is a mix of creativity, enthusiasm, an ability to choose objects based on a firm foundation of knowledge, and the use of self in a way that engages the child so that a relationship can be developed and intervention can promote growth. The "trick" is to appreciate the fact that the child has to be dealt with as a **whole person,** not as component parts or as an aspect of an occupational performance area. And, this must be done with each child individually, because each child is a unique human being.

The therapeutic relationship is important to the intervention process in any frame of reference. In some cases, it may be addressed specifically in the change process of the theoretical base, although, in many cases, it is not discussed at all. In specific frames of reference in which it is addressed, a particular type of relationship may exist that helps foster development. For example, in the sensory integrative frame of reference, as presented in Chapter 6, the therapist takes an active part in treatment and needs to engage playfully with the child. At the same time, she must allow the child to be self-directed in the treatment setting. In those situations in which the therapeutic relationship is not discussed, it is incumbent on the therapist to formulate a relationship that promotes growth and change and that is consistent in that frame of reference. The art of practice, as discussed here, relates broadly to all frames of reference.

Many characteristics color an effective therapeutic relationship. Perlman (1979) describes these characteristics as warmth, acceptance, caring/concern, and genuineness. Mosey (1981a) adds sympathy and empathy. It often is difficult to describe a therapeutic relationship because its uniqueness depends on its special components—the therapist and child. To say that it is an emotional experience based on feelings and interactions is to state the obvious. The therapeutic relationship involves not only sympathy but also empathy. Sympathy occurs when people share common feelings that often involve commiseration. Empathy involves the projection of one personality onto another in an effort to understand the feelings, emotions, and thoughts of another human being. Often, especially with entry-level therapists, sympathy is a strong initial part of the therapeutic relationship; however, it is important to move on to the point at which the therapist can be empathetic, because it is empathy that assists the therapist in being more effective in her interactions with the child.

Unconditional acceptance is an essential aspect of the relationship between therapist and child. The therapist accepts the child and his abilities "as is." This precludes a judgmental attitude about the child and his life style. Granted, the role of the therapist is to develop the strengths of the child and to remediate or minimize the deficits. The therapist, however, should not base her ability to care and interact on what the child is able to do or how he progresses. When a child cannot do particular tasks or has experienced previous failures, he is less likely to try that activity again. The therapist needs to let the child know that the *attempt* to do something is more important than the activity itself.

The manner in which the occupational therapist uses the legitimate tools of the profession is part of the art of practice. As adapted by the occupational therapist, the nonhuman environment becomes a component in the art of practice. Some frames of reference delineate the therapeutic nonhuman environment. For example, the biomechanical frame of reference, as presented in Chapter 8, describes as part of the nonhuman environment the use of specific equipment to promote positive change in the child. Other frames of reference do not address the specific environment but may make implications about or give guidelines for effective types of environments. To use any frames of reference effectively as presented in this book, the therapist must create a safe therapeutic environment. To raise this legitimate tool to the level of art, the therapist must use her understanding of the frame of reference, along with her creativity, to manipulate the environment so that it engages the child and promotes growth.

It takes time and experience to develop the art of practice. It is not something that can be presumed of an entry-level therapist, although, like some painters or musicians, some therapists have an innate talent for the art of practice. It is safe to say that the art of practice is not just skilled application of the frames of reference; rather, it is a combination of knowledge, self-confidence, self-understanding, self-acceptance, and awareness. It is hoped that the entry-level therapist becomes involved actively in exploring this process to become an artful practitioner.

### References

Crepeau, E. B. (1991). Achieving intersubjective understanding: Examples from an occupational therapy treatment session. *American Journal of Occupational Therapy, 45,* 1016–1025.

Gilfoyle, E. M. (1980). Caring: A philosophy for practice. *American Journal of Occupational Therapy, 34,* 517–521.

Mosey, A. C. (1981a). *Occupational therapy: Configuration of a profession.* New York: Raven Press.

Mosey, A. C. (1981b). Introduction: The art of practice. In B. Abreu (Ed.). *Physical disabilities manual* (pp. 1–3). New York, NY: Raven Press.

Peloquin, S. M. (1989). Sustaining the art of practice in occupational therapy. *American Journal of Occupational Therapy, 43,* 219–226.

Peloquin, S. M. (1990). The patient-therapist relationship in occupational therapy: Understanding visions and images. *American Journal of Occupational Therapy, 44,* 13–21.

Perlman, H. H. (1979). *Relationship: the heart of helping people.* Chicago, IL: The University of Chicago Press.

# 13

# Alternative Applications of Frames of Reference

PAULA KRAMER / JIM HINOJOSA

Effective practice involves the therapist's ability to match the client with the most appropriate frame of reference within the context of his life. After a patient is referred to occupational therapy, the therapist does a preliminary screening. This helps her determine the appropriate frame of reference, and thereby, the evaluation tools that should be used for the particular client. Sometimes, this can be one specific frame of reference, but at other times, one frame of reference is not adequate enough to deal with the complexity of problems presented by the child or his family. This chapter discusses the alternative ways that frames of reference can be applied, including the use of frames of reference alone, in sequence, in parallel, and in combination. In addition, the chapter discusses the development of new and unique frames of reference.

## Single Frame of Reference

To be comfortable with and understand how to use frames of reference, the entry-level therapist must first work with *one frame of reference at a time.* An important distinction needs to be made here: the therapist does not use only one frame of reference with all clients. For instance, with any given child, an entry-level therapist must first concentrate on the one frame of reference that fits that particular child's needs. With another child, that same therapist may need to use another frame of reference that is more suitable.

Entry-level therapists often are not fluent with theories relevant to pediatric practice. In the clinic, their primary concern, is how to help the child. This concern tends to focus them on **what** they are doing rather than on the reasons **why** they are doing something—that is, whether the practice is (or is not) effective. To become truly competent, however, novice therapists must take the time to familiarize themselves with all aspects of the frame of reference. To do this, entry-level therapists almost always have to start by using one frame of reference with each client. As discussed in Chapter 4, the frame of reference provides a **blueprint for practice** based on theoretical material.

When a therapist begins to use a frame of reference, she first should become comfortable with the entire frame of reference by concentrating on the theoretical base. Once the theoretical base is clearly understood, then the other sections of the frame of reference (function/dysfunction continua, evaluation, postulates regarding change, and application to practice) are easier to understand. The theoretical base, therefore, holds the key to understanding the important concepts for intervention. All important concepts are defined. Assumptions are stated in that section and the significant relationships between concepts and postulates are presented and described. The function/dysfunction continua, evaluation, postulates regarding change, and application to practice all flow from the theoretical base.

By studying one frame of reference at a time, the therapist can become comfortable with the theoretical material and its transition into application. Through her understanding of this material, the therapist develops the ability to use each function/dysfunction continuum systematically as a means to identify the child's strengths and limitations. Based on her findings relative to the function/dysfunction continua, the therapist then can determine what areas (if any) require intervention. Intervention is applied sequentially, using the postulates regarding change as illustrated in the application to practice. At this point, the therapist creates an environment to bring about a desired response from the child. This empirical approach to intervention based on theory differentiates the skilled, competent professional from the highly technical practitioner. The skilled, competent professional bases her intervention on a firm theoretical base that allows for a careful evaluation of the intervention process and its efficacy.

When one frame of reference is used properly, as outlined in this text, consistency in intervention is ensured. Concepts and postulates, as well as postulates regarding change, agree, and consistency exists in that one segment flows from the other. As long as the therapist works with one frame of reference, all actions agree, and the theoretical principles and the application to intervention are congruent. This consistency could not be achieved if a therapist took only one concept or postulate from one section and then proceeded to application. For example, in the neurodevelopmental frame of reference, **handling** is a major concept. By itself, handling does not comprise the entire frame of reference. If the therapist uses handling without the other therapeutic constructs from the theoretical base or the postulates regarding change, it is just a technique and not a way to apply the neurodevelopmental frame of reference.

It is important to note that when only one frame of reference is used, it ensures that concepts and postulates and postulates regarding change are all consistent and that the end result will be a more cogent intervention process. If, during the course of intervention, the therapist notices that something is not working, then she can go back to the frame of reference, and particularly to the theoretical base, postulates regarding change, and the application to practice sections, which should provide some insight for modifying the plan for intervention. An example of how successful a single frame of reference can be is found in Chapter 16.

Once a therapist becomes competent in using a frame of reference and is comfortable in her thorough understanding of its application, she may tend to use it exclusively with all children. Unfortunately, this would deter her from deciding, on an individual basis, which frame of reference is most appropriate for each client. At times, such exclusivity could create a certain "tunnel vision"—that is, the therapist may come to believe that the one frame of reference is superior to all others. In this case, she may identify with that frame of reference and begin to refer to herself as a "neurodevelopmental therapist" or a "sensory integration therapist," for instance, instead of an **occupational therapist.** When this occurs, the therapist may be overlooking the individual needs of the child and, instead, be working from a strong belief dedicated to one specific frame of reference. The dangers of this are twofold: (1) the child may not receive intervention that meets his needs, and (2) the therapist may not recognize the extent of her knowledge base in terms of other frames of reference. This may preclude any chance of meeting her client's needs.

# Multiple Frames of Reference

In the real world, many children cannot have their needs met through only one frame of reference. The problems of real children often are more complex than those of "paper patients" (i.e., the classic textbook case). It would be easier if one frame of reference could address all the problems of a particular child, but, in reality, frames of reference are limited by the scope of their theoretical bases. For example, in the sensory integrative frame of reference, activities of daily living (ADL) are not addressed comprehensively in the theoretical base. The theoretical base for sensory integration suggests that when a child has developed end-product abilities, he is then able to accomplish age-appropriate skills, which should allow him to perform ADL. Although this may happen for some children, other children require additional direct intervention to bring them up to an age-appropriate level in these specific tasks. This requires the use of an additional frame of reference, perhaps one that addresses specific skill acquisition. Such an additional frame of reference would have to focus on teaching the child specific skills to perform ADL successfully. In these situations, the occupational therapist must resort to more than one frame of reference.

To construct a relevant plan of intervention for a child who has multiple problems in the real world often requires more than one frame of reference (Mosey, 1986). When a frame of reference is used in the pure sense, as each chapter in this book suggests, then it may deal with some of the child's most significant problems at the time, but it frequently is not adequate for the entire course of treatment. Whenever the therapist considers the use of combined or sequenced frames of reference, it is necessary to develop a basic understanding of what each frame of reference entails, along with its unique approach to intervention.

## Frames of Reference in Sequence

Frames of reference can be used in sequence—that is, one frame of reference is used primarily and another frame of reference is used for a separate and more discrete problem. For example, a child who has cerebral palsy may be treated first with the neurodevelopmental frame of reference. After seeing the child for several months, the therapist observes that the child also appears to be having visual perceptual problems. She evaluates the child appropriately based on the visual perception frame of reference. In this situation, the therapist decides to continue with the neurodevelopmental frame of reference but, in addition, decides to use the visual perception frame of reference. Each frame of reference addresses different performance components and draws from different theories. Furthermore, each is based on different developmental perspectives and a belief that change occurs in different ways. The study of these two frames of reference leads the therapist to understand that neither is congruent with the other in its approach to the change process. They are not in conflict, however, when applied separately. Conflict is when constructs or postulates do not agree because they are contradictory from a theoretical perspective. In this situation, each frame of reference views the change process in a different way, therefore, neither one is compatible with the other should the therapist attempt to integrate them. The therapist decides, therefore, to use these frames of reference in sequence, with the neurodevelopmental frame of reference as her basic approach. She decides to begin each session with the neurodevelopmental frame of reference, and toward the end of the session, switches to the visual perception frame of reference. Each aspect of the intervention is clearly delineated, grounded in the theoretical base of each frame of reference. This clear demarcation is evident in the environment that the therapist creates for change and her use of legitimate tools. During the neurodevelopmental portion of the treatment session, the child and therapist may be on a mat, with the therapist using rolls, balls, and therapeutic handling in play activities. During the visual perception portion of the treatment session, the child may sit at a table and participate in drawing activities. The techniques and activities of intervention from each frame of reference are not integrated. The therapist is always aware of the frame of reference used at any given point in the session.

The characteristics of sequential intervention require that one frame of reference be designated as primary, followed by others that address discrete problems in a set order. Each frame of reference maintains its own integrity, and the therapeutic goals are separate. The intervention and the legitimate tools are distinct and are clearly tied to each unique theoretical base.

## *Frames of Reference in Parallel*

Frames of reference can be use in parallel—that is, two frames of reference are used at the same time to address similar or related problems from different perspectives. Each frame of reference is used separately in different treatment sessions or even in separate intervention processes. Although these frames of reference may not share the same theoretical perspectives, they do not conflict. Two frames of reference often used in parallel are the neurodevelopmental and biomechanical frames of reference. A therapist may treat a child who has cerebral palsy by using the neurodevelopmental frame of reference. She has selected this frame of reference to enhance the child's movement abilities and to assist the child in developing as many normal patterns as possible. During the course of treatment, the therapist reasons that the child would benefit from adaptive equipment. She selects the biomechanical frame of reference to determine what equipment or devices might provide proper positioning for the child, so that motor skills are improved.

The primary tool of the neurodevelopmental frame of reference is therapeutic handling, whereas the biomechanical frame of reference relies on specific devices and therapeutic equipment to position the child. This is not meant to oversimplify either frame of reference but, rather, to point out that they do not conflict with one another and that they work toward similar goals and, therefore, can be used well in parallel fashion. In this case, the neurodevelopmental frame of reference addresses the child's primary motor development, while the biomechanical frame of reference is used to address the child's static positioning needs. The neurodevelopmental frame of reference guides the therapist's regularly scheduled treatment sessions, whereas the biomechanical frame of reference provides proper seating equipment that positions the child throughout the day. Separately, each frame of reference addresses separate aspects of the child's motor performance; jointly, the two frames of reference facilitate intervention. (An example of frames of reference used in parallel is illustrated in Chapters 16 and 17).

## Frames of Reference in Combination

Frames of reference can be used in combination in an integrative way. This can be done when the constructs of the theoretical base are consistent in that they agree about how change occurs. To use frames of reference in combination requires a skillful, experienced therapist who clearly understands each frame of reference. The therapist has to examine each frame of reference to determine whether its basic postulates are congruent with those of the other frames of reference. To use the postulates regarding change together, the basic concepts should be consistent in that they all state the same or similar things.

An example of this is demonstrated in the case study of Joshua in Chapter 18, which illustrates the frames of reference for sensory integration and neurodevelopmental treatment used in combination. Both are developmentally oriented and propose that specific skills and abilities are achieved in a normal sequence. When frames of reference are used in combination, the techniques of both frames of reference are integrated during each session. The coping frame of reference (Chapter 9) is an example of how one frame of reference can be used frequently in combination with others.

The main characteristic of combined intervention is that two separate yet integrated frames of reference address the child as a whole. Both frames of reference are consistent with each other, and the therapeutic goals are integrated. The intervention is a blend that involves the combined use of various legitimate tools.

A skilled, competent therapist who combines two frames of reference over time may begin to view them as one. This is truly the use of two frames of reference in combination. To make this into one "new" frame of reference, the therapist must reconstruct the theoretical base, carefully exploring the concepts, postulates, and assumptions from each to interweave them into a unified theoretical base that is internally consistent. From that point, she must reformulate the entire frame of reference. This process is intense and requires postprofessional education and scholarship.

# Formulation of Original Frames of Reference

The formulation of new and original frames of reference is an ongoing process for occupational therapy, because, as discussed previously it is a dynamic profession, and the endemic problems change continuously. This section discusses the need for new frames of reference and serves as an overview for the process of developing new frames of reference. Additional information can be found in discussions of applied scientific inquiry for occupational therapy (Mosey 1989; 1992).

Over time, knowledge increases and technology advances. This creates change not only in society but also in the problems with which occupational therapists are concerned. One example is the recent technological strides made in neonatal intensive care that have resulted in the survival of more low-birthweight babies. This new population, with its unique needs, requires specialized intervention, which has been handled in several ways. Some therapists have modified or reformulated traditional frames of reference around the specific problems of low-birthweight infants. Other therapists have begun to evolve new frames of reference, based on new theoretical information, to work with this specific population. Each case requires advanced knowledge and skills.

As society changes, the profession adapts, mandating the search for new approaches and solutions to problems. This situation requires that occupational therapists develop new frames of reference. Infants born addicted to cocaine or those born with HIV infection are examples of "new" client groups. Another reason that might stimulate the development of new frames of reference is the need to change or add new legitimate tools, or when the context or setting for therapy is changed.

A change in knowledge also precipitates the need for new frames of reference. This "new" knowledge may result from the refinement of theory, the development of new theories, or new research findings that modify the theoretical bases of old frames of reference. This may also occur when a therapist finds that specific postulates regarding change from a frame of reference no longer work, or when she is unable to find one that addresses a particular dysfunction.

The process of developing and articulating a frame of reference is complex. It requires a strong, scholarly knowledge base combined with advanced clinical reasoning skills. It follows the sequence discussed in Chapter 4, concentrating first on raw theoretical information, which is woven into a comprehensive and cohesive theoretical base. From this sound foundation, the therapist formulates the rest of the function/dysfunction continua, identifies behaviors indicative of function and dysfunction, specifies evaluation procedures and tools, writes postulates regarding change, and outlines an application for practice. Throughout this process, the therapist is concerned about the systematic ordering of concepts and constructs combined with internal consistency so that a clear design can be formed to link theory to practice.

## Summary

With experience, therapists become more adept at identifying client problems and figuring out ways to deal with different deficits. The novice therapist begins her understanding of the intervention process by using a single frame of reference for each client. After she becomes comfortable with the theories that guide pediatric practice, the therapist can experiment with different ways to use various frames of reference, including sequential, parallel, and combined uses. The sophisticated, scholarly therapist eventually may move toward formulating a new frame of reference to guide intervention in new areas of practice.

### References

Mosey, A. C. (1986). *Psychosocial components of occupational therapy*. New York, NY: Raven Press.
Mosey, A. C. (1989). The proper focus of scientific inquiry in occupational therapy: Frames of reference (Editorial). *Occupational Therapy Journal of Research, 9*, 195–201.
Mosey, A. C. (1992). *Applied scientific inquiry in health professions: An epistemological orientation*. Rockville, MD: American Occupational Therapy Association.

# 14

# Influence of Settings on the Application of Frames of Reference

MARY MUHLENHAUPT

Pediatric occupational therapy services are delivered in various settings, ranging from home-based programs, public and private schools, to hospitals, clinics, and other agencies. Each setting belongs to a larger system, such as a family unit, a community based health care network, an urban school district, or a university-affiliated medical center. The larger system has an established philosophy, objectives, and governing regulations to provide direction and rationale for its existence. These factors are stated formally *and* implied. Based on the system's orientation, a model of thinking, operating procedures, resources, rules, and standards exist to define the setting as well as the services available to consumers in the system. Although these considerations may seem remote in relation to the daily practice of occupational therapy with children, they provide a structure that grounds a program's occupational therapy services. Ultimately, the influences that distinguish the system have implications for all phases of the occupational therapy process, from initial referral, to initial screening, to the selection of the appropriate frame of reference, to treatment implementation, through discharge planning, and termination of services.

In addition to knowledge regarding frames of reference used in pediatric occupational therapy services, an understanding of the systems and settings in which therapy services are provided contributes to the development of programs that represent "best practice." The frames of reference used in occupational therapy intervention are reinforced when applied in a system and setting whose orientations and beliefs are similar or complementary, and whose resources are adequate to support the intervention program. In contrast, treatment based on a particular frame of reference may not fit in another location based on differing or opposing values, beliefs, and resources. A good "fit" between system and frame of reference in terms of function and dysfunction is an important element. To illustrate, the neurodevelopmental frame of reference is used to guide occupational therapy intervention in a regional medical center's pediatric head injury clinic. In this situation, the occupational therapist's colleagues, physicians, and other allied health professionals share and value the focus of occupational therapy evaluations and interventions. Staff members understand the treatment goals and strategies used by coworkers, a factor that facilitates communication and planning among professionals and provides an opportunity for reinforcement of neurodevelopmental treatment strategies by other services, such as speech therapy. The occupational therapist collaborates with the speech pathologist to develop appropriate plans for carry-over activities to develop upper extremity motor functions consistent with the neurodevelopmental treatment frame of reference. Following this interchange, rather than present an auditory processing card game in a chair-and-table position, the speech pathologist may incorporate alternate positioning strategies for upper body weightbearing, weightshifting, and reaching as the child selects a response from an array of cards located across the table or floor surface.

Another situation concerns an urban home-based occupational therapy program for a seven-year-old boy who has mild learning disabilities. Based on the child's learning disabilities, the referring physician has suggested that occupational therapy be provided by using a sensory integration frame of reference. Because of the family situation and because the therapy concerns are not educationally related, a particular therapist, who has experience with this frame of reference, has been asked to provide the intervention at home rather than in the school. The therapist must use public transportation to travel to the family's home, and to travel with numerous supplies and large pieces of equipment is not realistic. Furthermore, the family's apartment lacks the needed space to allow for many types of sensory integration treatment activities. Both parents work, and the child is supervised after school by a care provider who speaks limited English. The family has requested that the therapist work with the care provider to support the boy's developing independence in many self-care tasks at home. The planned application of the sensory integration frame of reference conflicts with the practice setting and the family concerns. The frame of reference chosen for intervention needs to be compatible with the practice setting, the needs of the child, and the concerns of the family. The therapist must choose another frame of reference appropriate for this child or the setting for intervention must be changed.

Characteristics of children's therapy programs may be anticipated and "expectations of practice" may be developed with some degree of reliability, depending on the system and setting in which the service is provided. How does program location influence the type of occupational therapy service provided to children? How do expectations of practice develop, and what effect do they have on occupational therapy services and on the individual therapist in the system? To help answer these questions, the concepts of general systems theory can be applied (von Bertalanffy, 1968) to occupational therapy programs and to pediatric medical, health care, and educational systems.

Webster's New Twentieth Century Dictionary (2nd ed., p. 1853) defines a system as "a set or arrangement of things so related or connected as to form a unity." General systems theory, as discussed by von Bertalanffy, focuses on understanding an animate or inanimate object by examining its "wholeness" rather than by breaking it into isolated and independent parts. This theory is concerned with how the components of a system work together to contribute to its maintenance and function.

Von Bertalanffy describes the open system as a complex of interacting elements characterized by relationships with its internal *and* external environments. Interdependence between elements is an important concept in this approach. By definition, elements in an open system must be interdependent with one another and with the external environment. In relating this idea to pediatric health care practice, the occupational therapist and the therapy program have a reciprocal relationship with other personnel and programs provided by the agency.

Another important systems concept is **equifinality** (von Bertalanffy, 1968). Equifinality is a desirable outcome that results when each element of the system uses its unique capabilities in concert with the demands of the environment to achieve an organized state. In practice, the therapist applies and adapts occupational therapy principles to support the agency's mission when developing the therapy program. The way in which therapy beliefs and approaches are integrated with those of the system contributes to the life and definition of the system. Without a fit between the two, the system (including all its component parts) does not function in an orderly and effective way and, therefore, does not reach its potential. Through internal and external resources alike, the open system receives feedback to stimulate further activity, evaluate its function, and adjust its course of action, as needed, toward equifinality.

To extend even further Webster's definition and von Bertalanffy's principles of general systems theory to pediatric therapy practice, the local public elementary school can be used as an example of equifinality. Parents, occupational therapists, classroom teachers and physical education instructors are some of the elements in this system. Using their unique resources, each contributes to the education of children in the program (**input**). The way that each group uses these resources in its work, combines knowledge and expertise, and collaborates to develop a quality education program all impact on the school's operation and influence its ability to serve children and the community (**interdependence leading to system maintenance or disarray**). Shared values, beliefs, and objectives among these elements contribute to harmonious relationships and facilitate the school's ability to achieve its stated mission. Communication among the elements of the system guarantees optimal function of the system and its components. The successful result of this school experience is seen when students graduate with the requisite skills and abilities to continue in junior high school education programs (**output**).

## Locus of Pediatric Practice

Pediatric occupational therapy practice may be organized according to system models that reflect differing orientations, values, beliefs, and treatment foci. The values, beliefs, ideals, and biases that characterize and define a system model—its approach toward a problem and its resolution—are passed to occupational therapy practitioners during academic and clinical experiences. These attributes become part of the entry-level professional's identity, providing subtle yet obvious directions that characterize and influence thinking, choice of frames of reference, and approach to problems encountered in work situations. Professional identities may be refined and modified by experience and knowledge gained in practice and through advanced postprofessional education. These additional insights sometimes alter the practitioner's treatment approaches and lead to a deeper understanding of system characteristics.

Medical and educational model perspectives are discussed here as the two most common perspectives for practice. The names of these perspectives do not necessarily correspond exactly with the types of settings in which pediatric occupational therapy programs are found. For instance, medical model thinking is not restricted to application in hospital and clinic-based practices. Influences from the medical model perspective are adopted by the practitioner and, from there, she may develop a school-based occupational therapy program grounded in the medical model perspective. Similarly, educational model perspectives also are rooted in the therapist's orientation and may be found in home-based practice or in occupational therapy programs in the hospital environment. Therapists must consider approaches used in practice carefully, selecting and applying frames of reference that are compatible with the overall principles and objectives that characterize the treatment system. When system models are understood, analysis can be made of possible and probable influences on (1) an agency's philosophy and objectives, (2) a therapist's thinking approach, and, subsequently, (3) the ways in which an occupational therapy program may be designed and applied in a specific system. Using this information, the therapist may integrate various principles of evaluation, program planning, and intervention with the sponsoring agency's mission.

## Medical Model Perspective

The belief that the whole organism's function and operational behavior depend on the integrity of its underlying parts is a central concept in medical model thinking (Starr, 1982). The presenting problem is examined by breaking the organism into its component parts and analyzing those underlying functions believed to contribute to the expression of observed behaviors. Testing is diagnostic to identify and define symptomatology within elements of the whole organism. Environmental conditions that support or impede performance are not a central concern. Therapists in a medical model tend to select frames of reference based on neurophysiology and neuropsychology, or on neuromotor and other theories that explain causal relationships.

Frames of reference in systems based on medical model thinking tend to be concerned with the identification of pathology, or dysfunction, in any of the neuromuscular systems that contribute to the child's task performance. For example, when a child has a problem with self-care tasks, such as shoe tying, the therapist should select a frame of reference concerned with neuromuscular function that enables the child to learn and master shoe tying. The frame of reference chosen should not actually teach the task but, rather, the underlying components. The frame of reference selected should guide the therapist to evaluate the way in which the child receives and processes tactile and proprioceptive stimuli; it also should address how that information is used as feedback to initiate, monitor, and adjust motor activity in the eyes, arms, hands, and fingers. Muscle strength, endurance, and the ability to plan automatically and carry out coordinated sequences of motor activity also should be examined.

Based on the frame of reference, the medical model intervention focuses on those components that reflect dysfunction and those believed to contribute to problem behavior. Once the dysfunctional components are resolved, the child's development continues and he can participate in expected activities. Intervention does not focus on skill mastery or on the external environment that influences human performance. Ideally, the desired outcome of the treatment process is the ability to perform tasks spontaneously across environments and in novel situations, not the acquisition of location-specific skills and behaviors. With this frame of reference, the practitioner does not implement a training program in which the patient practices a given task or routine to develop mastery. Instead, the intervention plan is designed to remove the pathological processes identified through the diagnostic evaluation.

Based on a medical model perspective, occupational therapists select frames of reference designed to correct pathological responses. In these frames of reference, the performance components often focus on more than the occupational performance area. For example, the neurodevelopmental frame of reference may be selected when the child has motor difficulties. Consistent with this frame of reference is the therapist's attention to subtle motor behaviors.

When applying frames of reference within a medical model system, the priorities are on underlying processes in the child that contribute to his observable behavior and not on environmental elements that influence performance abilities. To support programs that address this priority, space and equipment are needed for child-centered evaluation and intervention procedures. Because treatment does not focus on environmental components, locations for medical-model interventions are chosen solely with the intervention in mind. For example, a spacious environment with a supply of various sized positioning aids and an obstacle-free area for the therapist to use when handling the child in various movement planes is well-suited for therapy based on the neurodevelopmental frame of reference, which is consistent with the medical model perspective. In contrast, a crowded preschool classroom with an abundance of creative play materials and arts and crafts supplies would not facilitate this intervention. In this regard, frames of reference consistent with a medical model perspective do not generally use interventions that can be integrated easily into natural settings, such as an infant's home, without disrupting the established routine.

Another characteristic of the medical model is that it uses many professionals with varied educational backgrounds. The medical system has evolved from a "general practitioner approach" to the segregation of knowledge into specialties (Rosenberg, 1989). Many different professions, each with a perspective toward a defined aspect of human function, contribute to care under the medical model. An illustration is the pediatric hospital clinic that may include a neurologist, an orthopedist, an audiologist, a nutritionist, and an internist.

Pediatric professionals in a medical model practice arena function within departments in the agency, sharing with their peers similar values, beliefs, and interests in a specific domain of child function and behavior. The institution has a vested interest in providing the continued training needed by all staff members to maintain updated knowledge about research and treatment advances, and these events frequently are scheduled for staff members' participation. As a result of these offerings, department members frequently acquire a similar knowledge base about interventions relevant to the population served by the agency. In practice, this departmentalized arrangement provides the occupational therapist with supervision and direction concerning patient care. It gives her ample opportunity to interact and collaborate with other therapists who "speak the same language" and share similar interests. When an occupational therapist works with a child who poses a treatment challenge, she may involve another department colleague to review the case and treatment regimen, so that additional or revised treatment strategies can be suggested. This peer support is particularly valuable to an entry-level therapist. The collaborative opportunity is also rewarding for the therapist who enjoys a mentoring relationship with other colleagues.

Team process in the medical model is based on principles of multidisciplinary function (Bailey, 1984). In practice, this approach is characterized by numerous disciplines, each assessing a component of the other's function by identifying pathology and outlining a plan of care to be managed by that discipline. Selection of the frame of reference that guides evaluation and intervention is determined by the individual practitioner. Evaluation procedures often are completed in a specialized environment, such as the professional office or a "testing laboratory" in an elementary school building. Each discipline carries out its intervention isolated from the other disciplines.

In this perspective, a young boy who has cerebral palsy may visit the outpatient department in a community based rehabilitation center. In addition to an appointment with a physiatrist, evaluation sessions are scheduled with the psychologist, the occupational therapist, the physical therapist, and the speech pathologist. Each professional completes assessment procedures during individual sessions with this child with his mother present. On another date, after each evaluator has had the opportunity to collect and analyze assessment data, the professionals convene with the physiatrist to present and review their collective findings. The physiatrist, functioning as team leader, summarizes the information presented and authorizes a plan of rehabilitation services for the child. In a meeting between the physiatrist and the boy's parents, evaluation outcomes and the plans for occupational, physical, and speech therapy rehabilitation are presented. Afterward, the family develops a schedule of visits with the therapists and the therapy program begins.

What follows demonstrates how medical model thinking may be applied to occupational therapy practice in a public school setting:

> Kevin, an eight-year-old boy, cannot copy letters from the blackboard legibly. His teacher also reported that Kevin often was fidgety and had difficulty remaining in his seat during classwork periods. Following a review of his educational record, the school's occupational therapist met Kevin in the classroom and advised him that they were going to work in another area of the school. During testing sessions outside the classroom, the therapist examined underlying sensory and motor processes believed to contribute to the handwriting task. Analyses of Kevin's body posture and control, ocular mobility, and tracking skills during various therapist-directed testing procedures were completed. Components of sensory integrative processing and visual perceptual function were measured through administration and interpretation of the Sensory Integration and Praxis Tests (Ayres, 1989) and the Test of Visual Perceptual Skills (Gardner, 1988).
>
> Test results indicated a deficiency in tactile system functions that the therapist interpreted as being related to the referring problem, poor handwriting. A subsequent program of occupational therapy intervention included treatment sessions that included play activities that emphasized deep pressure and touch sensory experiences, graded proprioceptive input, and calming movement stimuli. The therapist structured the sessions to encourage Kevin to initiate his own interaction gradually with various tactile stimuli, using and interpreting the sensory information as part of the session's adaptive tasks. In fact, during the course of his occupational therapy intervention, Kevin did not engage in any writing or drawing activities other than finger painting or forming shapes with his finger in a wet sand tray.

In this example, the chosen treatment program, based on sensory integration theory and practice (Fisher, Murray, & Bundy, 1991), does not appear to the casual observer to be related to a handwriting problem. Using this frame of reference, the occupational therapist plans intervention activities to develop mature central nervous system function by modifying tactile hyperresponsivity and enhancing Kevin's discriminatory capabilities. The focus is on changing the underlying neural functions that influence Kevin's ability to control and integrate sensory and motor systems. The structure and nature of the environment in which the handwriting performance is expressed are not evaluation or treatment concerns for the occupational therapist. The instructional materials, the teacher's directions or intervention approach, and the tools used are not addressed by the occupational therapist.

## Educational Model Perspective

An educational model perspective is based on learning theories that relate behavioral changes to the person's experience and interaction in a situation (Hilgard & Bower, 1966; Snelbecker, 1974). According to the frames of reference developed from these theories, behaviors change as a result of learning that occurs from experiences and interactions in the environment. Furthermore, through an activity's design, planned activities may foster desired changes. Behavioral change in this context does not refer to developments that result from innate predispositions, such as the physical and emotional maturation observed in the adolescent age span.

Describing a person's behaviors and performances in a given environment and how changes in that environment affect behavior are important concerns in this model. Both sensory and physical environmental conditions are the subjects of examination. In addition to identifying the current level of performance, the determination of skills needed to move forward to the next level of expected performance and alterations or adjustments needed in the environment to enable or discourage desired change are necessary components in the evaluation process.

Whenever a frame of reference is used that is consistent with an educational perspective, occupational therapy assessment information is presented in terms of end-product performance by using behavioral statements. This is a departure from the medical model, which aims to define dysfunction in terms of the underlying neuromuscular processes believed to affect behavior.

Behaviors are defined as levels of achievement in positive terms, even though they relate to dysfunction or disability in a child's performance. Rather than define a problem by highlighting what the child cannot do, the frames of reference that use educational model thinking translate the child's dysfunction into statements of baseline performance abilities relevant in the environment. These statements do not reveal a disability until the child's developmental and chronological age are considered, along with the environmental expectations. As examples, consider the following statements about dysfunction:

1. John has developed penmanship skills commensurate with third-grade-level expectations.
2. John expresses visual-motor skills typical of a 7-year-, 6-month-old child.

An occupational therapist who uses educational model thinking selects frames of reference based on learning and behavioral theories. Intervention in these frames of reference may involve practice and training activities. These strategies do not account for the cause of dysfunction, because this is not a concern in a frame of reference grounded in learning theories. Rather, the strategies are directed toward improving the fit between the person and the environment so that the desired performance can be expressed and used in a functional activity. (Additional examples of this perspective are discussed in Chapter 7 in this book).

In the case of a child who has difficulties in visual perceptual processing, the therapist evaluates areas of learned perceptual skill (size, form, and space concepts) and visual memory functions. Once the deficit areas are identified, a plan for intervention can be formulated. If, for example, a weakness in visual sequential memory is revealed, a program of practice and training activities that requires the child to retain and recall visual stimuli may be implemented. Following a timed period for visual stimuli (a series of three objects), the child may be asked to identify the matching series in an array of a similar ordered group that serves as a distractor. In the next step, the child may be asked to construct a duplicate set of three objects using a sample assortment of similar and matching objects. Repetition of entire activities, or steps within the activities, can provide other opportunities for experiential learning. Over time, verbal directions and assistance from an adult in the environment also may be reduced to develop the child's skill and independence as the practice activities continue and learning becomes evident.

This example demonstrates how treatment based on educational model perspectives and learning theories uses the environment and not the child's internal functions and processes to design, structure, and implement intervention. The intervention strives for change by focusing on the disparity between the child's performance and the demands from the human and nonhuman environments. Treatment is directed toward the development of specific skills needed for successful adaptation and performance in the environment. Training activities used in intervention are clearly related to the problem behaviors identified through the assessment process. Evaluation measures rate the child's end-product performances and are concerned with whether the observed behavior is suitable (according to the expectations for success within the given environment).

# Settings—Descriptions, Definitions

This section discusses pediatric occupational therapy as practiced in hospitals, clinics, home-based settings, and school-based settings, as well as in private practice. These practice settings share some common features and, in addition, present concerns unique to the location in which the service is provided. For example, in one hospital setting, funding requirements and administrative or management structures necessitated specific types and frequencies of documentation, intervention schedules, and service implementations. Third-party reimbursers could fund only clinic-based therapy sessions during which the therapist worked with the child on an individual basis. These insurers could deny coverage when the child received therapy services in a group. Specified therapy in a home-based program required a minimum frequency of visits each month, and occupational therapy could be provided only in conjunction with other health care and rehabilitation services.

Many pediatric occupational therapy settings offer various services. For example, a hospital center may offer on-site therapy for in-patient and out-patient groups alike, whereas some hospital staff may travel into the community to provide services to children and their families in the home environment. Another hospital may offer hospital-based and home-based services, using employed staff members and contracted persons or agencies in the community for additional coverage to augment the staff. Recognizing these variables, the descriptions and definitions of pediatric service settings that follow should not be considered as all-inclusive or exclusive in nature.

## Hospital-Based Settings

General hospitals and pediatric or adult rehabilitation hospitals sometimes include occupational therapy service programs for children. Services in any one agency may be offered for in-patients, out-patients, or both groups. Patients seen by hospital-based therapy staffs may be admitted for chronic or acute rehabilitation, depending on the hospital's focus. Frequently, treatment plans prescribe more than one therapy service to meet the patient's needs.

Typically, the occupational therapy service is located in the rehabilitation department, led by a physiatrist and other medical specialists, such as a neurologist or orthopedist. Occupational therapy departments in hospitals often are closely aligned with other therapy services, such as physical and speech therapies. Frequently, these disciplines share common physical space in the hospital, not only for the convenience of the patients who receive the services but also for efficiency when equipping departments with supplies and materials. The close physical proximity facilitates communication among therapists who often see the same groups of patients admitted for rehabilitation.

Hospital departments generally are staffed by a group of center-based therapists employed by the facility; however, some hospitals may contract to outside personnel agencies or health care worker pools for extra staff coverage. Therapy departments generally are managed by one person who is considered the "director." This person may or may not be an occupational therapist.

Sharing among disciplines is facilitated when staff members come together for routine meetings to review patient care and to discuss treatment outcomes. Beyond this, the approach to assessment and intervention does not generally encourage crossdiscipline interaction; usually, each staff member maintains responsibility for a discipline-specific assessment and intervention plan.

## Clinic-Based Settings

Various health care and medical disciplines coexist in the pediatric clinic. For the most part, the clinic represents an out-patient arrangement in which children and families are seen on a routine basis to monitor a condition or to follow up on a specific concern or procedure that may have been completed in the hospital program. Frequently, this agency makes referrals for additional services needed in the home or community. Many clinics are situated inside a hospital facility and are under hospital management and supervision; however, some are free-standing, community-based sites without any hospital or medical center affiliation.

Occupational therapy services in a clinic frequently are directed at monitoring a child's rehabilitation and referring the family and child to appropriate resources in the community. The therapist in a clinic may see children on her caseload infrequently, corresponding to the periodic appointments with other specialists based in the clinic. Children who visit the clinic may be followed for ongoing rehabilitation by other therapists in the hospital or in the community. These "treating therapists" communicate to the clinic team through written progress reports, by telephone, or by accompanying the child and family to the clinic visit.

The clinic therapist may be asked to develop specific recommendations for the child's management in the home, school, or community. Clinics also may include specialized technology centers that work in cooperation with representatives from equipment suppliers. These persons are available for consultation regarding products available for specific needs.

## Home-Based Settings

Occupational therapy services may be provided in a child's home under the supervision and management of a hospital, clinic, public school, home health agency, or private practice. Each of these administrative structures implies a service provision that includes elements associated with the particular supervising agency. Despite these differences, home-based therapy programs have common administrative features.

Home-based programs eliminate the family's need to access transportation services and therefore are more convenient in many cases. For children who require specialized nursing care, positioning, and transportation for travel outside the house, home-based services may be the only realistic option. Many children also function optimally only in the familiarity of their home environments rather than in a contrived situation characteristic of clinical settings.

The home-based therapist has an opportunity to address simultaneously family, child, and environment-centered factors that influence the child's development and adaptation. When providing home-based services, the occupational therapist can assess real situations with the challenges and resources that are a part of the family's everyday life. Treatment interventions and strategies to foster the child's development can be planned realistically to meet everyday needs of the child and his family because the therapist works directly in the environment in which caretaking and nurturing activities occur.

Therapists who provide home-based services are exposed to a unique relationship between child and family, and between family and therapist. Given the fact that the therapist enters the home on a routine basis, an element of closeness to the family develops that can be both advantageous and disconcerting with regard to program planning and implementation. Because of the "special" relationship between caregiver and home-based therapist, information that has not been shared with the doctor or others involved in the child's intervention may be offered to the therapist. Care must be taken to respect and protect that trust. At the same time, the occupational therapist must consider the health and safety of both child and family and refer problems to appropriate sources when additional assistance is warranted.

Collaboration with professional peers involved with the family is difficult to maintain when home-based services are provided. Agencies may offer or require team home visits on a periodic basis. This gives family members and others the opportunity to speak together about the treatment program and any progress made. All concerned can observe a particular activity or event that challenges the caretaker or others involved in the child's life.

## School-Based Settings

Occupational therapists have been working with children in public and private schools for many years; however, federal regulations passed in 1975 have brought massive changes to the way therapists, educators, and families now consider school-based therapy programs. Initially called The Education of the Handicapped Act (EHA) (Federal Register, 1977), Public Law 94-142 was renamed in 1990 to become the Individuals with Disabilities Education Act (IDEA) through amendments in Public Law 101-476 (1990). The IDEA legislation mandates that schools provide all children with an educational program tailored to their unique learning needs, regardless of the nature or extent of their disabilities. When the support of specialized services such as occupational or physical therapy is required for the student to benefit from a special education program, the school system must provide those services as well. Therapy services used in this way (to support special education programs) are called **related services.**

Occupational therapists who provide related services participate in a system that is in sharp contrast to the traditional medically based settings of practice. In addition to the acquisition of knowledge related to both the educational system in general and current special education laws and regulations, specialized skills and abilities are needed for the therapist to be an effective member of the educational planning team (AOTA, 1989a). The translation of occupational therapy knowledge and intervention for effective use in public school programs challenges many practitioners.

As public concern for persons who have disabilities grows and efforts toward mainstreaming and providing education in a cost-efficient way continue, children who have a wide range of educational strengths and needs enter the system. Frequently, unusual medical circumstances or social situations complicate a child's condition. Therapists are challenged to develop new frames of reference consistent with the educational perspective to address the multiple needs of children who have chronic and severe disabilities. In many cases, the decisions about type and degree of therapy support services are not obvious to any member of the planning team. In these situations, parents, educators, and therapists must work together to evaluate the child's level of performance, to identify strengths and weaknesses, and to plan a program that focuses on the development of necessary functional performance abilities so that the child can achieve a realistic degree of self-sufficiency. This shift from a specific aspect of human function to a global picture of function within the school environment represents another departure from the concerns that once characterized services based in the medical model.

## Private Practice Settings

Pediatric occupational therapy in private practice represents a growing arena for provision of services. The American Occupational Therapy Association Member Data Survey indicates that 9.4% of registered occupational therapist who have a pediatric practice interest currently work through a private practice, and 38.8% of those therapists indicate that they are self-employed (American Occupational Therapy Association. Personal correspondence. December, 1991). Private practices provide occupational therapy services in homes, schools, clinics, offices, or other locations. Many of the descriptions already presented that concern these settings at other levels also apply to the private practitioner. In addition, several unique issues influence the provision of pediatric services through private practice.

A private practice is a business and the managing therapist must be competent enough to develop and maintain the administrative aspects; she should also be an expert pediatric therapist. The practice may provide office-based services, home- or community-based services, or services that combine sites. When the practice is office-based then suitable space must be accessible for families and children in the area. Regardless of the service location, budgets must be developed, materials must selected and purchased, and adequate insurance coverage must be secured. Advertisement and contacts within the community are necessary to ensure referrals and to sustain the practice.

A group private practice may include additional occupational therapy personnel as well as other health-care providers. In addition to self-generated referrals, a therapist who maintains a private practice may offer her services to another service, such as a home health-care agency or a colleague's private practice. In this situation, the agency or colleague contracts with the private practitioner to provide consultation, evaluation, or intervention services on a temporary or long-term basis.

A feature common to private practice is the absence of any public interest or control in the structure or operation of the agency. As a result, the philosophies, priorities, and staffing patterns are directed by the person who owns the practice. This enables a private practice to offer various services to meet diverse needs. In addition, a practice may shift its focus to meet changing needs in the community as they become apparent. In situations in which this alteration may be needed on a temporary basis, the practice may respond without consulting a board of directors or convening any other advisory group to determine the appropriate response.

Assistance from financial and legal advisors is necessary. The therapist may find helpful resources by consulting with established private practitioners and other health care management experts. Because of varying state fiscal and legal considerations, assistance from consultants in the region is desirable.

## Concerns Based on Settings: Implications for Practice

It is important that pediatric therapists define and understand the settings in which they provide services so that effective programs may be planned and implemented. The frame of reference chosen should be consistent with the philosophy of the setting. As discussed earlier, the agency's philosophies, goals, and objectives provide a framework that influences the services offered in individual programs. Persons who provide services in the program need to be familiar with this framework and accept the agency's orientation. Without this commitment, a unifying foundation of beliefs among team members is missing, and those who work with the child and family may find that their philosophies and practices conflict. In this situation, inefficient service provision inconsistent with the program's global objectives frequently results.

To illustrate, a therapist who works in a preschool program that believes strongly in early intervention and prevention concepts of care must have specialized skills and attitudes. A belief that early intervention can prevent or delay dysfunctional performance is important for this therapist. In addition, she needs to demonstrate expertise in screening children to identify which behaviors represent early developmental irregularities or suggest the potential for future atypical development. Expertise in developing in-service programs and consulting with teachers so that they too can learn to identify appropriate children for referral to occupational therapy services are important.

Financial resources in an agency or system may influence the occupational therapist's selection of a frame of reference for intervention and resultant treatment protocol. An approach that depends on specific positioning aids and adaptive equipment pieces, such as the biomechanical frame of reference, may meet limited success in a program that has no available supplies to construct specialized seating, lying, or standing supports or that cannot fabricate splints to facilitate grasp and handling of materials. The therapist in this situation may choose to work closely with program administration to create ways of securing the funds to implement the intervention activities in a biomechanical frame of reference. Grant applications or cooperative payment options with community agencies are two possibilities.

# Professional Roles Related to Settings—Ethics

Ethics related to standards of correct and appropriate behaviors are unique to the development of a profession. The American Occupational Therapy Association's Code of Ethics (American Occupational Therapy Association, 1988) sets guidelines for the conduct of all occupational therapy practitioners and students, to maintain high standards of behavior. These ethical principles relate to the practitioner's competence, compliance with laws and regulations, and appropriate relationships in the professional context.

In addition to principles in the Occupational Therapy Code of Ethics, the American Occupational Therapy Association (AOTA) has developed official documents that reflect current practice with minimum levels of competency in various areas of occupational therapy service (e.g., Standards of Practice, Position Papers, Guidelines, and Statements). These documents delineate practice, define issues and concerns, and provide guidelines related to occupational therapy for groups of persons or for a particular treatment concern. For example, documents related to the areas of practice covered in this text include *Guidelines for Occupational Therapy Services within School Systems* (1989a) and *Guidelines for Occupational Therapy Services in Early Intervention and Preschool Services* (1989b). All of the AOTA's official documents are reviewed periodically and updated as needed to represent contemporary thinking and practice approaches.

Individual states have their own laws or standards that regulate occupational therapy practice. These state regulations may refer to specific practice areas (certification by the state education department to work as a school-based therapist) or they may apply to all areas of occupational therapy in the state (state licensure of occupational therapy practice). Such regulations require specific referrals for occupational therapy treatment from physicians or others and include guidelines related to acceptable supervision practices between registered occupational therapists and certified occupational therapy assistants.

Occupational therapists face many situations in practice that require ethical behavior to determine appropriate courses of action. The selection of an effective treatment approach for a particular patient has been identified as a common ethical dilemma that faces the practicing therapist (Hansen, 1988).

This concern may be applied to pediatric practice in the example of a therapist who is asked to determine the appropriate frame of reference to treat a twelve-month-old infant who exhibits a developmental delay of 5 to 6 months. The therapist practices in a pediatric service system based on a family-centered philosophy. In this approach, needs of the family, or other care provider are considered in intervention so that proper attention can be given to the child's nurturing and development. The evaluating therapist involves the family or care provider in the assessment and treatment planning process. Ethical principles of occupational therapy practice also require that the therapist develop and communicate anticipated outcomes of the planned intervention program to the family or care provider and then accept their right to refuse participation in the program.

The Occupational Therapy Code of Ethics requires that occupational therapists adhere to laws and policies that guide the profession, including all published standards of practice, as well as to regulations that affect occupational therapy services in their particular state and those of the agency in which service is provided. It is the therapist's responsibility to obtain and study these documents so that current information is used to guide individual practice. Compliance with these ethical principles and professional standards is reflected in the therapist's daily behavior.

### References

American Occupational Therapy Association. (1989a). *Guidelines for occupational therapy services in the schools* (2nd ed.). Rockville, MD: Author.

American Occupational Therapy Association. (1989b). *Guidelines for occupational therapy services in the early intervention and pre-school services.* Rockville, MD: Author.

*American Occupational Therapy Association.* 1990 AOTA Member data survey. Custom data run, 1991. Rockville, MD: Author.

*American Occupational Therapy Association.* (1988). Occupational therapy code of ethics. Rockville, MD: Author.

Ayres, A. J. (1989). *Sensory integration and praxis tests.* Los Angeles CA: Western Psychological Services.

Bailey, D. (1984). A triaxial model of the interdisciplinary team and group process. *Exceptional Child 51*;17–25.

Federal Register. The Education for All Handicapped Children Act of 1975, P. L. 94–142, Vol. 42, No. 163, August 23, 1977.

Fisher, A. G., Murray, E. A., & Bundy, A. C. (1991). *Sensory integration theory and practice.* Philadelphia, PA: F. A. Davis.

Gardner, M. E. (1988). *Test of visual perceptual skills.* San Francisco, CA: Health Publishing.

Hansen, R. A. (1984). Ethics is the issue. *American Journal of Occupational Therapy. 42,* 279–281.

Hilgard, E. R., & Bower, G. H. (1966). *Theories of learning.* New York, NY: Meredith.

Public Law 101-476. Education of the Handicapped Act Amendments of 1990. # 20, USC 1400. October 30, 1990.

Snelbecker, G. E. (1974). *Learning theory, instructional theory, and psychoeducational design.* New York, NY: McGraw-Hill.

Starr, P. (1982). *The social transformation of American medicine.* New York: Basic Books.

Rosenberg, C. E. (1989). Community and DE communities: The evolution of the American Hospital. In: D. E. Long, & J. Golden (Eds.). (pp. 3–17). *The American general hospital communities and social contexts.* Ithaca, NY: Cornell University Press.

von Bertalanffy, L. (1968). *General system theory: Foundations, development, applications.* New York, NY: George Braziller.

# 15

# Influence of the Human Context on the Application of Frames of Reference

JIM HINOJOSA / PAULA KRAMER

Up to this point, this book has concentrated on various frames of reference for pediatric occupational therapy and material that the therapist should know to put them into practice. This chapter goes beyond the general application of the frame of reference to discuss another context for effective intervention. The **nonhuman context for intervention** already has been presented in terms of how setting influences choice and use of frames of reference. The **human context for intervention** presents other important issues for the therapist; however, even though it generally does not influence the choice of frames of reference, it does impact on the effectiveness of the intervention process. This chapter, therefore, discusses the influence of the child's family life and culture on intervention. Other aspects of the human context that affect intervention are the therapist's relationship with family members; and with other professionals.

## Family and Culture

Children do not operate in a vacuum but, rather, in the context of family and culture. Effective occupational therapy intervention for a child requires that the therapist be sensitive to the child's environment, including family and culture. When therapists conduct intervention without regard to the important people in the child's environment, the intervention may not be appropriate. Thus, these therapists may not be effective treating the whole person. *Intervention must be conducted in the human context of the child's life.*

Some frames of reference include the family and the human environment as aspects of their theoretical bases. These frames of reference go so far as to involve family directly or indicate their influence in the application to practice. Examples of this are the **human occupation frame of reference** (Chapter 9), the **psychosocial frame of reference** (Chapter 10) and the **coping frame of reference** (Chapter 11). Although the human environment is not specifically mentioned in the theoretical bases of other frames of reference, it still is important for the therapist to consider when designing and implementing a comprehensive intervention plan. It is vital that the child's culture and family be considered in the application of any frame of reference. For example, the neurodevelopmental treatment frame of reference does not address family issues in its theoretical base; however, practitioners who use this treatment frame of reference usually consider family support when implementing intervention. They recognize that their interventions will be less effective if they cannot be carried over into the child's home on a frequent basis.

The interrelationship between culture and family is circuitous. Culture provides a backdrop for the family and influences the values and beliefs of family members. Family provides the background for the child. For the developing infant, family defines culture. As the major setting for family, culture is discussed first.

## *Culture*

Culture refers to accepted patterns of behaviors shared by a group. These groups are defined by what they have in common—religion, ethnic background, nationality, or some other characteristic. Cultural groups also share common beliefs, customs, values, and attitudes. Aspects of culture that affect a child's development include family structure, marital status of the parents, parent/child rearing practices, and educational background (Krefting & Krefting, 1991). Cultural patterns influence the child's behaviors by defining what is acceptable or unacceptable, what rules prevail in physical interactions, and how to communicate.

Culture influences the kinds of toys, games, foods, and objects that are part of daily life (Hopkins & Tiffany, 1988). The background of the authors serve as an example of this point. The child of Mexican heritage who lives in the West eats beans and tortillas as a regular part of his diet. He may listen to Spanish or country-western music, as well as rock and roll. A common pastime may include tossing horseshoes, bicycle riding, and going to the playground. A little boy in this culture would not be expected to do kitchen chores or play with kitchen utensils. A child from a Jewish family in the Bronx may eat chicken soup with matzo balls as part of a traditional dinner. The music in the household could be classical or broadway music, as well as rock and roll. A young girl would be encouraged to pretend "cook" and "bake" as well as play with Barbie™ dolls. She would also play in the playground and ride a bicycle. The shared experiences of these two children include rock and roll music, playing in the playground and riding bicycles, all of which are part of the "American culture." The child's culture must be defined in terms of his family background yet combined with the culture of his community.

The effects of culture on intervention are multifaceted. Views on health and illness may be influenced by culture. The ways in which people feel and act toward persons who have disabilities reflect cultural views or biases. This may be true of family members and therapists alike. It is important for the therapist to respond to cultural identity. One way is to delineate how culture affects the selection of goals and the establishment of rapport (Levine, 1984). The perception of therapist and client may be "filtered through the screen of culture" (Hopkins & Tiffany, 1988, p. 108). For the pediatric occupational therapist, culture may outline the therapist-child-parent interaction. Consistent with the frame of reference, culture determines the choice of goals and the selection of legitimate tools and activities. "In every culture . . . some activities are regarded as proper, some inappropriate, and other unacceptable for specific ages, social status, economic class, men or women, times of day, days of week, or seasons of the year" (Cynkin & Robinson, 1990, p. 10). Culture also determines acceptable levels of performance so that the therapist can decide on expected outcomes.

## Family

A family consists of two or more persons who provide the environment in which the child develops and learns to become a member of society. Families usually include parents and children and may include other significant people. Current American society has many different family configurations, including the nuclear, extended, expanded, and single-parent households. The nuclear family consists of a couple who shares the responsibility for raising a child. The extended family is a group related through family ties or mutual consent who share some part in childrearing. The expanded family is a complex combination of family configurations, involving a nuclear family, children, and significant others from previous relationships (Mosey, 1986). The configuration of this relationship among these different people is defined by the current *and* previous relationships. The single-parent household is one in which an adult assumes all the parental responsibilities.

For the purpose of this book, the primary function of the family is to provide a supportive and nurturing environment for the child's development. Consistent with its culture, the family shapes the child's ideological system and provides opportunities to develop interpersonal relationships (Turnbull, Summers, & Brotherson, 1986). In a well-functioning, healthy family, the needs of all family members are recognized and supported. Each family is unique, and this must be considered by the therapist. When providing occupational therapy services to a child, the therapist usually is in contact with the parents, although the extent of this interaction generally is determined by the treatment setting and service delivery model. It also can be affected by the opportunities and willingness of the therapist and the parent to collaborate.

Despite the setting or service delivery model, the therapist should make an effort to develop open communication with the family. To work effectively with families of children who have disabilities, occupational therapists must strive to understand the way in which each family functions and the normal conflicts inherent in childrearing. The entry-level therapist needs to gain some experience and sensitivity about the parenting process, and she must understand that it is not always a positive experience, that conflict occurs naturally even in the healthiest families.

Working with families requires specific knowledge and skills about effective communication. In addition, the therapist has to understand the dynamics of family function and what potential influence she may have on the family. Although the therapist should have a strong knowledge base related to occupational therapy, she may not have as much information about family operations and interactions. Such information can be gained only over time, with the establishment of a relationship based on mutual trust. Each family has its own concerns and needs. To be responsive, the therapist must approach the family at **their level,** addressing **their needs and concerns.** *She has to be careful not to impose her values or concerns onto the family.* To provide the most effective intervention, the therapist must work together with family members.

She should approach them as partners in this endeavor. The communication between therapist and family should be nonjudgmental, to meet the needs of all participants. The goal of communication is to establish a collaborative relationship, one in which the issues related to the child and his family are discussed openly. This communication can provide the therapist with a clear perspective of the child's real-life world demands, how these things impact on the family, and what feedback occurs with regard to their own intervention and interactions.

It is beyond the scope of this text to discuss in-depth issues about working with families; however, the issues that follow have been identified as important whenever any frame of reference is applied in the context of the family:

- As the center of concern for the child, the family has the **real** power in the therapist/family relationship. Family members can facilitate or sabotage the intervention process.

- Therapists must be concerned with the expectations and responsibilities that they impose on families. Depending on the frame of reference chosen, therapists must be realistic about the role that the family plays in the intervention process. Furthermore, they need to recognize that family members are not experts in the use of the profession's legitimate tools.

- Therapists must be willing to accept that they do not have all the answers and be willing to adjust their interventions to meet the families' realistic goals. The therapist needs to be open enough to discuss this with family members. This may require an adjustment or change in the frame of reference.

- When interventions do not work, therapists must examine several areas. Reasons for failure may be the choice of the frame of reference; the cultural influence that impacts on the demands of the particular intervention; unrealistic expectations by either the therapist or the family; or, the "fit" between the personalities of the therapist and family members.

- Therapists must be aware of how some families see the position of authority implied by the role of therapist, and they must be careful not to abuse that power.

Many professionals are sometimes apprehensive about working directly with parents and other family members. Often, family issues are overwhelming. The therapist may not feel adequately prepared to deal with family reactions, or she may feel uncomfortable with parent distress, anger, or frustration. Ironically, she also may be overwhelmed by parental feelings of elation over achievements. To understand this range of emotion, recognition of these feelings may contribute to the therapist's ability to develop a working relationship with families.

# Professional Relationships

A child does not operate in a vacuum, and occupational therapists should not operate in isolation. Almost all children who receive occupational therapy services are in contact with other professionals. Effective occupational therapy intervention requires that the therapist interact and communicate with any other professionals involved with the particular child.

Just as the therapist must establish rapport to work with families, so must she develop lines of communication to collaborate effectively with other professionals involved with the child. Each professional who works with the child has a different educational background that lends a different viewpoint to the situation. The roles of each profession and, therefore, each perspective are distinct leading to unique concerns and goals for the child. Furthermore, these professionals often have different beliefs, values, and attitudes. Each person involved brings not only her own professional perspective to the work environment, but also her preconceived view, of the other professionals involved. The one thing that all may have in common is a philosophy about and perspective of the setting in which they are working.

Interaction among professionals requires mutual respect and support, as well as a mutual understanding of different roles and goals. To achieve this rapport, professionals must communicate with each other and be willing to learn from one another. They must recognize and solve problems that arise when professionals from multiple disciplines interact and, ultimately, participate effectively in teams (Bailey, 1989).

To participate successfully with other professionals, the entry-level occupational therapist must become secure in her own role. She must understand her profession and the uniqueness that she contributes to the intervention process. This requires a firm understanding of the frames of reference and how they fit with the overall concerns for the child. The therapist must feel equal with the other professionals on the team. She must also develop a reciprocal relationship in which she learns about the contributions and perspectives of the other team members and teaches them about hers.

This section of the chapter presents an overview of skills required to collaborate effectively with other professionals. The issues that follow are important when using any frame of reference in the context of a professional team:

- All team members have equal status and should work toward facilitating positive change in the child and his family. Any one team member can sabotage team function and, therefore, affect the intervention process negatively.

- Therapists must be willing to accept the fact that they do not have all the answers, and, must be willing to modify their interventions to meet unified team goals for the child and his family. Therapists need to discuss and negotiate this openly with other team members. The result may require an adjustment or change in the frame of reference.

- Therapists cannot see themselves as being all things to all children. They must be aware of the strengths and limitations of their profession and understand the important contributions that can be made by other professionals.

- Therapists should be concerned about whether they are speaking the same language as other team members. They should avoid professional jargon for the sake of clarity. Each frame of reference has its own jargon, which should be translated for mutual understanding by all team members.

- When interventions do not work, therapists must examine several areas. This requires communication with other team members and may require an exploration of overall goals for the child. All avenues need to be explored rather than looking for blame. Additional collaboration may be required to redefine the team's approach or another frame of reference may be used by the occupational therapist.

- Therapists must be aware of the possibility of "conflicting loyalties" (Purtilo, 1978). This occurs when a personal or professional view conflicts with the personal or professional views of other team members. Therapists must be aware that the overriding concern is how best to meet the needs of the child and his family.

Many entry-level occupational therapists initially feel insecure about working as a full-fledged team member. With experience, sensitivity, and self-examination of their own interactions, they rapidly can acquire the skills needed to be an effective team member. Occupational therapists can draw from their educational background to facilitate the group process and psychosocial functioning to understand the workings of the team and to become an important contributing member.

## Summary

Collaboration among occupational therapists, family members, and other professionals is essential to provide the most appropriate intervention services for the child and his family. A collaborative relationship is one in which issues are discussed openly, decisions are made mutually, and a foundation is built for effective working relationships. Intervention in the human context is influenced by human interpretation of values, beliefs, and needs. To that extent, intervention becomes subjective, because feelings color the definition of these systems. The occupational therapist must be aware, however, that although her feelings are important, the values and beliefs of the child and his family should take precedence.

### References

Bailey, D. B. (1989). Issues and directions in preparing professionals to work with young handicapped children and their families. In J. J. Gallagher, P. L. Trohanis, & R. M. Clifford (Eds.). *Policy implementation and PL 99-457* (pp. 97–132). Baltimore, MD: Paul H. Brooks

Cynkin, S., & Robinson, A. M. (1990). *Occupational therapy and activities health: Towards health through activities.* Boston, MA: Little, Brown & Company.

Hopkins, H. L., & Tiffany, E. G. (1988). Occupational therapy—a problem solving process. In H. L. Hopkins, & H. D. Smith (Eds.). *Willard and Spackman's occupational therapy* (7th ed.) (pp. 102–111). Philadelphia, PA: J. B. Lippincott.

Krefting, L. H., & Krefting, D. V. (1991). Cultural influences on performance. In C. Christiansen, & C. Baum (Eds.). *Occupational therapy: Overcoming human performance deficits* (pp. 101–122). Thorofare, NJ: Slack.

Levine, R. E. (1984). The cultural aspects of home care delivery. *American Journal of Occupational Therapy, 38,* 734–738.

Mosey, A. C. (1986). *Psychosocial components of occupational therapy.* New York, NY: Raven Press.

Purtilo, R. (1978). *Health professional/patient interaction.* Philadelphia, PA: W. B. Saunders.

Turnbull, A. P., Summers, J. A., & Brotherson, M. J. (1986). Family life cycle: Theoretical and empirical implications and future directions for families with mentally retarded members. In J. J. Gallagher, & P. M. Vietze (Eds.). *Families of handicapped persons* (pp. 45–65). Baltimore, MD: Paul H. Brooks.

# CASE STUDIES

# 16

# Case Study: Neurodevelopmental Treatment Frame of Reference

MARGARET KAPLAN / GARY BEDELL

Joey is a three-year-old boy diagnosed with cerebral palsy resulting in spastic quadriparesis. He previously received occupational therapy but was referred for a new occupational therapy evaluation before starting a preschool program. The pediatrician referral asked for an occupational therapy evaluation because of delays noted on the Denver Developmental Screening Test in the areas of fine motor, gross motor, and self-help skills. It was also documented that Joey had limited movement options because of hypertonicity.

Joey is the youngest child of a four-member, middle-class family that lives in a two-bedroom apartment on the lower east side of Manhattan. His one older sister is five years old and attends kindergarten.

## Background

From a review of Joey's medical records, the therapist learned that Joey was born at 28 weeks gestation, weighing 850 grams. He had spent 2 weeks on the ventilator in the neonatal intensive care unit (NICU). Reports from the NICU documented difficulties in oral, gross, and fine motor development. He had a grade IV intraventricular hemorrhage and bronchopulmonary dysplasia and was fed on nasalogastric (NG) tube for 1 month. At discharge from the NICU, Joey had progressed to being fed formula through a bottle with a small nipple, demonstrating a weak suck. He was discharged to home after 3 months in the hospital.

After discharge from the hospital, Joey was followed medically for persistent upper respiratory infections. In addition, occupational therapy and physical therapy had been provided in the home for 1 year.

The occupational therapist's initial interview with Joey's parents revealed that they perceived difficulties in managing him at home in several areas. Since birth, they had difficulty feeding him. At the time of the interview, they were feeding Joey soft, puréed food because he gagged or choked on solid food. They were especially concerned about his strong bite on the spoon and nipple of the bottle. When food was placed in his mouth, he tended to push it out with his tongue.

Joey's mother expressed concern about dressing Joey in the morning because he tended to be stiff and had spasms. She felt that his physical reactions may have been aggravated by her rushing in the morning to get both children ready for school. Joey was unable to walk and did not assist in self-care activities.

Joey's parents reported having difficulty moving him around in the apartment and in the community in his stroller because he had grown older and bigger. They felt that his limited mobility was a major problem. In addition to the stroller, Joey had an adapted chair with a tray in which he was placed for feeding and some play activities. When placed on the floor, his parents reported that he rolled or pulled himself forward on his stomach, using his arms to get around the apartment.

Although Joey was nonverbal, both parents felt that he communicated his needs and desires. He used facial expressions, eye gazes, and a variety of sounds. They reported that he was friendly and enjoyed being with other children. According to his mother, the high point in Joey's day was when his father arrived home from work in the evening and they spent some time playing together.

During the interview, Joey's father stated that he wanted to be involved in Joey's treatment program. He explained that he worked during the day and could not attend treatment sessions or meetings regularly. He expressed concern about Joey's future, asking whether the therapist thought Joey would be able to walk. Other concerns revolved around how much assistance Joey would need as he got older and what school he would be able to attend.

Joey's mother expressed feelings of being overwhelmed. She stated that she did not have enough time during the day to do everything that she felt

Joey and her family needed. She stated that her own needs were often at the bottom of her list of priorities.

In addition to discussing Joey, both parents talked about how pleased they were that Joey's sister was starting kindergarten. Both parents claimed that she was bright, and they were concerned that they were unable to spend enough time with her. They reported that the two children played together at times. They also expressed concern that their daughter sometimes appeared frustrated at the amount of time that they had to spend caring for Joey. In addition, she appeared to resent the family's limited ability to engage in community activities.

# Occupational Therapy Assessment

Because a chart review and interview with Joey's parents had identified problem areas, no other specific screening tool assessments were administered.

The neurodevelopmental treatment (NDT) frame of reference was chosen to address Joey's movement and tone problems that affected his gross motor, fine motor, and self-help skills. Other frames of reference can be used by other therapists to address problems in other areas (communication, social interaction, play, and skill acquisition). It should be noted that the NDT frame of reference was used within the context of a family-centered, team collaborative-approach. This encourages consideration of the varied needs of both child and family (Anderson & Hinojosa, 1984; Hanft, 1988; Hinojosa & Anderson, 1991).

The NDT frame of reference was selected because Joey's difficulties in movement and tone were primary areas of concern. This frame of reference also can be used to address feeding and mobility deficits, which also were concerns expressed by Joey's family.

Evaluation entailed observation of gross motor abilities and upper extremity function in the context of play and in the performance of daily living activities. Oral motor abilities were observed during mealtime.

## Gross Motor Abilities

Joey exhibited **hypotonicity** in his trunk, neck, shoulder girdle and pelvic musculature and **hypertonicity** in all four extremities. Hypertonicity was predominant in his upper extremity flexors and lower extremity extensors. He exhibited some evidence of a nonobligatory asymmetrical tonic neck reflex (ATNR) in the supine position and a nonobligatory symmetrical tonic neck reflex (STNR) in the prone position. No equilibrium reactions were elicited in any position. In prone and supported sitting positions, Joey exhibited some head righting reactions in the anterior-posterior direction. He had a left-sided preference in all positions and when he turned his head, rolled and reached for objects.

Joey could initiate rolling by hyperextending his head and neck. He could roll from the prone to the supine position and back by using associated movement patterns. It was noted that he lacked segmental movement control between his head, shoulders, and pelvis. He rolled with his lower extremities both in extension. Joey rarely chose to remain in the supine position, but when he did, he assumed a pattern of neck and trunk extension, lower extremity extension, and scapular retraction. Joey could bring his head and upper extremities briefly to midline with difficulty. He assumed supine as a resting position.

In the prone position, Joey was able to maintain prone on his elbows with them positioned directly below or slightly behind his shoulders. In this position, he was able to propel himself forward with movement initiating from the shoulders with head, trunk, and lower extremities in extension. This was his primary means of independent mobility. He was able to shift weight to either his right or left side to free one arm to obtain a toy. Joey was unable to attain or maintain quadruped or floor sitting positions independently because of poor postural alignment, absent equilibrium reactions, and postural tone dysfunction. Because of habitual lower extremity movement patterns of extension, his hamstring muscles were somewhat tight. When placed in a floor sitting position, his pelvis, therefore, was pulled posteriorly, resulting in weightbearing on the sacrum. Joey was able to maintain this position only briefly with a rounded back, his head forward, and his upper extremities in the "highguard" position of scapular elevation and adduction, humeral extension and adduction, elbow flexion, forearm pronation, and wrist and digital finger flexion. This habitual pattern was used whenever balance was challenged or control against gravity was required. Protective extension of the upper extremities was absent in this position.

Joey could attain sidelying by using an associated movement pattern described previously for rolling. He assumed this position to play with toys. Joey was able to flex his head and neck actively, although they usually were held in slight hyperextension. Gravity assisted the top lower extremity into slight hip and knee flexion. He seemed to prefer weightbearing on his right side and manipulating toys with his top left arm.

In bench sitting, with the therapist stabilizing his pelvis and maintaining it in a neutral position, Joey was able to maintain his trunk in a more upright position. When his weight was shifted in small ranges, he exhibited some head righting reactions in the anterior-posterior and lateral directions. Larger weight shifts resulted in the habitual highguard upper extremity pattern, lower extremity extension, and adduction with toe curling, accompanied by a fearful facial grimace.

Joey was unable to kneel or stand independently. When placed in a kneeling position, he could maintain the position only with the therapist's support at his pelvis and the use of a support surface in front of his trunk. When placed in a standing position, he required a support surface for his upper body anteriorly, and the therapist had to provide increased support at the hips, knees, and ankles to maintain stability and postural alignment. His habitual lower extremity pattern consisted of hip extension, adduction, internal rotation, knee extension, ankle/foot pronation, and toe curling.

## Upper Extremity Function

In the prone position, Joey was able to reach forward by using full range of elbow flexion/extension as well as a pattern of forearm pronation with the wrist in a neutral position. He was able to grasp small objects such as $\frac{1}{4}$-inch beads by using a raking pattern into his palm. He grasped larger objects (1-inch cubes and pegs) by using a palmar grasp with his thumb adducted. Joey used wrist flexion, resulting in digital extension, to release objects (**tenodesis pattern**). He was able to bring objects to his mouth when weightbearing at the elbow for stability, using elbow flexion, forearm pronation, and wrist flexion. Joey was unable to perform in-hand manipulation in prone or in any other position.

In the supine position, Joey could reach and swipe to the right and left by possibly using elements of the ATNR, although this reflex was not obligatory. He occasionally could grasp a toy after repeated efforts. If an object was presented at midline, he could bring his arms together by using an internally rotated, and elbow extended pattern. He could not externally rotate his arms to position his hands for grasp, and he was unable to form or shape his hands for efficient bilateral grasp of a ball or cup.

When sidelying on his right side, Joey reached more often with the top left arm and used the bottom right arm as an assist and to stabilize objects. He could maintain the sidelying position for longer periods than other positions. Gravity assisted his top hand in accommodating to the shape and size of objects. The release of bilaterally grasped objects was initiated from his shoulder. The arm was removed from the object by using an associated pattern of movement. Grasp of small objects (1-inch cubes) was accomplished using a palmar grasp with thumb abduction. He released smaller objects by using a tenodesis pattern. If given more support in sidelying, with a bolster or stuffed animal placed at his abdominals, Joey was able to use a digital grasp with slight abduction of his thumb.

Joey's most functional position for using his upper extremities was supported sitting in his adapted chair. In this chair, he leaned forward and used the tray for support. He preferred to use his left hand to reach and manipulate when weightbearing on the right forearm. He could manipulate objects bilaterally by weightbearing and stabilizing on both elbows. If given more support at the abdominals, Joey was able to be more upright and could use his arms more independently, without the tray as a support surface. With this support at the abdominals, Joey could reach unilaterally or bilaterally, depending on the size or shape of the object. He was able to reach and grasp objects on the tray by using a pronated forearm, his wrist in midposition, and a digital grasp with slight thumb abduction. For example, he could pick up 1-inch blocks and drop them into a container, pick up and throw a "Koosh"™ ball, and stack two to three blocks and knock them over. He could reach out and obtain a larger ball or stuffed animal about 6 inches in diameter by using a bilateral pronated reaching pattern. After contact with the ball, he could attain supination to a midposition.

Joey used a left palmar pronated grasp of a crayon, and could mark on paper and make vertical strokes toward his body.

## Activities of Daily Living

Activities of daily living (ADL) that were assessed included feeding and dressing.

### Feeding

Feeding was evaluated with Joey positioned in his adapted chair with tray. Joey was able to pick up a Graham cracker by using a raking grasp and then bring it to his mouth in a pronated pattern. He could bite off a few pieces of the cracker but then crumbled the rest, apparently because of difficulties with grading grasp pressure and in-hand manipulation of the cracker. He was able to grasp and pick up a spoon from a bowl of applesauce by using a palmar grasp with pronated forearm, but could not scoop the food onto the spoon. He could bring the spoon to his mouth by using an associated upper extremity pattern of horizontal abduction, scapular adduction, elbow flexion, forearm pronation, wrist flexion, ulnar deviation, and palmar grasp. He leaned toward the tray to bring his mouth to the spoon and jutted his head, neck, and jaw forward. When the spoon reached his mouth, a tonic bite reflex was observed that he released after a few seconds. He then removed the food from the spoon by using a modified suckling pattern of large up, down, anterior, and posterior tongue and jaw movements. Joey's tongue appeared large and thickened and tended to push some food out of his mouth. Inefficient lip closure also was observed.

Joey picked up a cup of juice by using both arms while stabilizing on his elbows on the tray. He approached a cup positioned at midline with arms in a pronated fashion. On contact, both upper extremities supinated to midposition and his hands shaped to fit around the cup. He bore weight on elbows, leaned forward toward the cup, and jutted his head, neck, and jaw forward. The oral-motor pattern used for spoon feeding was similar to that used for cup drinking.

### Dressing

Joey helped to position his extremities for dressing but needed assistance for all aspects of dressing. If the back of a loosely fitted shirt was brought up to his shoulders, Joey could remove it by leaning forward and grasping the shirt with a pronated pattern and pulling down by using a palmar grasp. He also could assist in lowering his pants if he was supported in standing. He could assist with raising his pants if they were raised to thigh level so that he could grasp them.

## Evaluation Summary

In this section, we relate Joey's motor performance to the function/dysfunction continua as outlined in the NDT frame of reference in Chapter 5.

### *Postural Tone*

Postural tone was hypotonic in Joey's head, neck, trunk, shoulder, and pelvis. Postural tone was hypertonic in all extremities. Tone was particularly increased in the upper extremity flexors and in the lower extremity extensors.

### *Stability-Mobility*

Joey performed on the dysfunctional end of the stability-mobility continuum. He was able to bear weight on the upper extremities for stability when performing fine motor and self-feeding tasks. He required support of equipment or therapeutic handling to provide the stability necessary to allow upper extremity function (mobility, reach, and grasp).

## Reciprocal Innervation

In the area of reciprocal innervation, Joey used his upper extremities primarily in midrange. Control of movement out of midrange was difficult. Attempts at active movements appeared to be labored and stiff.

## Postural Alignment

Joey had some head righting reactions in the sagittal plane (anterior-posterior direction) when in the prone position and in the sagittal and frontal (lateral direction) planes for small weightshifts in supported sitting. Postural alignment was poor, but it was improved with supportive equipment or therapeutic handling. For example, in unsupported floor sitting, his pelvis was tilted posteriorly, his spine was kyphotic, and his upper extremities were maintained in a highguard position. Postural alignment improved when his pelvis was stabilized in a neutral position and his knees were flexed, reducing pull on the hamstring muscles.

## Dissociation

Associated movement patterns were demonstrated during rolling. Joey initiated rolling with head and neck hyperextension that appeared to increase the extension in his trunk and lower extremities. Associated upper extremity patterns were noted during fine motor and feeding activities.

## Variety of Movement

Joey's choice of movement patterns was limited because of postural tone dysfunction, difficulty in moving out of midrange, associated movement patterns, and absent equilibrium reactions. Mobility and exploration of his environment therefore were limited. This influenced other areas of development such as cognition, play, and social skills.

## Full Range of Motion—Structural Deformities and Contractures

Joey had full range of motion (ROM) at the time of evaluation, but, because of limited movement options, associated movement patterns, and difficulty in moving out of midranges, he was at risk for developing future contractures and deformities.

# Team Conference

Soon after the occupational therapy evaluation was completed, a team conference was held among Joey's parents, occupational therapist, physical therapist, speech language pathologist, pediatrician, and future teacher. After a careful review of the evaluation findings, the occupational therapist (together with the rest of the team) decided that she would focus on Joey's self-feeding, dressing, and upper extremity functional skills.

## *Occupational Therapy Goals*

In collaboration with the team, the following are the goals set for Joey by his occupational therapist:

1. To improve Joey's ability to initiate weigh shifts and to control movement transitions in all developmental positions;
2. To increase Joey's repertoire of reach and grasp patterns with handling and facilitation;
3. To improve Joey's ability to maintain an upright position of his trunk with handling and facilitation;
4. To improve Joey's ability to reach away from body midline;
5. To improve Joey's ability to use active wrist extension and graded digital release with fine motor activities;
6. To improve Joey's ability to use a more digital grasp to pick up a spoon during his snack time; and
7. To improve Joey's ability to keep his tongue inside his mouth and use upper lip control when removing food from a spoon during his snack.

# Intervention

The course of occupational therapy intervention for Joey is described here in three phases: initial treatment, treatment after 6 months, and recommendations for treatment at the end of 1 year.

## *Initial Treatment*

Representative sections of a treatment session conducted at the beginning of Joey's course of treatment are presented to illustrate specific treatment concepts and techniques. This relates to the discussion of the sequence of intervention in the NDT frame of reference (see Chapter 5).

### Long-Term Goals

Listed below are two long-term goals and two possible objectives addressed during the first 6 months of Joey's treatment:

1. Improve Joey's ability to reach for and obtain toys and objects independently.
   A. Joey will be able to reach for and grasp objects (1- to 2-inches in diameter) by using a digital grasp pattern. Objects will be positioned on either side of Joey, within 45° of body midline, and between shoulder height and table top. The therapist will provide stability and facilitation at the elbow.
   B. Joey will be able to release objects (1- to 2- inches in diameter) for placement (such as, 1-inch into a shape sorter) by using digital extension. The therapist will provide stability and facilitation at the wrist.
2. Joey will be able to feed himself independently with a spoon when in his adapted chair.
   A. Joey will be able to remove the food from the spoon and keep it in his mouth while eating his snack with the occupational therapist providing occasional lip and jaw control for 25% of the activity.
   B. Joey will be able to hold the spoon by using a palmar grasp, scoop the food, and bring the spoon to his mouth, retaining an upright trunk position during his snack.

Intervention began with preparatory activities on the mat that encouraged more controlled movement transitions. Joey wanted to play with the ring toss game, so one post was positioned on each side at waist level and about 6 inches from his body. With Joey positioned in supine, the therapist encouraged him to turn to the side by using a key point on the bottom leg. Facilitation entailed a caudal weightshift by using a key point on the ankle and traction, followed by a rotation of the bottom leg to facilitate a lateral weightshift to the side. By using the thigh of the upper leg as the other key point, the therapist was able to guide Joey's upper body over the stabilized

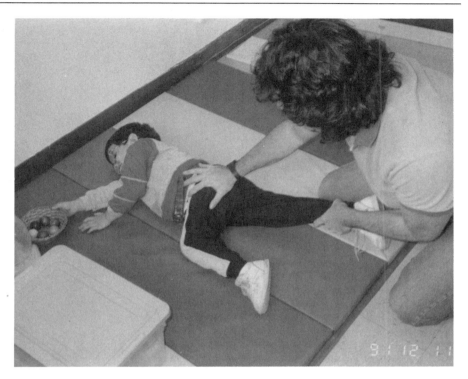

**Figure 16.1.** Supine to sidelying.

leg (Fig. 16.1). The movement was graded slowly so that the therapist could monitor Joey's reaction in his upper trunk, neck, head, and arms. Slow movement prevented the use of excessive extension and the associated upper extremity patterns that Joey used habitually. Because Joey initiated rolling with his head and neck hyperextended and used an upper extremity high-guard position, the therapist had to grade the direction and speed of the weight shift carefully to activate the head, neck, and trunk flexors and to promote forward reaching of the top arm.

In sidelying, the therapist had to change the key points of control. First, she provided pressure to Joey's abdominals to give added stability. Second, she placed her hand over the shoulder girdle of his top arm to facilitate more controlled reach (Fig. 16.2). This support was provided on both sides as Joey was engaged in the ring toss game.

To facilitate rolling from the sidelying to the prone position, the therapist had to use a key point at the pectoralis major on the weight-bearing side to facilitate a lateral weightshift and provide stability. The rest of Joey's body

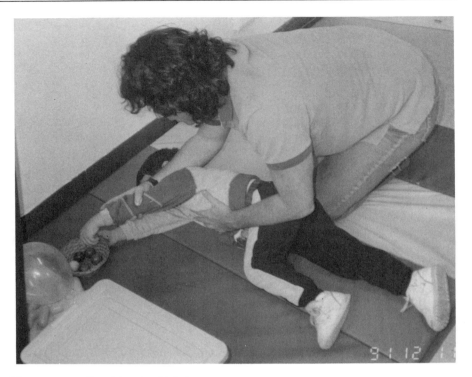

**Figure 16.2.** Reaching in sidelying.

then could propel over to the prone position. In that position, Joey was able to continue playing with the ring toss, weightshifting to one side and reaching with the opposite arm.

The next activity focused on righting and equilibrium reactions and upper extremity movements out of midrange into a more upright position—bench sitting. Transition from prone on elbows to bench sitting entailed movement through the quadruped position and supported kneeling. The therapist assisted Joey into prone on extended arms using facilitation at the right and left pectoralis muscles, weightshifting to right and left. A weightshift to his right freed the left elbow to extend. Then, the therapist was able to provide a weightshift onto the extended left arm, providing deeper tactile input to the left pectoralis muscle for more proximal stability. This position then freed Joey's right arm to extend.

Joey was able to maintain prone on extended elbows position briefly and then the therapist facilitated his transition to the quadruped position. The therapist maintained some support to Joey's upper body with the key point

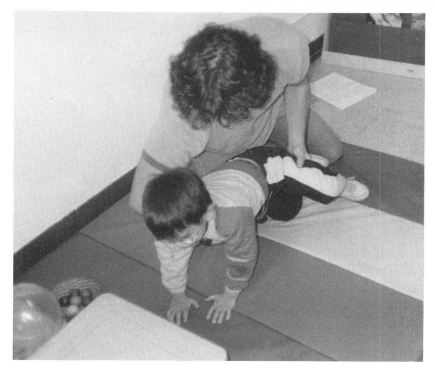

**Figure 16.3.**  Prone extension to quadruped.

between his chest and abdomen. She also facilitated a weightshift in a cephalolateral (**diagonal**) direction. This weightshift freed the opposite leg and facilitated hip and knee flexion. The therapist maintained her left hand on Joey's chest and moved her right hand to Joey's gluteus muscle. To free the left lower extremity, a caudolateral (**diagonal**) weightshift to the right was facilitated to promote hip and knee flexion. After left lower extremity hip and knee flexion was attained, the weight was shifted back toward the left side to promote weightbearing on the left knee (Fig. 16.3). In the quadruped position, Joey enjoyed rocking back and forth in a cephalocaudal direction with the therapist providing stability at the key points of chest, abdominals, and gluteus maximus (Fig. 16.4).

To move Joey into a sitting position, the therapist positioned a low bench parallel to Joey's body that provided for his hip/knee/ankle at approximately a 90°/90°/90° angle, with feet positioned securely on the floor. To make the transition to bench sitting from the quadruped position, the therapist facilitated a slight weightshift to Joey's right to free his left arm and hand so

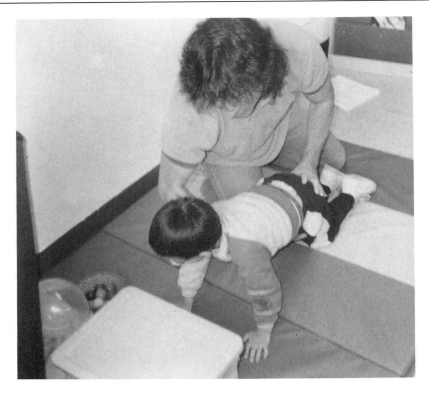

**Figure 16.4.**  Rocking back and forth in quadruped.

they could be placed on the bench (Fig. 16.5). The therapist then positioned herself behind the bench, with stability provided at Joey's left arm. The therapist used her right hand on Joey's right oblique muscles to guide his trunk in an upward rotation movement to bring his left hip up onto the bench (Fig. 16.6). To attain upright sitting, the therapist facilitated a weightshift using key points at both hips in a left posterior (**diagonal**) direction to elicit an equilibrium reaction (Fig. 16.7). This made it possible for Joey to be weightbearing on both hips and both lower extremities in a neutral, midline position (Fig. 16.8).

In upright sitting, the therapist stabilized Joey's pelvis in a neutral position and facilitated small weightshifts in all planes to elicit righting and equilibrium reactions. This was done slowly at first to give Joey a chance to regain and maintain balance. Speed was increased as he developed more movement control.

As Joey demonstrated more control in sitting, the therapist changed key points to one hand on his abdominals for stability and encouraged Joey to

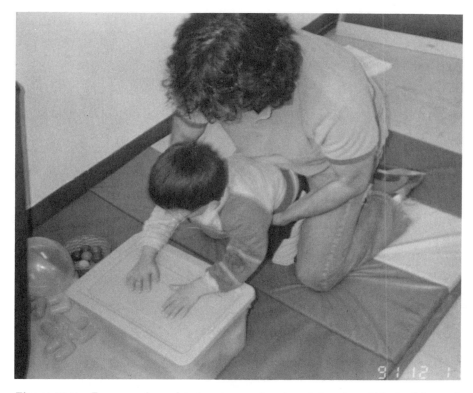

**Figure 16.5.** From quadruped to hands on a low bench (or closed bin in this case).

initiate the weightshift on his own by reaching for a ball held in front of him. The therapist used her own body to guide the weightshift. The ball was held at increasing distances from midline in all directions. Differently shaped and sized toys were used to increase Joey's repertoire of reach and grasp patterns.

When Joey engaged in activities that required a table surface, he leaned forward on the tabletop. To encourage more upright sitting, the therapist placed one hand on Joey's abdominals and one hand in midline on his back at the thoracic-lumbar articulation to facilitate extension for improved trunk alignment. To promote upper extremity reaching away from midrange, active supination, and wrist extension, the therapist positioned blocks on the right and left sides at shoulder height for Joey to grasp and place on the table. To obtain more control over supination and wrist extension, the key point was changed from the abdominals to the elbow. Joey then stacked the blocks in midline with the therapist moving the key point down to the wrist to prevent

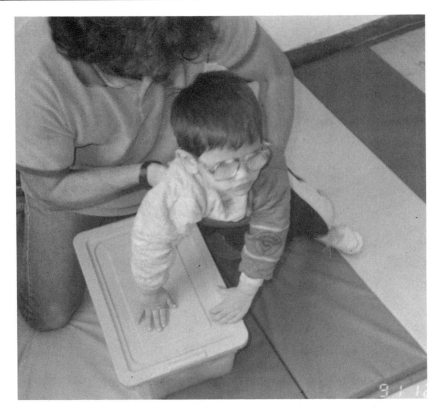

**Figure 16.6.**   Upward trunk rotation to get hips onto a low bench.

tenodesis release and to facilitate active wrist extension and graded digital release (Fig. 16.9). This activity was facilitated with both right and left upper extremities.

The last activity used during a treatment session was the spoon feeding of cereal, one of Joey's favorite foods. He was positioned in his adapted chair with a tray table and belt to stabilize his pelvis in a neutral position. To prevent Joey from leaning and jutting his head and neck forward, the therapist supported Joey's trunk in an upright position by placing her hand on Joey's abdominals (Fig. 16.10). Joey assisted in his feeding by using his right upper extremity to weightbear on the table. Joey used a left palmar grasp to pick up the spoon. The therapist facilitated a more digital grasp by providing stability at the wrist. This key point was used to guide Joey's arm and hand to scoop and bring the spoon to his mouth, using some forearm supination. The therapist provided stability at the jaw during spoon feeding because this

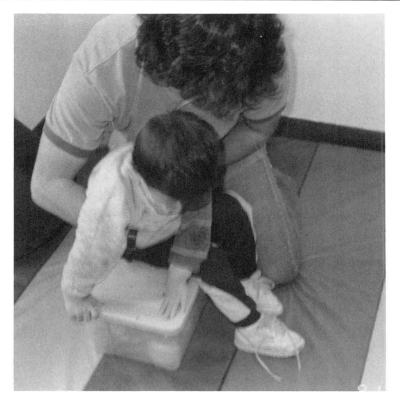

**Figure 16.7.**    Elicitation of lower extremity equilibrium reactions to obtain symmetrical sitting on a low bench.

seemed to improve Joey's ability to remove food from the spoon and to keep his tongue from protruding (Fig. 16.11). In addition, pressure on the upper lip at midline improved Joey's lip closure. This was continued until he finished eating the cereal.

Each session ended with a short conversation between Joey's mother and the therapist about how the session went, or a written note was sent to Joey's parents.

## Treatment After 6 Months

Joey was involved in the preschool program for 6 months and received individualized, direct occupational therapy services during that time. His ability to use equilibrium reactions to maintain postural control during movement transitions and during activities had improved. This was documented

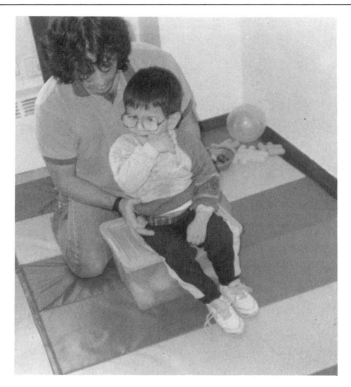

**Figure 16.8.**  Sitting with neutral pelvis.

by his improved ability to maintain an upright posture in bench sitting, as well as his ability to transition from a prone to a quadruped position and to bench sitting. Joey was able to initiate and control weightshifts in small ranges, using less head and neck hyperextension. He could transition from a prone to a quadruped position and pull up onto a low bench but continued to require handling to rotate his trunk and raise his pelvis up onto the bench for sitting. Joey continued to require support to maintain his pelvis in a neutral position. With this support, he could maintain his trunk and head in an upright position for longer periods without the therapist's support at the abdominals. He could initiate small weightshifts and head and trunk righting reactions when reaching for a toy out of midrange. This resulted in Joey being able to reach further away from the midline. Improvement also was seen in active supination and wrist extension when he reached for blocks and other objects.

In his adapted chair, Joey still required a seatbelt to stabilize his pelvis. He could maintain his trunk in an upright position without support at the

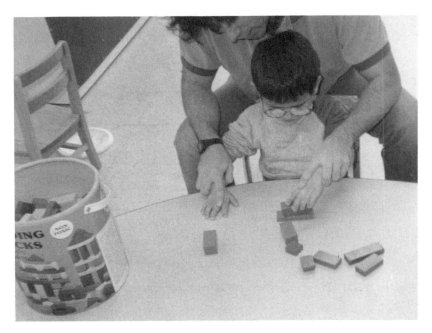

**Figure 16.9.** Facilitation of wrist extension and graded digital release.

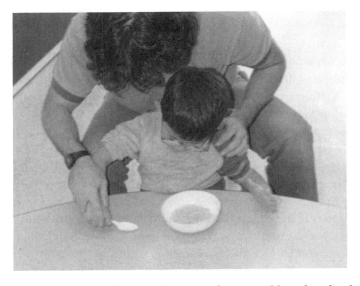

**Figure 16.10.** Facilitating the grasp of a spoon. Note that the therapist has changed the key point from the abdominals to the shoulder girdle.

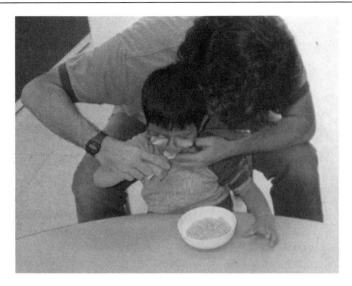

**Figure 16.11.** Providing jaw stability to improve ability to remove food from a spoon.

abdominals and back for a longer time. He still leaned forward occasionally when tired. Joey required support only at the shoulder girdle to facilitate active wrist extension and graded digital extension for the release of the cube blocks.

Joey was now able to remain upright during spoon feeding without jutting his head and neck forward, and no tonic bite was exhibited. Jaw stability was necessary only occasionally to prevent tongue protrusion and for approximation of lips. With support at the elbow, Joey could hold the spoon by using wrist extension and a digital grasp. He was able to scoop food with some active supination.

As his control of distal movement improved, Joey required less support and facilitation at his wrist and hand. The key point of control was changed from the distal one (wrist and hand) used at the beginning of treatment to a more proximal key point (elbow and shoulder). Treatment focused on encouraging Joey to initiate weightshifts and to move independently. Because he had developed more distal as well as proximal control, he could begin to use head, neck, and trunk righting reactions, which, at this point, were sufficient enough to realign his body following small displacements away from his center of gravity. He continued to require handling for support and to guide movements when he moved farther away from midrange.

Joey's teacher reported that he was able to participate in group activities in class for longer periods. He could maintain upright sitting on a bench with a table in front of him for a long enough period to participate in group activities such as songs, show-and-tell, and sensory activities. When he was tired, he would lean forward toward the table until his head and trunk were resting on it. His teacher also observed that Joey moved around the room more. At the beginning of the year, he remained wherever he was placed. After the 6-month program, if he was placed down on the floor or mat, he often rolled or crawled on his stomach to explore the classroom or to join other children. The teacher felt that this demonstrated improvement not only in motor skills and abilities but also in self-confidence, initiative, and adaptive coping abilities. She used an adapted chair for fine motor activities and observed an improvement in Joey's ability to manipulate pegs, puzzle pieces, blocks, and crayons.

### Six-Month, Long-Term Goals

The long-term goals identified during the first 6 months were applicable throughout the first year. At 6 months, the goals were modified in the following ways:

I. Improve Joey's ability to reach for and obtain toys and objects independently.
   A. Joey will be able to reach forward and grasp objects ($\frac{1}{4}$ to $\frac{1}{2}$ inch in diameter) by using a digital grasp pattern. Objects will be positioned on either side of Joey, within 90° of body midline, and between his shoulder height and the tabletop.
   B. Joey will be able to pick up small objects ($\frac{1}{4}$ to $\frac{1}{2}$ inch in diameter) by using a digital grasp and then release them for placement (such as stacking) by using active wrist and digital extension.
II. Joey will be able to feed himself independently with a spoon when positioned in his adapted chair.
   A. Joey will be able to grasp a spoon by using a digital pronate grasp and bring it to his mouth by using active wrist extension and forearm supination.
   B. Joey will be able to use a digital grasp to pick up a cracker, bring it to his mouth, and eat the whole cracker without crumbling it.

## Recommendations for Treatment at the End of 1 Year

To improve Joey's postural alignment and the upper extremity functional skills needed for his last year of preschool, the NDT frame of reference was continued. It was recommended that Joey receive direct occupational therapy intervention but that the services be provided in his classroom setting. His family, as well as the rest of the team, felt that this service provision would help meet Joey's needs to improve social and peer interaction skills and to minimize disruptions of the classroom routine. In addition, it was more likely that specific interventions could be carried over by the teacher and the teaching assistants. This offered Joey a greater chance to carry over movement patterns learned during occupational therapy to functional and preschool-related skills within the context of the classroom.

**Long-Term Goals For the Following Year**

Two possible long-term goals related to the NDT frame of reference for the following year included:

1. Joey will be able to reach and grasp $\frac{1}{4}$-inch diameter crayons on the table independently and position them for use in his hand.
2. Joey will be able to maintain an upright position and feed himself independently with a spoon in his adapted chair during the 20-minute snack period.

Furthermore, it was recommended that other frames of reference be explored to address Joey's other difficulties. Although he had improved his upper extremity functional skills, Joey still required increased effort and time for performance. This was especially true for perceptual motor activities and such tasks as writing, puzzles, block construction, and designs. Because of this, the NDT frame of reference can be used sequentially with an acquisitional frame of reference focussing on the use of adaptive technology. Computers and available adaptive software and hardware could be used by Joey to communicate his wants and needs, to perform homework assignments, and to access selected educational and perceptual motor programs. The NDT frame of reference could be used to improve Joey's postural alignment and upper extremity skills to activate the computer and adaptive hardware more efficiently.

Another frame of reference recommended to maximize Joey's independence and self-confidence in the classroom was the coping frame of reference. This can be used simultaneously with the NDT frame of reference. The coping frame of reference would be used to encourage even more independent functioning in the classroom. The therapist and teacher could observe Joey's coping styles and adapt their own styles to better fit his educational, functional and social/emotional needs.

Finally, it was recommended that an acquisitional frame of reference be explored that would focus on having Joey learning specific motor patterns needed to perform educational tasks. It could be used to develop specific skills needed in the classroom. Again, the acquisitional frame of reference would be used sequentially with the NDT frame of reference. For example, the occupational therapist might provide handling with Joey when the teacher taught a group of children how to perform a preschool fine motor skill. Often Joey was unable to use a smooth, well-coordinated upper extremity pattern when performing fine motor tasks in a group in his classroom. During these activities, the occupational therapist and teacher would have to decide whether it was more important for Joey to perform the activity independently and successfully in any way he was able, or whether he should be encouraged to perform these activities only when assistance or handling was provided to improve the quality of the motor pattern.

Another alternative was to use an acquisitional frame of reference to teach Joey adaptive methods for performing these activities or to adapt the activities so that he was able to perform them successfully without primitive or abnormal motor patterns.

## Summary

Joey seemed to be adapting well to preschool. His parents and the preschool education and therapy staff will probably need to plan for Joey's transition to kindergarten and elementary school. Some future occupational therapy concerns based on the NDT frame of reference follow. Because of delayed development of equilibrium reactions, postural tone dysfunction, and poor postural alignment, Joey probably will have difficulty in maintaining his balance during rapid weightshifts and movement transitions. This will continue to affect his ability to shift his weight when reaching for objects away from midline as well as his ability to move smoothly and quickly around a classroom or school, on and off the bus, and in and out of various chairs and seating equipment commonly used in schools. His ability to exercise fine motor control may continue to be affected by his need to use his arms for support in an upright position because of his tendency to stabilize at the neck and shoulder area to compensate for poor postural control. This may affect his ability to develop such fine motor skills as hand writing or to use the computer keyboard, to use scissors, or to develop the fine and in-hand manipulation skills needed for other school activities such as science experiments, art, or shop projects.

Other frames of reference may become necessary for Joey to accomplish school activities without a therapist being routinely available in the classroom. The occupational therapist will continue to assist him in the classroom, but she also wants to foster independence at home in his self-care activities. Joey's parents may need support and assistance in managing their son's developing need for independence as well as help in negotiating the educational system.

The NDT frame of reference will continue to be important for Joey so that he can continue to develop more proximal control, more efficient righting and equilibrium reactions, and better postural alignment. This can allow him a greater repertoire of movement patterns needed for mobility and upper extremity functioning in school.

The school years can be stressful for a child and his family because of increased societal and community demands for performance and because of increasing peer pressure. Joey's emerging self-confidence and curiosity should be supported by providing him with every possible opportunity to gain independence, to make mistakes, and to achieve success.

---

## STUDY QUESTIONS

1. Why was the NDT frame of reference selected for Joey?

2. How does Joey's habitual shoulder pattern (i.e., high guard position) affect his ability to reach for toys?

3. What other factors make it difficult for Joey to reach for toys?

4. How does the occupational therapist focus on Joey's habitual patterns and how does she attempt to improve his ability to reach for toys?

5. Why does the occupational therapist provide stability to the abdominals when Joey is bench sitting and reaching for toys? How? Could this stability be provided in other ways?

6. Why did the occupational therapist change the key point from the wrist to the elbow when Joey was spoon feeding?

7. Why did the occupational therapist give Joey support at the abdominals when he was spoon feeding? In what other ways could she provide this support?

8. How does the occupational therapist facilitate active support and wrist extension during reach and grasp? What are some other ways to do this?

---

## Acknowledgment

The authors wish to thank Ms. Yvette Comacho for giving permission to photograph her son, Brian, and Brian Comacho for his willingness to be photographed. Brian Comacho is not the child discussed in the chapter and was photographed only to demonstrate the treatment techniques discussed in this chapter.

## References

Anderson, J., & Hinojosa, J. (1984). Parents in a professional partnership. *American Journal of Occupational Therapy, 38,* 451–461.

Hanft, B. (1988). The changing environment of early intervention service: Implications for practice. *American Journal of Occupational Therapy, 42,* 724–731.

Hinojosa, J., & Anderson, J. (1991). Home programs for preschool children with cerebral palsy: Mothers' perceptions. *American Journal of Occupational Therapy, 45,* 273–279.

# 17

# Case Study: Biomechanical Frame of Reference

CHERYL ANN COLANGELO

This chapter is based on the case study presented in Chapter 16. The biomechanical approach is appropriate as a supportive or sequential frame of reference in the integrated treatment program for Joey. Joey is young and actively engaged with his environment. His age and current level of function indicate a need for a program of active therapeutic handling, as outlined in Chapter 16. The biomechanical approach can provide a means of practicing components of movement when therapeutic handling is not provided; it also can facilitate independence in specific skills with the help of external controls.

Joey's background information identified several needs that could be addressed by using the biomechanical frame of reference. These include feeding, mobility, and physical management in the context of his family. Because Joey has just started to attend a preschool program, physical management in the school is an area that needs attention. In addition, the occupational therapy assessment established relevant needs based on the function/dysfunction continua described in Chapter 8.

## Functional Range of Motion

Despite full passive range of motion (ROM), Joey's functional mobility is limited by the influence of reflexes, associated reactions, compensatory movements, and tight muscle groups.

The influence of the tonic labyrinthine reflex (TLR) reinforces an undesirable pattern of shoulder girdle retraction and lower extremity extension in the supine position, preventing flexion against gravity.

Tight hamstrings interfere with anteroposterior pelvic mobility, particularly in floor sitting; the resultant posterior pelvic tilt creates a rounded back. In this position, Joey cannot right his head without a great deal of neck hyperextension as well as effort. In addition, his shoulders assume a compensatory "high guard" position so that his arms and hands are not available for protective extension or object manipulation.

Associated reactions in response to the stress of postural demands (in the form of retraction/flexion in the upper extremities and adduction/extension in the lowers) also limit freedom of arm movement and independent repositioning of legs to provide a wider base of support in bench or chair sitting. In addition, Joey is at risk for developing future deformities, particularly at the hips.

## Ability to Maintain Righted Head and Control Neck Mobility

Although Joey generally has fair head control, the position and movement of his head and neck warrant attention in several situations. In the supine position, the influence of the TLR reinforces a pattern of neck extension with accompanying tone throughout the body.

In floor sitting, Joey's neck is either flexed forward or hyperextended as a result of the position of his pelvis and back. Neck hyperextension limits the ability to turn the head to the side, so that Joey cannot attend visually and his eye contact is impaired.

The jutting forward of Joey's head during self-feeding is a result of his inability to get the spoon to his mouth once his arm leaves the laptray to move through space. He, therefore, must bring his head to his hand. This head/neck position influences oral-motor control negatively.

## Ability to Maintain Righted and Stable Trunk

Joey's trunk control in floor sitting is poor. Floor sitting is a particular issue for a three-year-old because so much play, learning, and social interaction occur at floor level. Floor sitting also is significant for Joey because his potential for mobility through space is best attained on the floor. He is more likely to move independently from floor sitting to prone crawling.

Although Joey's trunk control is better in chair sitting because of reduced pull on his hamstrings, a high guard pattern occurs frequently in his arms, either as an associated reaction to postural stress or as a compensatory pattern to provide upper back extension. The need to lean on a laptray during manipulation stems not only from lack of shoulder stability—in itself, this is not significantly limited; Joey can weight shift and reach out fully in the prone position—but also from the inability of the trunk to support two lever arms as they are placed farther from the center of gravity.

## Ability to Place and Control Position of the Hands

In sitting, Joey cannot control his arms in space simultaneously for bilateral activities. Upper body dressing depends on the ability to move both arms through space in a controlled fashion. Perceptually, Joey needs to engage in bilateral activities to develop an integrated body scheme.

## Ability to Move Through Space Efficiently

Joey's drag-crawl consumes a great deal of energy, limiting the distance he can cover to explore or attain an object. It also reinforces a pattern of extension/adduction in his lowers that interferes with the development of sitting, creeping, and walking skills. Rolling, his other means of mobility, precludes maintained visual contact with a goal and reinforces a nonsegmental pattern of movement that Joey is working to modify during therapy sessions. At this time, however, rolling does provide Joey with unique vestibular stimulation through full rotations of his head through space.

Joey is unable to move through space in three planes; he is limited to the surface of the floor. He experiences passive movement in all planes when roughhousing with his father. As he and his father get older and as Joey gets bigger, this becomes a more difficult form of play.

It is difficult for other persons to move Joey from one place to another. He is outgrowing his stroller and frequently stiffens into extension from associated reactions when being carried. His stroller has a soft back and sling seat with a seatbelt that holds his waist rather than his hips. It provides him with little postural support. Joey either sags into the seat with a rounded back and protracted, internally rotated shoulders or, when excited, he extends his back and hips and then slides out of the stroller.

## Ability to Engage in Self Care Activities

### Feeding

The compensatory neck movements necessary to bring Joey's mouth halfway to the spoon when self-feeding are produced by cervical extension, particularly at the base of the skull. This position contributes to instability of the jaw as well as to swallowing difficulties. Although he can feed himself, enhancing Joey's hand-to-mouth patterns may have a positive impact on oral-motor function.

### Toileting

Joey is in diapers but is physiologically and cognitively mature enough for toilet training. Because he cannot sit independently on a potty and because of the time his physical management already demands, his parents decided to postpone this additional task.

### Bathing

Joey's mother had been bathing him in the kitchen sink, where she could support and contain him while preserving her back. He has outgrown the sink, as well as commonly available infant tub seats. In the tub, Joey feels unsafe when his mother attempts to support him with one hand and bathe him with the other as she leans over the side of the tub. Because of his posterior pelvic tilt, he falls back easily when startled or when he tries to help bathe himself. Bathing had been a pleasant, interactive sensory-motor activity, but it now has become an unpleasant chore for all concerned.

## Summary

The evaluation focused on those needs that the biomechanical approach could address. The goals are not so much "biomechanical" or even "occupational therapy", but, rather, they are *Joey's* goals, established by the team of therapists, parents, and teachers. The occupational therapist takes no ownership of the goals but provides a unique component in addressing them, and the biomechanical frame of reference offers a specific modality in the treatment/educational program.

Joey's goals include:

1. Functional use of head and arms in floor sitting:
   A. The ability to attend to language tasks while maintaining upright head and trunk;
   B. The ability to use his hands when provided with external trunk/hip controls;
   C. The ability to move from a floor sitting device to prone lying;
   D. The ability to move head and arms without external controls.

2. Liberation of arms in chair or bench sitting:
   A. Increased range of shoulder/elbow/forearm movements given artificial hip, trunk, and arm supports;
   B. Increased range of shoulder/elbow/forearm movements given hip supports only.
3. Efficient active movement through space:
   A. Ability to move rapidly through space with minimal associated reactions, using a wheeled device.
4. Experience passive or active movement in many dimensions of space;
   A. Ability to experience this movement with minimal increase in pathological tone (flexion in uppers, extension in lowers) in an adapted device;
   B. Ability to initiate or maintain the movement.
5. Improved head position during self-feeding to enhance oral-motor control.
6. Develop the ability to sit and void on toilet or potty.
7. Facilitate physical management at home based on the needs of the entire family.

# Application

Adults tend to engage in manipulative tasks primarily in a chair-sitting position. Children, particularly preschoolers, interact with objects and each other in various positions in space. They often choose the floor over a chair and a table as a support surface and assume a variety of positions from which to play. For this reason, a repertoire of support devices should be available to the preschooler who has a disability so that he can engage with his peers in age-appropriate activities. The devices need to meet two basic criteria: First, they must contribute to the functional goals established for, and with, the child; second, they must be manageable in terms of size and ease of use in the context of the environment.

Joey's equipment was meant to be used primarily at home and at school to carry over goals that were addressed by physical handling during therapy. Although it was his therapists' responsibility to provide devices to address physical goals, it was Joey's teachers and parents who would determine whether the devices "worked" in the context of his life. The therapist provided many options for positioning, and Joey's caretakers determined their appropriateness, choosing some and "discarding" others. Those devices selected for use were modified over time as Joey's postural skills improved. Rather than present a treatment plan in terms of short- and long-term goals, the section that follows describes each support system sequentially in terms of the seven general goals discussed previously.

## 1. Functional Use of Head and Arms in Floor Sitting

Two components of this first goal are (1) the ability to floor sit independently and (2) the ability to engage in play in supported floor sitting. Joey had to develop the postural skills necessary for independent sitting because much peer play occurred on the floor at school, and because floor sitting is a natural position from which to assume a quadruped position. In addition, until he could floor sit independently, Joey needed support so that he could interact with friends at their level (as opposed to prone lying when others sat). In long sitting, tight hamstrings were a significant deterrent to independence. In ring sitting, limitations in functional external rotation and abduction prevented contact between the lateral aspect of Joey's thighs with the floor, causing him to rock back on the base of his spine and compensate with trunk flexion.

To facilitate independent long sitting, Joey was seated on a therapy wedge, facing the downward slope. This took some stress off his tight hamstrings by opening the angle of his flexed hips by about 15°. With his pelvis then in a neutral position, Joey was able to maintain an erect spine and righted head; however, he lacked lateral stability. Flexor tone in his arms prevented him from maintaining full elbow extension to prop on either side of his body. If he began to lose lateral control, Joey became startled, and his arms retracted and flexed rather than providing protective extension. To make his arms available for support, cardboard building blocks (3 inches high) were placed on either side of his body, so that his hands could rest comfortably on them in a protective position. A nonskid pad was placed beneath each block. Joey was able to practice sitting independently this way during physically passive activities, such as storytime and calendar activities, as well as when watching television. The system was easy to set up and was introduced during "circle time" in school, when all the children sat on the floor.

After trying this adaption in school, Joey's teacher asked to discontinue its use. Although Joey was able to maintain sitting, it was somewhat precarious, and his teacher was distracted from teaching by the possibility that Joey might be knocked over by some of the more active children. Joey's therapists were not so concerned about him occasionally falling off onto the rug; falling to a soft surface while mastering a postural skill was part of his learning process; however, this possibility interfered with Joey's teacher's ability to do her job well; therefore, the wedge was discontinued in school.

Joey's parents were willing to set him up on the wedge at home for 15 to 30 minutes at a time as he watched television. This was generally reserved for weekend use, because Joey could not tolerate more postural demands placed on him after a full day at school.

Joey's need for support in floor sitting in school was met better through the use of a floor sitter. Basically, this is a chair without legs that has a large base to keep it from tipping. The back of the chair supported Joey up to his shoulders. His pelvis was stabilized by a belt that crossed his hip at a 45-degree angle. Joey was most stable when one leg was flexed and externally rotated while the other was extended and crossed over the ankle of the flexed leg. At first, the floor sitter provided low lateral trunk supports. These were placed so that they would not interfere with arm movements, and they prevented Joey from falling over laterally yet required that he exercise upper trunk control. In this device, Joey's arms were liberated for play. As he became more stable over time, the lateral trunk supports were removed. Because his pelvis was stable, he could then rotate his trunk to reach for toys without falling over. As the months passed, Joey became more skilled at transitioning from a sitting to a quadruped position during his therapy sessions. At that time, he was taught to open his Velcro™ seat belt to transfer independently from a sitting to a prone position, shifting his weight over his flexed, externally rotated side to leave the floor sitter.

The practical application of the floor sitter enabled Joey to play with his peers at school. The device complemented the following goals outlined in Joey's case study on neurodevelopmental therapy:

1. Maintenance of an upright position (**upper trunk control**)
2. Reaching away from the body midline
3. Initiation of weight shifts as he reached to the side and, later, when transitioning to a prone position.

## 2. Liberation of Arms in Chair or Bench Sitting

As was the case with floor sitting, the two areas addressed in chair sitting were (1) the ability to chair sit independently during physically passive activities and (2) the ability to engage the arms when in supported sitting.

Joey's adapted chair provided full support to his pelvis and thighs, a back height ending at shoulder level, and a 90-degree hip angle maintained by a seat belt at a 45-degree angle. He was provided with bilateral trunk supports slightly above his waist. These supports were very thin and lightly padded so that they would not interfere with Joey's humeral position and mobility when the laptray was not used. The laptray itself was placed 1 inch above elbow height. A modification was made on Joey's chair based on clinical observations. First, when Joey's therapist facilitated his abdominals during therapy, his sitting stability improved. Second, when Joey sat in his upright adapted chair, he often leaned on his laptray, using it partially for trunk support. By tipping Joey's adapted chair backward (two-inch-high blocks were placed beneath the front legs), these related issues were affected. First, when he tired, Joey leaned back against the slightly reclined back. Gravity then assisted his abdominals as he rested. Second, to sit upright, Joey had to come forward **actively,** calling in his abdominal musculature. With this more active way of sitting upright, Joey was less inclined to lean onto the laptray. Appropriately, the laptray became a support for his arms rather than his arms becoming a support for his trunk. Because he no longer needed to weight bear on his arms for stability, his range of active arm movements increased. Opportunities for mobility superimposed on stability were also provided in prone positions.

Joey's adapted chair maintained a stable, neutrally positioned pelvis through use of the seatbelt in conjunction with the 90-degree, seat-to-back angle. In bench sitting, Joey required facilitation techniques by his therapist to maintain a bench sitting position independently, with 90° of flexion at his hips, knees, and ankles. Joey still succumbed to the pull of the hamstrings on the pelvis. This caused a rounding of his back and shoulders and precluded reaching activities. When provided with slight hip extension and moderate hip abduction in sitting, Joey was able to maintain a neutral pelvis. By sitting Joey on a narrow therapy roll elevated on stable props (commercially available), Joey was able to sit as if on a horse—hips at 75–80° flexion, knees flexed, and ankles below the hips. Because his knees were lower than his hips, Joey's legs were abducted by the diameter of the roll. If a large roll was used to avoid elevation on props, the roll demanded too much abduction, and Joey's thighs would slide up to the top of the roll, rotating his hips internally and bringing his feet off the floor.

This elevated roll was used at a table in school to encourage an independent, upright position. Joey used this position during low-motor demand tabletop activities, such as language and visual discrimination tasks.

As Joey's endurance for unsupported sitting on the roll developed, modifications were made in his adapted chair, which was his primary unit for engaging in fine motor activities. Lateral trunk supports automatically became lower as he grew taller and, eventually, were removed altogether. Toward the end of the year, Joey began to feel comfortable with gross reach and grasp when on the roll, a measure of increased postural competence. He started to attempt upper body undressing. At this time, his adapted chair was returned to the upright position, with use of the seatbelt continued.

## 3. Efficient Active Movement Through Space

A scooterboard used for mobility allowed Joey to attain a desired object quickly and to move playfully, while enhancing components of movement. When crawling, Joey was unable to bring his elbows forward of his shoulders; active shoulder flexion was limited to 90° because of increased tone and limitations of mobility superimposed on stability. Crawling was accompanied by increased extension in his head, trunk, and lower extremities. Joey was provided with a scooterboard that supported him from below the sternoclavicular joint to just above his ankles. The front edge was cut away (like an ironing board) to leave the shoulders free for full movement. A slight wedge was placed beneath his chest so that less neck extension was needed to look forward from a horizontal plane. Joey's pelvis was stabilized by crossed straps. An abductor was placed from midthigh to midcalf to discourage the extension/adduction pattern in his legs and to keep the bottom half of his body centered on the scooterboard yet leave his upper trunk and arms free to move from side to side. The base of the scooterboard was selected for the high responsiveness of the ballbearing casters. With the weightbearing demands on his shoulders decreased, Joey was able to reach forward to propel himself. At first, Joey propelled himself by using a symmetrical tonic neck reflex (STNR) pattern of neck flexion/arm flexion and neck extension/arm extension. This was discouraged through the use of two activities: (1) Joey was taught to propel himself in circles, which encouraged lateral arm movements, and (2) he was engaged in activities with moving toys, such as trucks and balloons, that maintained his visual attention. The scooterboard provided a mobility option for Joey during gross motor activities in the classroom and hallway.

The therapy team considered an adapted tricycle. A commercially available tricycle with seatbelt, back support, footplates, and abductor would have met Joey's postural needs. Although Joey could not propel a tricycle initially, the passive reciprocal leg movements that he would have experienced during a training period could have contributed to separation of the two sides of his body. Practically, however, the tricycle's introduction was not warranted: classroom staff to carry out training was limited; Joey's parents had no use for a trike in their urban community; and Joey was happy with his scooterboard mobility.

## 4. *Experience Passive or Active Movement in Many Dimensions of Space*

Several convenient and inexpensive options were available for the school to provide variety of movement experiences for Joey. The emphasis was not on postural demands but on the experience of movement through space with minimal pathological tone. A preschooler swing-chair was modified by adding a hip strap at a 45-degree angle to keep Joey's hips from extending. A pillow was stuffed between the front bar and Joey's body to keep him upright.

To provide movement in various planes, an inexpensive camping hammock was hung on the swing set with both ends attached on the same hook. Joey was placed in this net swing, straddling it so that one side of the swing supported his back and the other side ran up front, between his legs. He was supported in this way in a flexed position, with extensor overflow inhibited. In addition to swinging and spinning, Joey was able to experience simultaneous bouncing when the hammock was suspended by a loop of elastic cord. Joey was able to control some of his movement through space by pulling on one end of a rope tied to a pole or held by an adult. This "special" equipment was appropriate for all the children in the preschool program.

## 5. *Improved Head Position During Self-Feeding to Enhance Oral-Motor Control*

Joey's habit of jutting his head forward when self-feeding compromised his oral-motor control. With his neck in that position, it was more difficult for him to bring his lips together, to control his swallow, and to stabilize his jaw. Some of this neck position was a result of decreased head control during two fine motor activities (chew/swallow and hand-to-mouth). Another contributing factor was his inability to direct the spoon to his mouth because of a pattern of horizontal abduction, retraction, elbow flexion, forearm pronation, wrist flexion, and ulnar deviation.

In the absence of therapeutic handling, Joey was provided with external controls to help him carry over feeding skills. Initially, a semicircular neck ring was attached to the back of Joey's adapted chair to provide additional neck stability. His hand-to-mouth pattern was modified in several ways. His laptray was elevated to axilla level. This eliminated the need for Joey to lift his arm off the tray to get his hand to his mouth. Humeral wings were attached temporarily to the tray to position his shoulders in slight protraction and horizontal adduction A simple splint was strapped to the ulnar border of his hand to stabilize his wrist in a neutral flexion and neutral lateral deviation.

Under these circumstances, Joey had to control only elbow flexion/extension and slight forearm rotation to bring the spoon from the bowl to his mouth and back. With stress decreased and hand-to-mouth accuracy increased, Joey was better able to maintain his head in a neutral position.

Therapeutic feeding continued during direct treatment. Joey rapidly shed the need for the neck ring. Following that, the humeral wings were removed. When Joey showed a consistent ability to accomplish hand-to-mouth movement without neck compensation in the absence of neck and humeral supports, the laptray gradually was lowered. Joey did not have enough forearm mobility to get the spoon to his mouth with his elbow supported on the lowered laptray, but he did learn to control antigravity shoulder movements to bring his spoon to his mouth once he had mastered the other components of movement, one step at a time.

## 6. Develop the Ability to Sit and Void on Toilet or Potty

Joey's preschool had purchased an adapted potty chair that provided height adjustment of seat-to-floor, depth of seat adjustment, a seatbelt at 45-degrees, lateral trunk supports, and a laptray. Although he sat safely and comfortably in this chair once the depth and height were adjusted, his teacher complained that his flow of urine inevitably was directed into the air rather than into the potty. The problem stemmed from the size of the hole in the seat. Children usually abduct their legs to straddle a toilet seat so they do not fall in. Lacking active abduction, Joey slid down slightly into the hole, forcing his legs into further adduction and his pelvis into a posterior tilt, creating the fountain effect. To get Joey's pelvis into an anterior pelvic tilt, he was provided with an abductor, and his laptray was pulled slightly away from his body. When Joey leaned forward to rest on the laptray, his pelvis assumed a more functional position.

## 7. Facilitate Physical Management at Home Based on the Needs of the Entire Family

This goal includes the provision of devices to ease the caretaking process, as well as to make suggestions about positioning that could enhance Joey's development of components of movement.

Once Joey's program of supportive devices was established in school, the team was anxious to see carry over at home, particularly in the area of self-feeding. The family had indicated a sense of being overwhelmed by Joey's physical needs. Rather than introduce changes in what Joey's parents were comfortable with, the first several months were devoted to suggesting devices to address their stated needs.

Joey had outgrown his stroller. Transportation needs now required some sort of durable medical equipment. Three choices were (1) a larger stroller with minimal adaptations, (2) a larger stroller fully outfitted with seating insert, or (3) a wheelchair. Joey's potential for self-propulsion in a wheelchair had yet to be established. This would make it difficult to determine whether he might need a manual or powered device for mobility. Although he certainly had the potential to propel a manual chair briefly, functional speed and endurance were questionable. The possibility for assisted ambulation was not altogether ruled out. In short, it was too early to make a decision that would be so costly. A stroller large enough to accommodate Joey was a reasonable temporary alternative. The addition of an expensive and cumbersome insert for the stroller to correct Joey's posture was discussed in terms of therapeutic value and family needs. Ideally, Joey needed to sit in a well-supported position as much as possible to carry over therapeutic goals. Practically, Joey's parents were experiencing stress; an adapted insert adds weight to the stroller and adds time to packing it and unpacking it from the car; it takes up space in an apartment. Joey was properly positioned 5 hours per day at school, although he spent less than 1 hour per day, on average, in his stroller. At home Joey used his adapted chair or relaxed on the floor or couch. When visiting, he preferred the floor. The conclusion was to order a large, collapsible stroller with tightly stretched upholstery, a seatbelt, and a footplate.

A toddler chair that hooks onto almost any table and is collapsible and portable is available in toy stores and inexpensive. It has a hard seat and hard back. This was recommended to Joey's parents for use when visiting friends and eating out. It was adapted for Joey with a hip strap and a cardboard back insert with lateral trunk supports.

The recommendation of a bath set that was lightweight (with adjustable hip angle and recline angle) provided Joey with full support in the tub. He was able to engage in water play, and his parents were able to bathe him with no risk to their backs.

As Joey developed motor skills and his parents experienced less stress from his physical management, they shared in more of his school program. They identified which parts of the program were reasonable for them to carry over. Within months, they asked for an adapted potty (when Joey became consistent with his potty training at school), and they brought in his adapted home chair for modifications to provide a consistent feeding program. They also reported making spontaneous adjustments to Joey's positioning based on input from school. For example, when Joey was resting or playing in a supine position, his parents placed pillows beneath his neck and knees to reduce extensor tone, and they encouraged him to sidelie when engaging in fine motor play on the floor. By the end of the school year, his parents were experimenting with positioning and adaptations on their own. Having integrated the principles of intervention into his daily life, Joey's parents brought back to the school ideas that could be implemented for Joey, as well as for other children in his class.

## STUDY QUESTIONS

1. In the adaptations suggested for the school (such as the swing and hammock), explain how the use of this equipment is related to the frames of reference.

2. Describe the interrelationship of these two frames of reference for Joey.

3. Explain how the two frames of references are being used with Joey. Identify areas of consistency and areas of inconsistency.

4. Can you suggest other strategies in this frame of reference that could be used in the situation in which the teacher was not comfortable using the wedge in the classroom?

5. In the situation mentioned in Question 4, can you suggest other strategies for working in collaboration with the teacher?

# 18

# Case Study: Combined Sensory Integrative and Neurodevelopmental Treatment Frames of Reference

SUSAN NESBIT

Joshua was referred to occupational therapy at 8 months of age. A pediatric neurological examination on discharge from a neonatal unit revealed a baby with subtle movement problems: too much extension, head lag when pulled to sit, and poor control of upper extremities when reaching and grasping. Tremors of the tongue also were observed. Private occupational therapy was recommended to supplement Joshua's participation in a child development program, and he has been receiving occupational therapy once a week since then.

Occupational therapy focused on improving Joshua's gross and fine motor deficits. This chapter concentrates on 1 year of Joshua's occupational therapy history, beginning at the age of 3 years and 9 months, when he was referred for a comprehensive evaluation because of coping problems in school.

Joshua is now 4 years, 9 months old. He is the oldest child in a middle-class family of four that resides in a large suburban home in northern New Jersey. Joshua's father is a computer consultant and his mother, a nurse, currently is a full-time mother and homemaker. Joshua's brother is 1 year, 11 months old.

Joshua is enrolled in a private preschool program, three mornings per week. Reportedly, he has difficulty following the school routine and does not relate well with his peers. It is also reported that he cannot control his behavior with other children.

## Medical Background

Joshua was delivered vaginally at 28 weeks gestation, weighing 1265 grams. The pregnancy was remarkable for spotting throughout the first trimester and cervical dilation at 24 weeks gestation, requiring hospitalization and bed rest until delivery. Joshua's nine-week hospitalization was notable for the use of an oxyhood for 48 hours, gavage feeding, and jaundice. Head ultrasound studies were within normal limits.

Joshua's developmental milestones were within normal limits. Walking was at the later end of normal limits, with independent walking occurring at 18 months. Joshua has worn orthotic shoe inserts for pronation of his feet since then.

# Occupational Therapy Assessment

At the age of 3 years, 9 months, Joshua was referred for a comprehensive evaluation to assess his occupational functioning. The primary presenting problem was difficulty in coping at school.

Based on observation and chart review, the occupational therapist determined that two frames of reference would best assess Joshua's status. These two frames of reference were used simultaneously. The sensory integrative frame of reference was chosen to assess Joshua's ability to organize sensory information in the brain and central nervous system (CNS). In other words, does Joshua's CNS have the ability to organize input efficiently, enabling him to make adaptive responses? It was hypothesized that poor sensory integration may be influencing Joshua's quality of gross motor and fine motor skills detrimentally. Because of the quality of Joshua's tonal and movement abilities, the occupational therapist thought that the neurodevelopmental treatment frame of reference also should be used. These two frames of reference could be used simultaneously because they are consistent in their developmental orientation and in the way that they view children.

The occupational therapy evaluation included the Miller Assessment for Preschoolers (Miller, 1982) as well as clinical observations for a set time period. Joshua's chart also was reviewed for the psychological, speech and language, audiological, and learning reports. These comprehensive reports contained significant information for the therapist to enhance her understanding of the child.

The psychological report indicated that Joshua had taken the *Wechsler Preschool and Primary Scale of Intelligence* (1967). He received a full scale score of 100, a verbal scale score of 98, and a performance scale score of 102. Intratest scatter suggested uneven skill development and possible learning difficulties. Although most of Joshua's scores fell within the average range, he had relative weaknesses in areas that tap word knowledge and visual-motor speed. The psychologist felt that emotional variables may have accounted for some of these weakness; therefore, the results might be only a minimal estimate of Joshua's potential cognitive functioning.

The speech pathologist reported that Joshua's overall receptive language skills were mildly impaired. Weaknesses were evident in his understanding of single words at the isolated level. Expressive language skills were mildly impaired as well. Difficulties were noted on tasks that involved cause-and-effect relationships, identification of similarities and differences among related items, and sequencing of pictorial stimuli to produce an integrated story. Articulation skills were judged to be well within normal limits, and overall intelligibility was considered adequate during connected speech. Simple phrase repetitions were noted in Joshua's conversational speech, although rate and vocal quality were unremarkable.

The audiological report indicated that Joshua possessed hearing within normal limits bilaterally. Middle ear analysis findings suggested the absence of significant middle ear dysfunction bilaterally.

The academic evaluation also reported that Joshua's academic achievements were within the average range. In other words, basic concepts considered necessary for success in a school setting were within average range. Specifically, the report stated that Joshua was familiar with some early reading and mathematical concepts.

## Evaluation Based on the Sensory Integrative Frame of Reference

The sensory integrative frame of reference was used to assess Joshua's sensory integrative abilities by looking at his sensory modulation level, functional support capabilities, and end-product abilities. First, sensory modulation was assessed in the various sustems.

**Tactile System.** Joshua demonstrated hypersensitivity to touch. He reacted negatively to touch during the second tactile test on the *Miller Assessment for Preschoolers.* Aversive responses included giggling, frequently trying to peek, rubbing his hand after being touched, and asking, "Are we finished yet?"

**Auditory System.** Joshua responded inappropriately to sound input, demonstrating hypersensitivity to sound. He was afraid of sudden, loud noises, requesting a parent to hold his toes. This reflects the unusual responses often seen in children with sensory modulation dysfunction. Joshua also seemed to have difficulty habituating to continuous, steady sounds. He heard every noise, loud or soft, and had difficulty filtering out the unimportant auditory information.

**Relationship to Gravity.** Joshua disliked being on surfaces that moved or that had the potential to move. Although he agreed to being placed in a sitting position on a large ball, he did not move onto his back easily from the sitting posture. He asked for help stepping up and down from surfaces higher than 8 inches. He jumped off a 16-inch stabilized roll but was unable to jump from higher surfaces, displaying a reluctance to climb onto higher stationary surfaces.

**Movement Level.** Joshua demonstrated an atypical amount of movement; he appeared to move constantly.

**Oral Arousal.** Joshua responded normally to food and drink.

**Olfactory Arousal.** Joshua responded normally to odors.

**Visual System.** Joshua oriented normally to changes in his visual field.

**Attention Level.** Joshua exhibited an inappropriate attention level. He appeared to be aroused constantly by stimuli, especially auditory stimuli.

**Postrotary Nystagmus.** Joshua became overly dizzy after rotary movement.

**Sensitivity to Movement.** Joshua tolerated very little rotary movement without excessive vertigo or nausea.

**Proprioceptive Sensitivity.** Joshua demonstrated poor awareness of joint and muscle movement. On the *Miller Assessment for Preschoolers,* he had difficulty drawing a dotted vertical line, with vision occluded, from the bunny to the house. His "hops" were far from the center line.

**Emotional Arousal.** Joshua exhibited overarousal. He became upset by things that typically are considered trivial by other children of comparable age. He became upset by a little scratch, for example. Also, he became extremely anxious when he was in the same room with a pet, such as a cat.

## Functional Support Capabilities

After assessment of Joshua's sensory modulation in the various systems, the occupational therapy evaluation focused on functional support capabilities.

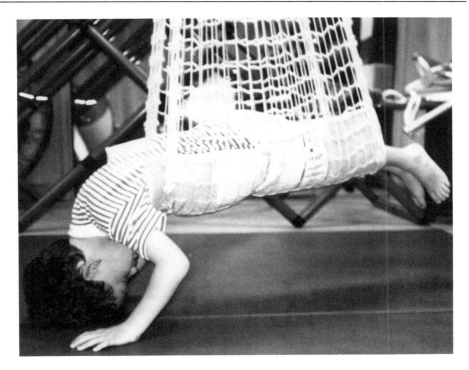

**Figure 18.1.** Difficulty moving volitionally against gravity.

**Tactile Discrimination.** Joshua was administered the two tactile tests from the *Miller Assessment for Preschoolers.* A test for stereognosis evaluated Joshua's ability to identify objects by touch with vision occluded, and Joshua identified all objects correctly. On a test for finger localization, however, Joshua was unable to identify the fingers touched. Joshua reacted negatively to touch during the latter test, and this may have had a detrimental influence on his performance.

**Cocontraction.** Joshua exhibited difficulty in simultaneous contraction of flexor and extensor muscles. He also had difficulty stabilizing his proximal joints adequately during weightbearing. Stability and mobility also were assessed using the neurodevelopmental treatment (NDT) frame of reference.

**Muscle Tone.** Joshua exhibited low muscle tone. Postural tone was assessed further by using the NDT frame of reference.

**Balance and Equilibrium.** Joshua seemed to have difficulty catching his balance when falling. Righting and equilibrium reactions also were assessed with the NDT frame of reference.

**Developmental Reflexes.** Joshua seemed to have mild to moderate difficulty with volitional movement against gravity (Fig. 18.1). This possibly was caused by a lack of integration of the developmental reflexes (in addition to his low muscle tone). Variety of movement was assessed with the NDT frame of reference.

**Lateralization.**   Joshua preferred his right hand for writing and manipulation. He also demonstrated a right-eye and right-foot preference.

**Bilateral Integration.**   Joshua used both hands together in bilateral activities. He used his right hand to write as he stabilized the paper spontaneously with his left hand. He crossed the midline of his body with his right hand to draw on the left side of the page. Joshua also used his right hand to hold scissors when cutting a straight line across the paper held in his left hand.

## End-Product Abilities

End-product abilities comprise the final areas assessed during the occupational therapy evaluation related to the sensory integrative frame of reference.

**Praxis.**   Joshua appeared to have difficulty in motor planning and in coordinating complex movements that required an adaptive response. For example, Joshua had difficulty catching and throwing a 12-inch-diameter soft ball. This activity seemed difficult because of inadequate sequencing and timing, as well as poor awareness of joint and muscle movement.

On the *Miller Assessment for Preschoolers,* Joshua had difficulty on the sequencing test, being unable to pick up the blocks in order. On the test for motor accuracy, he drew lines that were too long.

**Form and Space Perception.**   Joshua displayed adequate form and space perception. He copied a circle, a horizontal line, a vertical line, and a cross. He readily engaged in and seemed to enjoy drawing. He used broad strokes to color within lines. Joshua's familiarity with early reading and mathematical concepts has been noted previously in the academic evaluation.

On the *Miller Assessment for Preschoolers,* Joshua performed well in the areas of block design and stacking (a block tower). He copied the two designs presented to him and stacked 11 blocks. Joshua also solved picture puzzles and completed a test of figure-ground perception successfully.

**Behavior.**   Generally, Joshua was cooperative. He often required redirection to the task at hand, however, because of distractibility and impulsivity. During the assessment, it was noted that Joshua was adept at using his verbal skills to evade activities in which he did not want to participate, showing resistance to activities that either frightened him or that were difficult. He talked freely about various subjects. He was very active verbally and motorically during the evaluation sessions. He understood all verbal directions given.

**Academics.**  As previously discussed, Joshua's academic achievements were within average range.

**Language and Articulation.**  Joshua's mild receptive and expressive language deficits had been noted previously in the speech pathologist report.

**Emotional Tone.**  Joshua seemed to have difficulty with emotional tone. He demonstrated tactile and auditory defensiveness. He had difficulty in relating to gravity. Joshua also seemed to be organized compulsively when putting toys and equipment away.

**Activity Level.**  Observations indicated that Joshua frequently would became unmanageable and could not control his behavior.

**Environmental Mastery.**  Joshua was not always able to respond to environmental demands. He often demonstrated inappropriate emotional tone and increased activity level.

## Evaluation Based on the Neurodevelopmental Treatment Frame of Reference

The neurodevelopmental frame of reference was used to assess further Joshua's quality of movement in gross and fine motor activities.

**Postural Tone.**  Joshua appeared to have mild to moderately low muscle tone in his trunk and all extremities. Joshua easily rolled to either side from a prone and a supine position when on the floor. He had slight difficulty with antigravity extension and moderate difficulty with antigravity flexion in various playing positions. He lacked the amount of antigravity extension and flexion needed to competently perform high-level activities (hopping and riding a bicycle).

**Range of Motion.**  Formal measurement of Joshua's range of motion (ROM) was not done, but it was apparent that he had excessive joint ROM throughout his body. Excessive range was noticeable in elbow and wrist extension, as well as in his lower extremities. In one stance, Joshua displayed moderate to severe bilateral foot pronation with heel eversion.

**Variety of Movement.**  Joshua exhibited poor integration of the asymmetrical tonic neck reflex (ATNR), the symmetrical tonic neck reflex (STNR), the tonic labyrinthine reflex (TLR) in the prone position, and the TLR in the supine position. These reflexive responses were not persistent; however, they seemed to affect his ability to move volitionally against gravity.

**Righting and Equilibrium Reactions as They Relate to Postural Alignment.**  During activities that demanded static or dynamic balance, Joshua did not elongate the muscles on the weight-bearing side of his body. He thus had difficulty regaining his balance when falling on such equipment as a jungle gym or a suspended swing. One additional factor that may have aggravated Joshua's motor problems was the fact that his pronated feet may have interfered with his development of good balance reactions in standing.

**Stability and Mobility (Gross Motor Skills).** Although Joshua used minimal upper trunk rotation spontaneously, he tended to keep his trunk stiff. Thoracic trunk extension was inadequate. He had the flexibility to move his spine in all directions but appeared to lack the hip extension control and abdominal control necessary for proper spinal alignment.

Joshua was ambulatory and he walked on flat surfaces with no problem. He assumed standing from the floor with no assistance by half-kneeling with his right leg up first. He was able to alternate between half-kneeling with his right leg up and half-kneeling with his left leg up only with assistance. As he played, he was observed to move spontaneously from squatting to standing and back again. He assumed quadruped and kneeling positions with no difficulty. Because of poor motor planning, Joshua had difficulty creeping and walking slowly forward and backward on his knees. Lordosis and raising of the medial border of his scapulae were observed. In a quadruped position, Joshua tended to lock his elbows, especially when his hips were higher than his shoulders.

Joshua was able to run and jump forward without difficulty. When jumping, he recruited extra extension by posturing with his elbows behind his shoulders. He jumped over a balance beam and was able to jump a distance of 20 inches; however, he had difficulty jumping backward and sideways. He was only able to stand on one leg and hop with considerable assistance. He skipped without alternating legs.

During most activities, Joshua maintained a wide base of support. For example, when standing or walking he preferred to keep his legs far apart. This is typical of a child with low muscle tone, balance problems, or gravitational insecurity.

Joshua had noticeable lack of muscular development in his upper trunk and shoulders. He did not maintain weight on his arms easily, and, whether weightbearing or not, his scapulae were prominent and tended to lift away from his thoracic wall medially.

Joshua was able to walk on his hands forward for a short distance with support at his hips in wheelbarrow activities. He collapsed on his forearms when walking backward on his hands.

**Stability and Mobility (Fine Motor Skills).** Joshua demonstrated a general instability in his upper extremity movements consistent with his low muscle tone. He often required the additional stability of a surface when completing two-handed activities. For example, when assembling construction toys or joining beads, Joshua braced his arms on the table surface. When additional support was not available, he tended to elevate his shoulders to "fix."

Joshua was able to isolate finger movements on each hand and to coordinate thumb-to-finger opposition with visual cuing. He had difficulty with fine motor tasks that offered resistance. He often used two hands to complete tasks that typically require one hand. Joshua was able to complete basic tasks (stringing $\frac{1}{2}$-inch beads and building a tower using 1-inch cubes). Joshua rolled clay into a snake shape and a ball, shaping his hands around the clay.

Other frames of reference were used to address the quality of such developmental skills as writing, cutting, undressing, and dressing. These skills are not discussed in this chapter but did concern the occupational therapist.

## Summary of Evaluation Findings

Although Joshua had acquired developmental milestones, both gross and fine, he exhibited moderate difficulties in the quality of his movement. The motor difficulties he demonstrated were part of a cluster that commonly fits together. They included low muscle tone, excessive joint ROM, poor cocontraction, and gravitational insecurity.

The evaluation findings indicated that Joshua would benefit from occupational therapy twice each week, using the frames of reference of sensory integration and NDT simultaneously. Because Joshua's muscle tone and quality of movement affect his abilities and resultant skills, and because his sensory deficits also affect his abilities and resultant skills, and because each problem exacerbates the others, it was felt that all areas needed to be addressed concurrently. This emphasized even more the need to use two frames of reference simultaneously to meet Joshua's needs.

A sample of the occupational therapy goals and objectives related to the sensory integrative frame of reference includes:

**Goal:**  To improve Joshua's relationship to gravity for a greater sense of self-confidence when moving through space.

    **Objective 1**: Joshua will use symmetrical arm movements to propel himself forward on a scooterboard a distance of at least 6 feet.

    **Objective 2**: Joshua will climb up and down a four-foot-high jungle gym without assistance.

    **Objective 3**: Joshua will swing prone in a suspended therapy net continuously for 3 minutes, pushing with his hands on the floor and without feet contacting the floor.

A sample of the occupational therapy goals and objectives related to the NDT frame of reference includes:

**Goal**: To enhance righting and equilibrium reactions for improved safety during play.
    **Objective 1**: Joshua will maintain balance for 2 minutes when seated on a moving piece of equipment.
    **Objective 2**: Joshua will be able to half-kneel and play with a toy on the floor without losing his balance.

# Application of the Frames of Reference to Practice

As recommended, Joshua has received occupational therapy once weekly. Postulates regarding change from the sensory integrative and NDT frames of reference were used simultaneously to guide treatment.

## Sensory Integrative Frame of Reference

General postulates regarding change apply to all identified function/dysfunction continua. As stated, *if the therapist provides a situation in which the child can act on his environment, then the child will be more likely to produce adaptive responses.* Based on this general postulate regarding change, various toys and pieces of equipment were selected for use during the treatment sessions. Joshua was encouraged to explore these activities. Examples of toys and equipment that encouraged Joshua to explore his environment were:

- Containers filled with rice and beans
- Shaving cream–like substances
- Soft foam balls
- Therapy rolls
- Ramps and other inclined surfaces
- A jungle gym and other irregular climbing structures
- Unstable surfaces
- A wheeled riding toy propelled by his hands
- A scooter board
- Suspended equipment such as a platform swing

*If intervention involves several sensory systems and requires intersensory integration, then it will be more powerful and more likely to bring about an adaptive response.* For example, a suspended, carpeted platform swing provided Joshua with input from the tactile, proprioceptive, and vestibular systems

*If the therapist provides a situation that requires an adaptive response that is developmentally appropriate, then the adaptive response is more likely to occur and more likely to promote growth.* Initially, suspended equipment was hung close to the floor so that Joshua could start and stop the movement with his hands or his feet. Gradually, the suspended equipment was raised to require a more complex adaptive response.

*If the therapist provides the child with a sense of emotional safety, then the child will be more likely to engage in the therapy process.* For example, Joshua was made aware that the mats would prevent his getting hurt if he fell during the gross motor activities. He also was guided physically through the activities, as necessary, and was praised for good work or for good attempts.

*If the therapist provides the child with constant feedback during the therapy session, then the child will gain a greater understanding of what he is doing or what he has done.* For example, spoken language was used to guide Joshua's behavior.

*If the activity presented to the child is challenging yet achievable, then it will facilitate an improved adaptive response.* For example, Joshua was pushed **slowly** to attempt activities that ordinarily provoked fear in him. This one-step-at-a-time approach empowered Joshua to engage in gross motor activities that he previously had avoided.

*If the child is self-directed during therapy, then feed-forward and corollary discharge will occur.* Joshua was allowed to choose from among several appropriate activities, thus he remained motivated and self-directed. He seemed to enjoy therapy.

*If the therapist provides activities that involve controlled change and variety, then the child is more likely to make an adaptive response rather than develop a learned behavior.* A scooterboard activity that first provides acceleration down a ramp, followed by forward propulsion across the floor, followed by pivoting around on one hand, is an example of an activity that involves constant change.

Specific postulates regarding change apply to one function/dysfunction continuum. As noted in the assessment, Joshua exhibited deficits in sensory system modulation, and this continuum will be used to illustrate intervention by using specific postulates regarding change. Joshua had difficulty modulating tactile, auditory, and vestibular input. Modulation of vestibular input was addressed, using the appropriate specific postulates regarding change.

*First, if modulating input is given to one system, then influence is seen in all systems because they are interdependent.* Through linear acceleration and deceleration on the scooterboard, for example, direct input was provided to the otoliths of the vestibular system to enhance Joshua's ability to relate to gravity overall.

*Second, if the child's sensory diet is modified, then sensory system modulation is more likely to occur.* Joshua's vestibular diet was increased. For example, the therapist provided Joshua with a variety of movement experiences, using several pieces of suspended equipment, each piece of equipment moving in a different way with varied intensity.

*Third, if the child is overreactive, then the usual adaptive response will reflect survival needs and not integration; therefore, the sensory system input will have to be modified for the child to produce an adequate adaptive response.* Vestibular input was intensified slowly to make the activities challenging rather than threatening. This slow change allowed for an adequate adaptive response.

*Fourth, if the sensory system modulation level is normalized, then functional support capabilities and end-product abilities will be facilitated.* By the end of the first year, Joshua had made great strides in his ability to modulate vestibular input— for example, facilitating balance and equilibrium (a functional support capability) and displaying more socially appropriate behavior (an end-product ability).

## *Neurodevelopmental Treatment Frame of Reference*

To make Joshua's therapy efficacious, postulates regarding change from the NDT frame of reference were used simultaneously with the postulates regarding change from sensory integrative frame of reference to address specific concerns. One example from the function/dysfunction continua of postural tone, variety of movement, and righting and equilibrium reactions as they relate to postural alignment is described here, followed by two examples from stability and mobility.

*If the child's movement is not automatic because of poor muscle control, then the therapist needs to provide graded therapeutic input that consists of various combinations of tactile and proprioceptive stimulation provided at different rates and speeds. Children with low muscle tone frequently benefit from input at distal key points. Children with low muscle tone benefit from slow, controlled movements in limited ranges.* To walk forward on a six-inch-wide balance beam, for example, Joshua was slowly facilitated from his hands, with arms outstretched, to encourage weightshifting with trunk rotation, allowing for the unweighted leg to be placed forward.

*If the therapist adapts the environment to take into account the child's developmental level, needs, and interests, then the maximum amount of stimulation will be provided to encourage motor skills.* For example, Joshua wanted to swing prone in a suspended net, an activity typically enjoyed by children of comparable age but that fright-

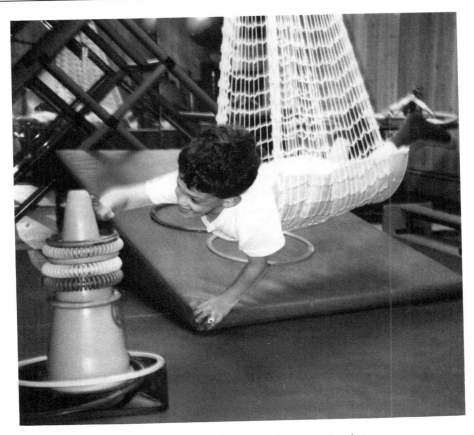

**Figure 18.2.**   Placing a ring on a traffic cone enhances extension.

ened him. Along with providing vestibular input and opportunity to integrate the TLR in prone position, this activity is good for enhancing shoulder and upper extremity stability because weightbearing and weightshifting are required to propel in the net. Stability in the neck and trunk also are enhanced when moving against gravity in a horizontal position. To make the activity interesting and less fearful, an incline mat was placed initially under the net, allowing Joshua the choice of being nearer to the mat at the raised end or farther from the mat at the tapered end. This positioning also changed the effect of weightbearing. For weeks, Joshua chose to spin in circles, making a game of being near and far from the mat. He gradually added linear movement to reach for an object or to put a ring on a traffic cone, thus enhancing extension and promoting integration of the TLR even more in a prone position (Fig. 18.2). Eventually, he was able to push himself far over the tapered end of the mat and high off the ground by using improved extension from head to toe.

*If the therapist handles the child in a way that facilitates mature righting and equilibrium reactions in all developmental positions, then the child is able to use these reactions to maintain normal postural alignment to engage in activities.* When standing on a tiltboard to swing a bat at a soft foam ball, for example, Joshua was facilitated from the pelvis to encourage increased weightbearing in the downhill leg and flexion of the hip and knee in the uphill leg. Despite his low muscle tone, facilitation from a proximal key point despite low muscle tone, enhanced Joshua's ability to maintain balance when hitting the ball with the bat.

*To promote stability or mobility, the therapist must provide a sequence of intervention, beginning with preparatory activities. These activities may include techniques to promote stability through postural alignment of the body before active movement. Furthermore, stability may be facilitated by intermittent application of compression directly to the muscles surrounding a joint.* At the beginning of each treatment session, Joshua chose some preparatory activity, such as wheelbarrow walking, crab soccer, or hands-and-knees balancing on rolls. An example of an activity that provides a lot of compression to the upper extremities is pressing clay when in a hands-and-knees position on rolls. For example, Joshua's hands were on an eight-inch-wide roll with his knees on a ten-inch-wide roll. Because his hips were higher than his arms, more weightbearing was provided to the arms than to the legs. To make the activity more challenging, Joshua pressed clay on the mat in front of his right hand, returning his right hand to the roll, pressing clay on the mat in front of his left hand, returning his left hand to the roll, and starting again with his right hand. Good postural alignment was maintained by the position of the rolls in relation to each other. The back roll was positioned so that Joshua's knees stayed under his hips. Facilitation was used as necessary.

*If the therapist facilitates effective movement patterns and the child has ample opportunity to repeat these movement patterns, then these patterns become integrated into the child's repertoire of motor behaviors.* Facilitation was used repetitively during each treatment session to assist Joshua in walking forward on a six-inch-wide balance beam and in batting at a soft foam ball when standing on a tiltboard. Joshua now walks forward unassisted on a six-inch-wide balance beam and forward with facilitation on a three-inch-wide balance beam. He also now balances unassisted on a tiltboard with uphill hip and knee flexed. (Fig. 18.3).

## A Typical Therapy Session

Postulates regarding change guide Joshua's treatment. A typical therapy session, approximately 6 months postevaluation, illustrates how these postu-

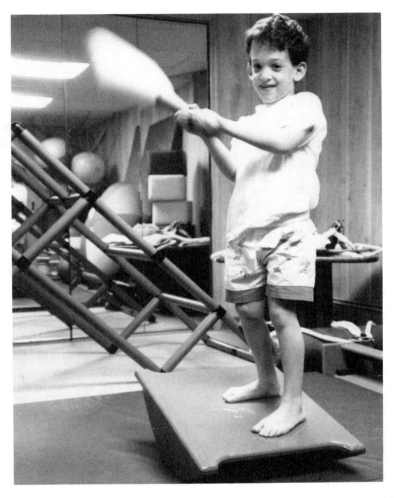

**Figure 18.3.**    Balancing unassisted on a tiltboard with uphill hip and knee flexed.

lates regarding change are blended. The postulates regarding change are implicit and are not highlighted here. In general, therapy was self-directed and Joshua picked the activities and media.

Joshua entered the therapy session and eagerly put on his shorts. He asked for the suspended bolster swing with the incline mat placed underneath. He straddled the bolster swing and pushed against the mat with his feet to make the swing move. In front of Joshua were large foam blocks that he swung into and knocked down. When asked to stand on the bolster swing, which was elevated 13 inches from the floor, he assumed this position only after

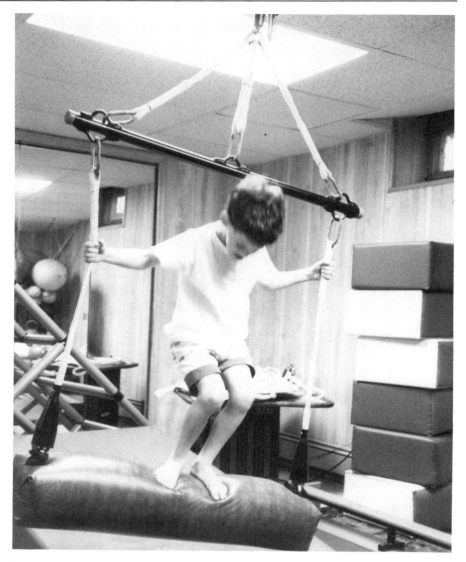

**Figure 18.4.** Standing on the bolster swing momentarily with minimal movement; looking down at feet.

hesitation and an attempt to negotiate a different activity. He stood on the bolster swing only momentarily and with minimal movement, looking down at his feet (Fig. 18.4). He also attempted to clutch the therapist with one hand.

Joshua agreed to use the suspended platform swing, but not the therapy net. The platform swing was elevated ten inches from the floor. Joshua sat and permitted the therapist to push him slowly. He then begin to play with movement transitions between squatting and semistanding when the swing was slightly mobile.

Joshua asked to crawl through the barrel. After crawling in and out several times, he lay prone and gently rocked the barrel from side to side. When the therapist pushed the barrel slowly so that Joshua moved closer toward a supine position, he said, "I'm scared." Joshua then was encouraged to rock the barrel from side to side a few more times.

Joshua asked for the scooterboard. He propelled himself forward with symmetrical arm movements and then pushed off the wall with his hands. The water that ran through the heating system suddenly made a noise and Joshua ran to his father. He whimpered and was held by his father for a few minutes.

A ten-inch roll was placed on the mat and Joshua sat on the roll facing the therapist. While his legs were supported with the knees slightly flexed but not blocked, Joshua leaned toward the left, put his left hand on the mat behind the roll, picked up a large vegetable magnet with his right hand, sat up, switched the magnet to his left hand, leaned to the right, put his right hand on the floor behind the roll, put the magnet on a raised, vertical cookie sheet, and sat up. This procedure was repeated approximately 10 times, and then the pile of vegetable and fruit magnets was switched to his right side and the adapted cookie sheet was switched to Joshua's left. The entire process was repeated again.

Joshua went to the jungle gym and climbed up and down two rungs, one rung higher than the previous week. When encouraged to climb higher, he said, "I'm finished with gross motor." Joshua then sat at the table, with his feet flat on the floor. The "fun box" was placed next to the table. Joshua chose a large, jointed plastic snake. He held the snake's tail and attempted to keep his wrist in a neutral position while slowly making the snake slither. Joshua moved his whole arm and did not separate hand from forearm movements. He also moved the snake quickly, and it slipped to a vertical position. With hand-over-hand assistance from the therapist, Joshua kept the snake horizontal and slowed down his movements. He slithered the snake for approximately 1 minute.

Next, Joshua picked a spray bottle from the fun box. He attempted to squeeze the trigger with the second and third fingers as the thumb and fourth and fifth fingers held the bottle steady. The dehumidifier automatically turned on and Joshua tensed. He asked his father to hold his toes, and after some discussion about the noise, he agreed to continue working as long as his father continued to hold his toes.

For the final activity of the session, a plastic eight-ounce cup was placed upside-down on the table. Joshua asked for the magic markers that smell, and he colored the bottom of the cup, completely filling the space by mixing the colors together. He then covered the colors by squeezing Elmer's Glue over the surface. He was told that he could peel off the colored disk next week and take it home.

Joshua took off his shorts and put on his pants with his father's help. He said that he was ready to go home to tell his mother and brother what he had done that day.

## Responses to Intervention

One year has passed since the assessment, and Joshua is now 4 years, 9 months old. He has made great strides in therapy, and the highlights of his progress are described next.

Joshua no longer seems to be hypersensitive to touch. He plays with objects of various textures and consistencies. Joshua also no longer seems to be hypersensitive to sound. He does not display fear of sudden, and loud noises, and he now can attend to a task with sounds occurring that once frightened him (hearing the water go through the pipes, the dehumidifier turning on, and cars driving past the office).

Joshua exhibits an improved relationship with gravity. He has accomplished the three objectives listed in the summary of evaluation findings for this goal. He uses symmetrical arm movements to propel himself forward on a scooterboard a distance of at least 6 feet. He climbs up and down a four-foot-high jungle gym without assistance, even leaning backwards with a smile (Fig. 18.5). He swings prone in a suspended therapy net continuously for 3 minutes, pushing with his hands on the floor and without his feet contacting the floor. In addition, Joshua now lies supine over a twenty-four-inch therapy ball. He rolls in a barrel, moving through prone and supine positions. He stands on the bolster swing as it moves; and he also hugs the bolster swing, hanging on the underside like a sloth (Fig. 18.6). Joshua is beginning to propel himself forward on rollerskates, although he moves with small steps and he does not lift his feet off the ground. He most recently started to ride a scooterboard in the prone position down a four-foot-long ramp with a thirteen-inch-high platform, without clutching the sides of the ramp. When assisted onto a suspended trapeze bar, however, he demonstrates

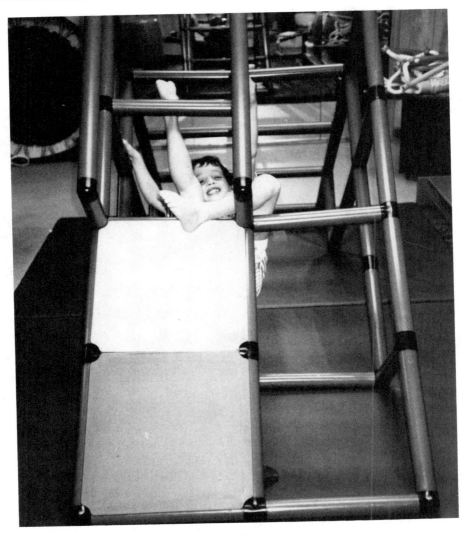

**Figure 18.5.**   Leaning backward with a smile.

fear when attempting to hang upside-down with arms extended fully over-head. He puts his legs up on the bar only when assisted, and he giggles excessively as he leans backward and lets go of the bar. Physical contact is maintained throughout this activity.

Joshua now initiates activities that incorporate rotary movement. He no longer becomes overly dizzy, nor does he experience excessive vertigo or

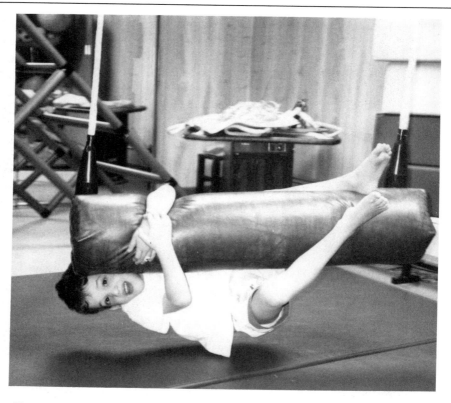

**Figure 18.6.**   Hanging like a sloth on the bolster swing.

nausea. Joshua still is extremely anxious, however, when he is in the same room with animals such as cats.

Joshua has less difficulty catching his balance when falling. He shows improved ability to elongate the muscles actively on the weight-bearing side of his body, and his trunk is less stiff. Because of improved trunk rotation, he has accomplished the two objectives listed in the summary of evaluation findings for the goal of enhancing righting and equilibrium reactions. He is able to maintain balance for 2 minutes seated on a moving piece of equipment. He is able to half-kneel and play with a toy on the floor without losing his balance; however, he has difficulty maintaining a half-kneeling position on a mobile surface.

Joshua has less difficulty moving volitionally against gravity. He now is able to maintain adequate neck and trunk extension without fatigue when swinging prone in a suspended therapy net, but he does have difficulty in assuming a prone extension posture without linear acceleration. Although developmental or primitive postural reflexes seem better integrated, muscle tone remains low.

Joshua now jumps backward and sideways. He also no longer needs to move constantly from one activity to another. He is less distractible and impulsive on an individualized basis.

Joshua continues to have difficulty with motor planning and coordinating complex movements that require an adaptive response. His ability to catch a ball has improved but remains problematic because of inadequate sequencing and timing, as well as poor awareness of joint and muscle movement.

Joshua continues to need the additional stability of a surface when completing two-handed activities, and he elevates his shoulders to "fix" when additional support is not available. He occasionally uses two hands to complete tasks that typically require one hand. Pencil grasp is age appropriate but still tight.

## Implications for Future Intervention

Joshua can continue to benefit from occupational therapy. He enters kindergarten in the next academic year, and the need for therapy can be reassessed at that time. Therapy will continue to focus on Joshua's relationship to gravity and righting and equilibrium reactions, as well as joint stability during gross motor and fine motor skills. Examples of objectives can be updated as follows:

**Goal**: To improve Joshua's relationship to gravity for a greater sense of self-confidence when moving through space.

**Objective 1**: Joshua will lift his feet off the ground when propelling himself forward on rollerskates.

**Objective 2**: Joshua will hang upside-down from a suspended trapeze bar with arms fully extended overhead, without physical contact once the position is assumed.

**Goal**: To enhance righting and equilibrium reactions for improved safety during play.

**Objective**: Joshua will be able to half-kneel and play with a toy on a mobile surface without losing his balance.

# Summary

Two frames of reference were used beneficially in combination for Joshua's treatment. In therapy, Joshua no longer becomes unmanageable, and he is capable now of controlling his behavior. He continues to have difficulty, however, with behavior in a group, and this is a current concern at school.

Joshua continues to display mild difficulties in vestibular processing and praxis. Difficulties in these areas are likely to interfere with Joshua's fine motor skills (writing, cutting, and coloring) and gross motor skills (sports and playground activities).

Play and socialization skills can be hindered by inefficient sensory perception and dyspraxia. Perhaps most significant is the potential effect such difficulties could have on Joshua's self-concept, self-esteem, and self-confidence. Children who have "invisible handicaps" such as those displayed by Joshua are at risk for being misunderstood and mislabeled. If his difficulties are misinterpreted, the child may become frustrated or withdrawn.

Joshua has many strengths, including perseverance and motivation. His strong inner drive to learn and good cognitive and language skills continue to help him progress in therapy as well as in the classroom.

## STUDY QUESTIONS

1. Why were the sensory integrative and NDT frames of reference used together?
2. Discuss the consistency between the two frames of reference.
3. Write additional goals and objectives for both frames of reference based on the assessment administered when Joshua was 3 years, 9 months old. Indicate which goals relate to sensory integration and which relate to NDT.
4. Discuss how the postulates regarding change address the function/dysfunction continua from which the additional objectives or behaviors are derived.
5. What additional frames of reference can be used simultaneous with or subsequent to the sensory integrative and NDT frames of reference.
6. Explain how the additional frames of reference can be used for evaluation and intervention.

### References

Miller, L. J. (1982). *The Miller Assessment for Preschoolers*. Littleton, CO: Foundation for Knowledge In Development.

Wechsler, D. (1967). *Wechsler Preschool and Primary Scale of Intelligence*. San Antonio, TX: Psychological Corp.

# Index

Page numbers in italics denote figures; those followed by "t" denote tables.

Academic ability, 109
  evaluation of, 127
  function/dysfunction continua for,
    123
Acceptance of child, 444
Achievement, 309, 314
Activities
  adaptation of, 31
  analysis of, 29–30
  integration of, 82
  meaningfulness of, 317–318
  play or leisure, 17–18, 21–22
  purposeful, 31–32
  work/educational, 16–17, 21
Activities of daily living
  assessment of, 332–333
  definition of, 16, *17*
  development of habits for, 341–342
  in neurodevelopmental treatment
    frame of reference, 71
  OT interventions and, 20–21, *21*
Activity groups, 32
  to foster peer interaction, 389
  parent/child, 388
  therapeutic, 357–358, 388, 390–391
Activity level, 110
  evaluation of, 127
  function/dysfunction continua for,
    124
Adaptive equipment, 77, 82–83. *See also*
    Biomechanical frame of reference
Adaptive responses, 87, 92–94, 136
  facilitation of, 137–158
Affective state
  assessment of, 416

effect on movement and posture, 250
enhancement of, 424
function/dysfunction continua for,
  410–411
influence on coping, 404
Alerting, 181
Anterolateral system, 94–95, 99
Anxiety, 110
Apraxia, 107
Arm control
  assessment of, 73, 263–265, *264*
  function/dysfunction continua for,
    254
  interventions for enhancement of,
    295–296
Arousal, 181
Articulation, 110
  evaluation of, 127
  function/dysfunction continua for,
    123
Assessment. *See* Evaluation
Assistive devices, 28. *See also* Bio-
    mechanical frame of reference
Assumptions, 40
Athetosis, 58, 63, 79, 248
Attachment relationship, 353–355, *354–*
    *355*
  definition of, 370
  function/dysfunction continua for,
    370–371
  insecure, 354, 370–371
  interventions related to, 386–388
  postulates regarding change for, 379–
    380
  secure, 353–354, 370

Attention
  selective, 181
  visual. *See* Visual attention
Attention deficit disorder, 102
Attention level, 102
  evaluation of, 125
  function/dysfunction continua for,
    117–118, 121
Auditory defensiveness, 100
Auditory discrimination, 120
Auditory stimulation, 301
Auditory system, 89, *91*
  dysfunction of, 100
  function/dysfunction continua for,
    115
Autonomic nervous system arousal, 96,
  *98*
Autonomy, 317
Ayres, A. Jean, 87–89. *See also* Sensory
  integration


Balance, 105, *107*
  activities for development of, 144–145
  evaluation of, 126
  function/dysfunction continua for,
    121
Bayley Scales of Infant Development,
  332, 334
Behavior
  as end-product of sensory integra-
    tion, 109
  ethical, 471–472
  evaluation of, 127
  indicative of function/dysfunction,
    43–44, 123
  occupational, 308–309, 313–322. *See
    also* Human occupation frame of
    reference
  psychosocial frame of reference re-
    lated to, 351–393
Beliefs, 403
  assessment of, 415–416
  enhancement of, 423–424
  function/dysfunction continua for,
    410
Bilateral integration, 106
  activities for development of, 153
  evaluation of, 126

function/dysfunction continua for, 122
Biomechanical frame of reference, 233–
  305
  application to practice, 272–300
    central stability, 272–294
    functional skills, 294–300
  assumptions of, 251
  case study of, 511–523
  evaluation for, 257–267
    arm control, 263–265, *264*
    eating, 266–267
    head control, 259–260, *259, 261*
    mobility, 265–266
    range of motion, 258–259
    toileting, 267
    trunk control and stability, 260–263,
      *261, 262*
  function/dysfunction continua for,
    252–256
    arm control, 254
    eating, 255–256
    head control, 253
    mobility, 255
    range of motion, 252
    toileting, 256
    trunk control, 253–254
  goals of, 234, 250
  outline of, 302–304
  postulates regarding change for, 267–
    272
  summary of, 300–302, *301*
  theoretical base of, 235–251
    development of motor responses
      that maintain posture, 235–238,
      *238*
    effect of damage/dysfunction on
      postural reactions, 246–251
    motor patterns develop from sen-
      sory stimulation, 235
    postural control and skill develop-
      ment in developmental posi-
      tions, 238–246
''Bird-feeding,'' 299
Bobath, Berta and Karel, 49–50, 83
Boulding, K.E., 309–310
Brainstem, 91–92
Bruininks-Oseretsky Test of Motor Pro-
  ficiency, 126, 332, 377
Budgeting frustration technique, 390

Caring, 382
Carolina Record of Infant Behaviors, 333
Case studies, 483–546
  of biomechanical frame of reference,
    511–523
  of combined sensory integration and
    neurodevelopmental treatment,
    525–546
  of coping frame of reference, 430–433
  of neurodevelopmental treatment,
    485–508
Categorization, 182, 212
Center of gravity, 233, 234
Central nervous system. *See also* Sen-
    sory integration
  hierarchical organization of, 92
  plasticity within, 93
  sensory integration and, 91–93
Cerebellum, 92
Cerebral cortex, 92
Cerebral hemispheres
  lateralized functions of, 106
  left hemisphere problems
    in children with sensory integrative
      dysfunction, 88
    language dysfunction due to, 110
  right hemisphere problems, 88
Cerebral palsy, 15
  case study of
    biomechanical frame of reference,
      511–523
    neurodevelopmental treatment,
      485–508
    neurodevelopmental treatment for,
      49
  postural tone in, 56, 58, *59*
Chairs, 278–290, *279–288*
Change process, 322–323, *322–323*
Children's Self-Assessment of Occupa-
    tional Functioning, 334
Chunking, 211
Clinic-based practice, 466–467
Clinical reasoning process, 158–160,
    174–175
Cocontraction, 104, *105*
  evaluation of, 126
  function/dysfunction continua for,
    121
Code of Ethics, 471–472

Cognitive functioning, 12
Cognitive integration, 12
Communication skills, 320, 330
  evaluation of, 332
  interventions for enhancement of,
    342–343
  for working with family, 478–479
Community environment, 368, *368*
Compatibility, 352
Competence, 309, 314–315, 363–364
Compression
  intermittent, 80, *80*
  light joint, 80
Computers, 28
Concepts, 40
Conscious use of self, 28–29
Contractures, 68–69
Coping
  assessment of, 413–420
  definition of, 395, 396
  effect of disabilities on, 405–406
  effectiveness of, 395, 396, 408–410
    interventions based on, 427–429
  goal of, 396
  maladaptive, 409
Coping ability, 365–366
  assessment of, 378
  function/dysfunction continua for,
    374–375
  interventions related to, 389–391
  postulates regarding change for, 381
Coping frame of reference, 395–434
  application to practice, 426–433
    case studies, 430–433
    direct vs. indirect strategies, 426–
      427
    integrating coping into treatment,
      429–430
    intervention based on levels of cop-
      ing effectiveness, 427–429
  assessment for, 413–420, 418t
    intervention planning and, 417–420
  assumptions for, 396
  in children with special needs, 405–
    406
  coping process, 396–402, *398*
  coping resources, 400, 402–405
  function/dysfunction continua for,
    406–413

Coping frame of reference—*continued*
  beliefs and values, 410
  coping style, 407–410
  demands and expectations, 412–413
  developmental skills, 411
  human supports, 411–412
  material and environmental supports, 412
  physical and affective states, 410–411
  outline of, 433–434
  positive orientation of, 395
  postulates regarding change for, 420–426
    enhancing coping resources, 422–425
    modifying demands, 420–422
    providing contingent feedback, 426
  summary of, 433
  theoretical base of, 396–397
  use with other frames of reference, 395
Coping Inventory, 378, 414–415
Coping process, 396–402, *398*
  determining meaning of event, 399
  developing action plan, 399–400
  evaluating effectiveness, 400–401
  example of, 401–402
  implementing coping efforts, 400
Coping resources, 400, 402–405
  assessment of, 414–417, 418t
  enhancement of, 422–425
  external, 400, 405
    human supports, 405
    material and environmental supports, 405
  function/dysfunction continua for, 406–413
  internal, 400, 402–405
    beliefs and values, 403–404
    coping attributes, 403, 404t
    coping style, 402
    developmental skills, 404–405
    physical and affective states, 404
    reactivity, 403
    self-initiation, 403
    sensorimotor organization, 402
Coping style, 402
  assessment of, 414–415

definition of, 402, 407
enhancement of, 422–423
function/dysfunction continua for, 407–410
Coping transactions, 396, 398–399
  assessment of, 413–414
Copying graphic designs, *201*, 201–202
Cranial nerves, 99–100
Culture, 476–477
  definition of, 476
  effect on interventions, 477
  influence on nonhuman environment, 26–27
  influence on occupational performance areas, 19
  interrelationship with family, 476
Cylert, 141

Day hospital programs, 383–384
Definitions, 40
Deformities, 68–69
Development, 4–7
  coping related to, 404–405
    assessment of, 416
    function/dysfunction continua for, 411
  of depersonalized controls, 390
  enhancement of, 424–425
  environmental changes affecting, 6
  motor, 51–57
    abnormal, 55–57
    normal, 5–7, 51–55
  performance components and, 14–15
  rates of, 5–6
  reductionist vs. nonreductionist views of, 4–5
  sequential nature of, 4–5, 93–94
  theories of, 4–7
Developmental Eye Movement Test, 230
Developmental Profile of Young Infants and Children, 332
Developmental Test of Visual Motor Integration, 126, 332
Dissociation, 53–54, 66, *67–68*
  assessment of, 73
  lack of, 56–57, 66, *67*
  postulate regarding change related to, 75

Dorsal column medial lemniscal system, 94, 99, 104
Dyspraxia, 88, 111–113. *See also* Praxis
    developmental, 107–108
    evaluation for, 128

Early Coping Inventory, 414–415
Eating. *See* Feeding
Educational activities
    definition of, 17
    OT interventions and, 21
Educational model, 463–464
Effort, 249–250
Ego strength, 364
Emotional arousal
    evaluation of, 125
    function/dysfunction continua for, 119
Emotional discrimination, 121
Emotional tone, 103, 110
    evaluation of, 127
    function/dysfunction continua for, 123–124
Empathy, 443–444
End-product abilities, 97t, 106–111
    activities for development of, 154–158
    evaluation of, 126–127
    function/dysfunction continua for, 122–124
    postulates regarding change for, 130–131
Environment
    community, 368, *368*
    within context of postulates regarding change, 46
    home, 367
    human, 475–482
        culture, 476–477
        family, 477–479
    in human occupation frame of reference, 310–311, 316, 343
    influence on temperament, 353, 379
    internal vs. external, 6
    nonhuman, 26–28, 444
    safety of, 366–367
    school, 367
Environmental demands
    appropriateness of, 412–413
    assessment of, 413
    grading of, 420–421
    modification of, 420–422
Environmental interaction, 366–368
    function/dysfunction continua for, 375
    interventions related to, 386–388
    postulates regarding change for, 381–382
Environmental mastery, 110, 310
    evaluation of, 127
    function/dysfunction continua for, 124
    interventions for enhancement of, 338
Environmental stimulation
    effect on movement and posture, 250
    visual perception and, 213–214
Environmental stressors, 351
Environmental supports, 405
    assessment of, 417
    enhancement of, 425
    function/dysfunction continua for, 412
Equifinality, 457
Equilibrium reactions, 53, 105, *106, 234, 235*–236
    activities for development of, 144–145
    definition of, 235–236
    development of, 236
    evaluation of, 126
    external forces provoking, 236
    function/dysfunction continua for, 121
    postural alignment and, 65–66
    protective reactions and, 236
Erhardt Developmental Prehension Assessment, 332
Ethics, 471–472
Evaluation, 45
    biomechanical, 257–267
    for coping frame of reference, 413–420, 418t
    for human occupation frame of reference, 331–335
    for neurodevelopmental treatment, 69–74
    for psychosocial frame of reference, 375–379
    sensory integrative, 124–128, 170–173

Expectations
appropriateness of, 412–413
assessment of, 413
Exploration, 309
Eye-hand coordination activities, 206, *206*

Facilitation techniques, 79–81
combined with inhibition techniques, 81
improved body alignment due to, 81
intermittent compression (pressure tapping), 80, *80*
purpose of, 79
tapping, 79–80
Family, 475–479, *478*
definition of, 477
expanded, 477–478
extended, 477
function of, 478
guidelines for working with, 479
interrelationship with culture, 476
nuclear, 477
therapist's communication with, 478–479
Feeding
biomechanical interventions for, 299
evaluation of, 266–267
function/dysfunction continua for, 255–256
Fight-flight-freeze response, 92, 96, 99
Financial resources, 470–471
Flexion response, 146–149, *148–152*
Form constancy, 199
Form perception, 109
evaluation of, 126
function/dysfunction continua for, 123
Frames of reference, 3–4, 25, 37–48
alternative applications of, 447–454
appropriate selection of, 449
art of practice and, 442–444
articulation of, 439–442
biomechanical, 233–305
components of, 37–48
application to practice, 47–48
evaluation, 45

function/dysfunction continua, 42–44
postulates regarding change, 45–47
theoretical base, 38–42
coping, 395–434
effect of financial resources on selection of, 470–471
human occupation, 307–349
incongruent vs. conflicting, 451
influence of human context on application of, 475–482
family and culture, 475–479
professional relationships, 480–481
influence of settings on application of, 455–472
legitimate tools for, 25–33
multiple, 449–453
combinations, 452–453, 525–546
parallel, 451–452
sequential, 450–451
neurodevelopmental, 49–86
original formulation of, 453–454
performance components and, 15
psychosocial, 351–393
purposes of, 3–4, 37
sensory integrative, 87–175
single, 447–449
visual perceptual, 177–232
Friendship development, 355–358, *356*
function/dysfunction continua for, 371–373
Function/dysfunction continua, 42–44
behaviors and, 43–44
for biomechanical frame of reference, 252–256
for coping frame of reference, 406–413
as guideline for evaluation, 45
for human occupation frame of reference, 324–331
for neurodevelopmental treatment, 58–69
for psychosocial frame of reference, 369–375
sensory integrative, 114–124
visual perception, 191–195
Functional performance behaviors, 255–257
Functional skills
assessment of, 71–72

interventions for enhancement of, 294–300
Functional support capabilities, 97t, 104–106
  evaluation of, 126
  function/dysfunction continua for, 119–122
  methods used to facilitate adaptive responses in, 144–154, *145–153*
  postulates regarding change for, 130


Gallant reflex, 249
Games, 361–362, *364*, 389
Gangs, 362–363
Glutamate, 100
Gravitational insecurity, 100
Gravity responses, 95–96, 100, *101*, 233–234, *234*
  evaluation of, 125
  function/dysfunction continua for, 115, 120
Group therapy, 357–358


Habituation, 310, 316, 318–320
  age-appropriate habits, 328–329
  assessment of, 333–334
  definition of, 343
  function/dysfunction continua for, 328–329
  habit patterns, 308
  interventions for enhancement of, 340–342
  postulates regarding change for, 336
Hand control
  evaluation of, 263–265, *264*
  interventions for enhancement of, 295–296
Hand dominance, 106
Handling, therapeutic, 57–58, 74–79, 234, 449
Harnesses, *286*, 284–286
Hawaii Early Learning Profile, 332
Head control
  evaluation of, 259–260, *259, 261*
  function/dysfunction continua for, 253
  in sitting position, 287, *288*, 289–290

supports for feeding, 299
Headrests, 289–290
Helpfulness, 382
Hemiplegia
  neurodevelopmental treatment for, 49
  postural tone in, 58
High guard posturing, 61, *62*, 63, 72
Hip strapping, 276
Home-based practice, 467–468
Home environment, 367
Home Observation for Measurement of the Environment, 417
Hospital-based practice, 465–466
Hospitalization of child, 384
Human context, 475–482
Human occupation frame of reference, 307–349
  application to practice, 337–344
    environment, 343
    habituation subsystem, 340–342
    performance subsystem, 342–343
    volition subsystem, 338–340
  assumptions of, 323–324
  evaluation for, 331–335
  function/dysfunction continua for, 324–331, 344
    habituation subsystem, 328–329
    performance subsystem, 329–331
    volition subsystem, 325–327
  historical perspective on, 307–310
    general systems theory, 309–310
    occupational behavior, 308–309
  outline of, 344–346
  postulates regarding change for, 335–337, 344
  summary of, 343–344
  theoretical base of, 310–324
    assumptions, 313
    change process, 322–323, *322–323*
    occupation and occupational behavior, 313–322
    summary, 324
    systems theory, 310–313, *312*
Human supports, 405
  assessment of, 417
  enhancement of, 425
  function/dysfunction continua for, 411–412

Hyperactivity, 102, 141
Hypotheses, 41–42

Imagery, 182, 212
Information processing model, 179–180
Inhibition techniques, 79–81
    combined with facilitation techniques, 81
    improved body alignment due to, 81
    light joint compression, 80
    purpose of, 79
    traction, 80
Innervation. *See* Reciprocal innervation
Inpatient child psychiatric units, 384
Interest contagion technique, 390

Joint mobilization, 77

Kaufman Assessment Battery for Children, 127
Key points of control, 57, 78
Kielhofner, Gary, 307–308. *See also* Human occupation frame of reference
Knee "locking," 245
Kyphosis, 273

Labeling, 184
Language, 110
    evaluation of, 127
    function/dysfunction continua for, 123
Laptrays
    use in sitting position, 283–287
    use in supported standing position, 293–294
Lateralization, 106
    activities for development of, 153
    evaluation of, 126
    function/dysfunction continua for, 122
Learning
    information processing model of, 179–180
    process of, 32

of visual perception skills, 185–186, 204–205
Learning disabilities, 87–88
Legitimate tools, 25–33
    activity analysis and adaptation, 29–31
    activity groups, 32
    conscious use of self, 28–29
    definition of, 25
    manner of use of, 444
    nonhuman environment, 26–28
    purposeful activities, 31–32
    teaching/learning process, 32
Leisure activities, 17. *See also* Play
Limbic system, 92
Log rolling, 66, 67
Lordosis, 273

Matching, 186–187, *188. See also* Visual discrimination
    evaluation of, 198–202
    function/dysfunction continua for, 194–195
Material supports, 405
    assessment of, 417
    enhancement of, 425
    function/dysfunction continua for, 412
Medical model, 459–463
Memory
    eidetic, 198
    information coding and, 182
    semantic, 198
    short- vs. long-term, 182
    visual. *See* Visual memory
Meyer, Adolf, 308
Miller Assessment for Preschoolers, 200, 332
Mnemonic strategies, 183, 212
Mobility, 52–53
    assessment of, 72–73
    biomechanical interventions for, 295–299, *297–298*
    development of, 237
    evaluation of, 265–266
    function/dysfunction continua for, 255
    postulates regarding change related to, 74–77

Mosey, Anne C., 3, 37
Motivation, 310, 314, 317
  related to functional skills, 71
Motor development, 5–7
  abnormal, 55–57
  evaluation of, 257–267
  normal, 51–55, 237
    components of, 52–54
    control mechanisms for, 51
    dissociation of movement and, 53–54
    interplay between stability and mobility in, 52
    postural control in three planes and, 54
    postural reflex mechanisms and, 53
    principles of, 51
    sensory-motor-sensory feedback for, 51–52
    sequence of, 51, 54–55, 235–238
    variety of movement and, 55
Motor Free Visual Perception Test, 126, 197
Motor patterns
  definition of, 237
  development from sensory stimulation, 235
Motor performance, 12, 13
Motor restlessness, 100–101, 110
Movement Assessment of Infants, 73–74
Movement level, 100–101
  function/dysfunction continua for, 116, 120
Movement sensitivity, 102–103
  evaluation of, 125
  function/dysfunction continua for, 118
Movements
  abnormal, 55–57
  assessing quality of, 71–73
  associated patterns of, 56–57, 66
  compensatory, 246
  coordinated, 63, 65
  dissociation of, 53–54, 66, 67–68, 73
    lack of, 56–57, 66, 67
  dynamic, 52
  function/dysfunction continua for, 252–257
  skilled, 238

stereotypical, 68–69
synergistic, 56–57, 66
variety of, 55, 68–69, 73
Muscle tone, 53
  definition of, 104
  evaluation of, 126
  function/dysfunction continua for, 121
Muscles
  agonist vs. antagonist, 53
  cocontraction of, 104, 105, 121
  phasic vs. tonic, 250
Myofascial release, 78

Neck rings and collars, 290
Neonatal Behavioral Assessment Scale, 333, 334
Neurodevelopmental treatment, 49–86
  application to practice, 77–83
    handling, 57–58, 74–79
    inhibition and facilitation, 79–81, 80
    integration of activities, 82
    positioning and adaptive equipment, 82–83
    sequence of intervention, 77–78
    team for, 77
    training for, 77
    weightshifting and weightbearing, 81–82
  case studies of, 485–508
    combined with sensory integration, 525–546
  clinical applications of, 49
  definition of, 49
  evaluation for, 69–74
    assessment of functional skills, 71–72
    format for, 70
    outline for, 70t
    quality of movement, 72–73
    questions answered by, 70
    specialized assessments and, 73–74
    standardized evaluations, 70, 73–74
  function/dysfunction continua for, 58–69, 83
    dissociation of movement, 66, 67–68
    full range of motion vs. structural deformities and contractures, 69

Neurodevelopmental treatment—
  *continued*
  postural tone, 58, *59,* 60
  reciprocal innervation related to
    controlled coordinated move-
    ment, 63, 65
  righting and equilibrium reactions
    related to postural alignment, 65–
    66
  stability/mobility, 60–61, *61–62,*
    63
  variety of movement, 68–69
  historical evolution of, 49–50
  outline of, 84–85
  postulates regarding change for, 74–
    77, 83
  summary of, 83–84
  theoretical base of, 50–58, 83–84
    abnormal motor development, 55–
    57
    components of normal develop-
    ment, 52–54
    phases in motor development, 54–
    55
    principles of normal motor devel-
    opment, 51
    sensory input as means of bringing
    about change, 57–58
    sensory-motor-sensory feedback,
    51–52
    variety of movement, 55
Neurodevelopmental Treatment Association, 77
Neurological soft signs, 87
Neuromuscular performance, 12
Nystagmus, postrotary, 102
  evaluation of, 125
  function/dysfunction continua for,
    118, 120

Occupation, defined, 313
Occupational behavior, 308–309, 313–
    322. *See also* Human occupation
    frame of reference
  definition of, 313–314
  environment and, 316
  hierarchies and, 316–322
  use of play and work, 314–316, *315*

Occupational performance areas, 16–22
  activities of daily living, 16, *17,* 20–21,
    *21*
  cultural effects on, 19
  definition of, 16
  interventions and, 19–22
  play or leisure activities, 17–18, *18,*
    21–22
  temporal adaptation and, 19–20
  work activities/education, 16–17, 21
Occupational role, 314, 316
  play and, 363–365
Ocular motor skills, 178
Olfactory arousal, 102
  function/dysfunction continua for,
    117
Olfactory defensiveness, 102
Olfactory discrimination, 120
Oral arousal, 101
  function/dysfunction continua for,
    116
Oral defensiveness, 101
Oral discrimination, 120
Oral-motor assessment, 266–267
Orthotic devices, 77
Outpatient child psychiatry clinics, 383

Peabody Developmental Motor Scales,
    200
Pediatric occupational therapy
  art of, 442–444
  articulating frames of reference in,
    439–442
  child development and, 6–7
  domain of concern of, 10–22
    occupational performance areas,
    16–22
    performance components, 11–16
  educational model for, 463–464
  effect of societal changes on, 9–10
  ethical practice of, 471–472
  influence of human context on prac-
    tice of, 475–482
    family and culture, 475–479
    professional relationships, 480–481
  legitimate tools of, 25–33
  locus of practice, 458–459
  medical model for, 459–463

practice settings for, 10
  clinic-based, 466–467
  concerns based on, 470–471
  home-based, 467–468
  hospital-based, 465–466
  influence on frames of reference,
    455–472
  private practice, 469–470
  school-based, 468–469
Peer interaction, 355–358, *356*
  evaluation of, 377
  function/dysfunction continua for,
    371–373
  interventions related to, 389–391
  postulates regarding change for, 380
Perceptual motor skills, 321, 330
  evaluation of, 332
  interventions for enhancement of,
    342–343
Performance, 310, 316, 320
  definition of, 343
  evaluation of, 331–332
  interventions for enhancement of,
    342–343
  postulates regarding change for, 337
Performance components, 11–16
  cognitive integration and cognitive
    components, 12
  definition of, 11
  interrelation of, 11
  interventions and, 14–16
  psychological skills and psychological
    components, 13, *14*
  sensory motor components, 11–12
    definition of, 11
    motor skills, 12, *13*
    neuromuscular performance, 12
    sensory integration, 12
  subparts of, 11
Personal causation, 317, 325
  assessment of, 334
  interventions for enhancement of, 338
  postulates regarding change for, 335–
    336
Personal interests
  age-appropriate, 327
  assessment of, 334–335
  interventions for enhancement of,
    339–340

Personal standards, 318
Pets, 27
Physical state
  assessment of, 416
  enhancement of, 424
  function/dysfunction continua for,
    410–411
  influence on coping, 404
Piers-Harris Children's Self-Concept In-
    ventory, 334, 415
Play, 358–365, *359*, 360–361, *362*
  assessment of, 335
  benefits of, 358, 364–365
  constructional, 361, *363*
  definition of, 17–18, *18*, 358
  development of skills for, 309, 358–
    359
  function/dysfunction continua for,
    373–374
  games, 361–362, *364*, 389
  in gangs, 362–363
  group, 362–363, *365*, 390
  imaginary, 360–361, *362*
  interventions related to, 389–391
  occupational behavior and, 314–316,
    *315*
  occupational roles and, 363–365
  OT interventions and, 21–22
  parent/child activity groups for, 388
  with peers, 355–358, *356*
  postulates regarding change for, 380–
    381
  vs. recreation, 358
  roles and habits acquired by, *319*,
    319–320
  screening competency in, 377
  sensorimotor, 360, *361*, 391
  in therapeutic milieu, 386
  types of, 360–362
  use in neurodevelopmental treat-
    ment, 82
Play exploration, 18
Play history, 334, 378
Play performance, 18
Play scales, 334
Positioning, 82
Positioning log, 256
Postrotary nystagmus, 102
  evaluation of, 125

Postrotary nystagmus—*continued*
  function/dysfunction continua for,
    118, 120
Postulates, 40–41
Postulates regarding change, 45–47
  for biomechanical frame of reference,
    267–272
  for coping frame of reference, 420–426
  for human occupation frame of refer-
    ence, 335–337
  for neurodevelopmental treatment,
    74–77
  for psychosocial frame of reference,
    379–382
  for sensory integration, 128–131
  for visual perception, 203–204
Postural alignment, 53
  assessment of, 72
  effect of facilitation and inhibition
    techniques on, 81
  postulates regarding change related
    to, 74–75
  relation of weightbearing and weight-
    shifting to, 81–82
  righting/equilibrium reactions and,
    65–66
Postural control development, 54, 237–
    246
  influence of damage/dysfunction on,
    246–251
  in prone position, 240–242, *241*
  in sidelying position, 242–243, *243*
  in sitting position, *244*, 244–245
  in standing position, 245–246
  in supine position, 239–240, *240*
Postural reflex mechanisms, 53
Postural tone, 58, 60
  abnormal, 56, 58, 60
  assessment of, 71–72
  coordinated movement and, 63, 65
  normal, 53, 58, 60
  pattern of distribution of, 57–58
  postulates regarding change related
    to, 74–75
Posture and Fine Motor Assessment of
    Infants, 73–74
Poverty, 405
Practice settings, 10
  clinic-based, 466–467

concerns based on, 470–471
  home-based, 467–468
  hospital-based, 465–466
  influence on frames of reference, 455–
    472
  private practice, 469–470
  for psychosocial frame of reference,
    383–384
  school-based, 468–469
Praxis, 88, 92, 107–108, 111–113
  activities for development of, 155–
    158, *157–158*
  articulation problems and, 110
  definition of, 95, 107
  evaluation of, 126
  function/dysfunction continua for,
    122–123
  neural processes underlying, 107,
    *109*, 112
  process of, 111
  role of dorsal column medial lemnis-
    cal system in development of,
    94
Pressure-proprioceptive treatment, 141–
    142
Private practice, 469–470
Problem solving. *See* Process skills
Process skills, 320–321, *321*, 330
  evaluation of, 332
  interventions for enhancement of,
    342–343
Professional relationships, 480–481
Prone extension posture activities, 146,
    *146–147*
Prone position
  developmental sequence of motor be-
    haviors in, 240–242, *241*
  enhancing stability in, 273–276, *274–
    275*
  hand control in, 264–265, *265*
  head control in, 259
  trunk control in, 261
Prone stander, 291–294, *292, 294*
Prone wedge, 273–276, *274–275*
Proprioception
  definition of, 95, 105
  evaluation of, 126
Proprioceptive discrimination, 120
Proprioceptive sensitivity, 103

function/dysfunction continua for, 118–119
Proprioceptive system, 89, *91*, 95
Protective reactions, 236
Psychological functions, 13
Psychosocial frame of reference, 351–393
  application to practice, 382–391
    peer interaction, play, coping ability, 388–391
    practice settings, 383–384
    temperament, attachment, environmental interaction, 386–388
    therapeutic milieus, 384–386
  evaluation for, 375–379
  function/dysfunction continua for, 369–375
  outline of, 392–393
  postulates regarding change for, 379–382
  summary of, 391–392
  theoretical base for, 351–369
    ability to cope, 365–366
    attachment, 353–355, *354–355*
    environmental interaction, 366–368
    innate temperament, 352–353
    peer interactive skills, 355–358, *356*
    play, 358–365, *359*, *361–365*
    summary of, 368–369

Quality of movement, 72–73

Range of motion
  evaluation of, 258–259
  full passive, 68–69
  function/dysfunction continua for, 255
  with structural deformities and contractures, 68–69
Reactivity, 403
Reciprocal innervation, 53
  controlled coordinated movement and, 63, 65
  lack of, 65
  postulates regarding change related to, 75–76

Recognition, 186. *See also* Visual discrimination
  evaluation of, 198–202
  function/dysfunction continua for, 194–195
Reflex inhibiting postures, 50
Reflexes
  definition of, 235
  developmental, 105, *108*
    evaluation of, 126
    function/dysfunction continua for, 121–122
  in infancy, 235
  postural reflex mechanisms, 53
  tonic labyrinthine, 239, 263–264, *264*
  tonic neck, 105, *108*, 235, 239
Rehearsal
  elaborative, 211–212
  maintenance (repetition), 211
Reilly, Mary, 307–309
Relationships
  attachment, 353–355
  child peer, 355–358
  cultural, 476–477
  family, 477–479
  professional, 480–481
  therapeutic, 28–29, 442–444
Repetition, 211
Residential treatment facilities, 384
Responsibilities, age-appropriate, 386
Righting reactions, 53, 235–236
  definition of, 235
  development of, 236
  postural alignment and, 65–66
Ritalin, 141
Rituals, 384–385
Roles
  age-appropriate, 328–329
  definition of, 318
  internalized, 318–319
  interventions for development of, 340–341
  occupational, 314, 316
Rolling, 66, *67*
Rooting response, 236, 249
Routines, 384–385
Rules
  of reciprocal social interaction, 362
  in therapeutic milieu, 385

School-based practice, 468–469
School environment, 367
Scooterboards, 296, *297*
Self-image, 326
Self-initiation, 403
Self-management skills, 13
Semicircular canals, 95
Sensorimotor organization, 402
Sensory defensiveness, 110
   treatment of, 140–144
Sensory diet, 97–98, 131, *132*, 142, *143*
Sensory integration, 12, 87–175
   application to practice, 131–137, *132*
     general considerations, 133–137
     sensory diet, 131–132, *132*
     treatment environment, 132–133
   background of, 87–88
   case study of combination with neu-
     rodevelopmental treatment, 525–
     546
   clinical reasoning process for, 158–
     160, 174–175
   definition of, 87
   evaluation of, 124–128, 170–173
   function/dysfunction continua for,
     114–124
     end-product abilities, 122–124
     functional support capabilities,
      119–122
     sensory system modulation, 114–
      119
   goals of, 89–91, 131
   methods used to facilitate adaptive
     responses in, 137–158
     end-product abilities, 154–158
     functional support capabilities,
      144–154, *145–153*
     guidelines for, 138
     sensory system modulation, 140–
      144
     sequence of treatment, 139–140
   other end-product abilities and, 158
   outline for, 161–164
   postulates regarding change for, 128–
     131
   sensory integrative functions, 96, 97t
   summary of, 160–161
   symptoms indicative of problems
     with, 168–169

theoretical base of, 89–114
   basic concepts, 91–94
   end-product abilities, 106–111
   functional support capabilities,
     104–106
   postulates of, 113–114
   praxis, 111–113
   sensory system modulation, 96–
     103, *98*
   sensory systems, *91*, 94–96
Sensory Integration and Praxis Tests,
   88–89, *90*, 126, 377
Sensory-motor-sensory feedback, 51–
   52, 310, *311*
Sensory motor techniques, 49
Sensory system modulation, 96–103, *98*
   effect of sensory diet on, 97–98
   effects of problems with, 98–99
   evaluation of, 125
   function/dysfunction continua for,
     114–119
   methods used to facilitate adaptive
     responses in, 140–144
   overarousal to shutdown of, *98*, 98–99
   postulates regarding change for, 129–
     130
Sensory systems, 89, *91*, 94–96
   arousal problems of, 98–103, 103t
   facilitation and inhibition of, 93
   information processing component
     of, 99, 104
Seriation, 182, 212
Sidelying position
   developmental sequence of motor be-
     haviors in, 242–243, *243*
   enhancing stability in, 276–278, *277*
   hand control in, *262*, 264
   head control in, *259*, 260
   trunk control in, 262, *262*
Sitting position
   developmental sequence of motor be-
     haviors in, *244*, 244–245
   enhancing stability in, 278–290, *279–
     288*
   hand control in, 264–265
   head control in, 260, *261*
   long, 244–245
   ring, 244
   tripod, 244

trunk control in, 262–263
"W," 60–61, *61*
Skills
  age-appropriate, 330–331
  communication, 320
  evaluation of, 331–332
  function/dysfunction continua for, 329–331
  peer interactive, 355–358, *356*
  perceptual motor, 321
  process, 320–321, *321*
  splinter, 94
Slagle, Eleanor Clarke, 308
Sleep/wake cycles, 318
Social functions, 13, *14*
Sorting, 187–190, *189. See also* Visual discrimination
  evaluation of, 198–202
  function/dysfunction continua for, 194–195
Southern California Postrotary Nystagmus Test, 88, 125
Southern California Sensory Integration Tests, 87–88
Spasticity, 65, 78
Spatial orientation, 187
Spatial perception, 109
  evaluation of, 126
  function/dysfunction continua for, 123
  OT interventions for, 223–224
Special education programs, 383
Splinter skills, 94
Stability, 52–53
  assessment of, 73
  central, 272–293
  compensatory, 61–63
  development of, 237
  dynamic, 60–61, 63
  evaluation of, 260–263, *262*
  positional, 60–61, *61–62, 64*
  postulates regarding change related to, 74–75
  in prone position, 273–276, *274–275*
  in sidelying position, 276–278, *277*
  in sitting position, 278–290, *279–288*
  in supine position, 272–273
  in supported standing position, 290–294, *292, 294*

Standards, personal, 318
Standing position
  developmental sequence of motor behaviors in, 245–246
  hand control in, 264–265
  head control in, 260
  supported, 290–294, *292, 294*
  trunk control in, 262–263
Stimulant drugs, 141
Stress. *See also* Coping
  coping with, 396–397
  definition of, 396–397
  effect on movement and posture, 249–250
  reactions to, 397
Stressors, 397
Suck-swallow-breathe synchrony, 104
  activities for development of, 154
  evaluation of, 126
  function/dysfunction continua for, 119
Supine position
  developmental sequence of motor behaviors in, 239–240, *240*
  enhancing stability in, 272–273
  hand control in, 263–264
  head control in, 259
  trunk control in, 261
Supine stander, 290–294, *294*
Surface support, 250
Sympathy, 443–444
Systems theory, 309–310, 457–458
  applied to human occupation frame of reference, 310–313, *312*

Tactile defensiveness, 88, 99–100
Tactile discrimination, 104
  evaluation of, 126
  function/dysfunction continua for, 119–120
Tactile stimulation, 246
Tactile system, 89, *91*
  divisions of, 94–95
  function/dysfunction continua for, 115
  inaccurate interplay between divisions of, 99
Tapping, 79–80
Teaching process, 32
Team process, 461–462

Technology, 28
Temperament, 352–353
  assessment of, 334
  compatibility between parent and
    child, 352
  components of, 352
  definition of, 352, 369
  easy vs. difficult, 352
  environmental influence on, 353, 379
  function/dysfunction continua for,
    369–370
  interventions related to, 386–388
  postulates regarding change for, 379
Temperature, 250
Temporal adaptation, 19–20
Temporal organization, 342
Temporal orientation, 317
Test of Sensory Functions in Infants, 332
Test of Visual Perceptual Skills, 197, 332
Theoretical base for frames of reference,
    38–42, 448
  biomechanical, 235–251
  coping, 396–397
  human occupation, 310–324
  neurodevelopmental, 50–59, 82–83
  psychosocial, 351–369
  sensory integration, 89–113
  visual perception, 178–190
Theories, 38–42
  assumptions and, 40
  concepts and, 40
  definitions and, 40
  developmental, 4–7
  hypotheses and, 41–42
  integration with practice, 38
  postulates and, 40–41
  purpose of, 38
Therapeutic milieus, 384–386
Therapeutic relationship, 28–29, 442–444
  characteristics of, 443–444
  definition of, 442
  goal of, 442
  importance to intervention process,
    443
Three-dimensional tasks, 200–201
Toe clawing, 63, 64
Toileting
  biomechanical interventions for, 299–
    300

evaluation of, 267
function/dysfunction continua for,
    256–257
Tonic labyrinthine reflex, 239, 263–264,
    264
Tonic neck reflex, 105, 108
  asymmetrical, 235, 239
Toys, 27
  for sensory integrative frame of refer-
    ence, 133, 134–135
Transitional objects, 26, 27
Tricycles, 297–298, 298
Trigeminal nerve, 100
Trunk control
  evaluation of, 260–263, 261
  function/dysfunction continua for,
    253–254
Tufts Assessment of Motor Perfor-
    mance, 73

Uniform Terminology, 10, 15

Values, 317
  assessment of, 334, 415–416
  cultural, 318
  enhancement of, 423–424
  function/dysfunction continua for,
    326–327
  influence on coping, 403–404
    function/dysfunction continua for,
      410
  influence on interventions, 339
  postulates regarding change related
    to, 336
Vestibular stimulation, 441–442
Vestibular system, 89, 91, 95–96
Vigilance, 181
  function/dysfunction continua for,
    193
Vineland Adaptive Behavior Scales,
    333
Vision screening, 230–231
Visual attention, 181–182
  alerting, 181
  definition of, 181
  evaluation of, 196–197
  function/dysfunction continua for,
    191–193

OT interventions for, 205–211
  activity modification, 208–209
  activity selection, 208, *209*
  preparation, 205–206, *206–207*
  structuring, 206–207
  therapist verbalization and cuing,
    209–211, *210*
postulates regarding change for, 203
selective, 181
vigilance, 181
Visual discrimination, 183–185
  concrete to abstract, 185
  definition of, 183
  development of, 183–184
  evaluation of, 198–202, *200–201*
  familiar to novel, 185
  function/dysfunction continua for,
    120, 194–195
  general to specific, 184
  OT interventions for, 213–225
    constructional tasks, *219,* 219–220
    guidelines for graphic materials,
      216
    matching tasks, 217–218, *218*
    modifying environmental stimuli,
      213–214
    organization of visual array, 217
    positioning visual materials, 215–
      216, *216*
    starting points, 220–223, *223*
    two-dimensional tasks, 220, *221–*
      *222*
    visual presentations, 214–215, *214–*
      *215*
  postulates regarding change for, 204
  specific abilities for, 186–190
    matching, 186–187, *188*
    recognition, 186
    sorting, 187–190, *189*
  whole to parts, 184–185
Visual memory, 182–183
  evaluation of, 197–198
  function/dysfunction continua for,
    193–194
  OT interventions for, 211–213
    categorization, 212
    chunking, 211
    compensatory techniques, 212
    elaborative rehearsal, 211–212

environmental structuring, 213
games, 212–213
imagery, 212
maintenance rehearsal (repetition),
  211
mnemonic devices, 212
sequencing, 213
seriation, 212
postulates regarding change for, 203–
  204
Visual perception, 109, 177–232
  definition of, 177
  evaluation of, 196–202
    vision screening, 230–231
    visual attention, 196–197
    visual discrimination, 198–202, *200–*
      *201*
    visual memory, 197–198
  function/dysfunction continua for,
    191–195, 226
    visual attention, 191–193
    visual discrimination, 194–195
    visual memory, 193–194
  information processing model of,
    179–190
  learning skills of, 185–186
  OT interventions for, 204–225, 226
    teaching/learning, 204–205
    visual attention, 205–211
    visual discrimination, 213–225
    visual memory, 211–213
  outline of, 226–228
  postulates for frame of reference, 190
  postulates regarding change for, 203–
    204, 226
  processing skills for, 180–185
    visual attention, 181–182
    visual discrimination, 183–185
    visual memory, 182–183
  resources for activities/workbooks
    for, 232
  specific visual discrimination abilities
    for, 186–190, *188–189*
  summary of, 225–226
  theoretical base for, 178–190, 225–226
  visual skills and, 178
Visual system, 89, *91,* 178
  function/dysfunction continua for,
    117

Visual system—*continued*
  responses to stimuli of, 102
Vocational activities, 17
Volition, 310, 316–318
  assessment of, 334
  definition of, 343
  function/dysfunction continua for,
    325–327
  interventions for enhancement of,
    338–340
  postulates regarding change for,
    336

von Bertalanffy, L., 309–310, 457–
  458

"W" sitting position, 60–61, *61*
Wechsler Intelligence Scale for Chil-
  dren—Revised, 127
Weightbearing, 81–82, 237–238
Weightshifting, 81–82, 237–238, *238*
Wheelchairs, 298–299
Work activities
  definition of, 16–17
  OT interventions and, 21